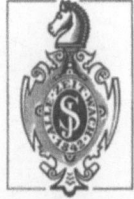

M. S. John Pathy · Paul Finucane

Geriatric Medicine:

Problems and Practice

With 67 Figures

Springer-Verlag
Berlin Heidelberg GmbH

M. S. J. Pathy, FRCP
Professor of Geriatric Medicine, University of Wales College of
Medicine, Cardiff, UK

P. Finucane, MB, MRCPI
Senior Lecturer in Geriatric Medicine, University of Wales College
of Medicine, Cardiff, UK

British Library Cataloguing in Publication Data
Geriatric medicine.
  1. Geriatrics
  I. Pathy, M.S.J. (Mahan Sankar John)
  II. Finucane, Paul
  618.97

Library of Congress Cataloging-in-Publication Data
Geriatric medicine : problems and practice / M.S. John Pathy, Paul Finucane (eds.).
      p.   cm.
  Includes bibliographies and index.
    ISBN 978-1-4471-1648-6   ISBN 978-1-4471-1646-2 (eBook)
    DOI 10.1007/ 978-1-4471-1646-2

  1. Geriatrics. I. Pathy, M. S. J. II. Finucane, Paul, 1955–
  [DNLM: 1. Aged.   2. Geriatrics.   WT 100 G366366]
RC952.G394   1989
618.97—dc19
DNLM/DLC
for Library of Congress   89–6013
                                                                      CIP

© Springer-Verlag Berlin Heidelberg 1989
Originally published by Springer-Verlag Berlin Heidelberg New York in 1989
Softcover reprint of the hardcover 1st edition 1989

Filmset by Tradeset Photosetting Ltd, Welwyn Garden City, Herts AL7 1BH
Printed by The Alden Press, Osney Mead, Oxford
2128/3916-543210 (Printed on acid-free paper)

Preface

As medical students, we are taught that the successful practise of medicine hinges on our ability to analyse the clinical presentation of disease and thereby to apply the correct diagnostic label. Such a label-orientated approach is often inadequate when dealing with elderly people, where acute medical breakdown often presents with a complex amalgam of physical dysfunction, cognitive impairment and social incompetence. As underlying causation is often multi-factorial, accurate assessment and management relies on the identification of problems rather than disease labelling. Precision of diagnosis is no less important than in the young, but a problem-orientated approach is particularly relevant to the disorders of old age.

That physiological competence declines with age is undoubted, but insidious physical and intellectual deterioration is too often ascribed to ageing when reversible pathology exists. Disease is best understood by seeing man in the world in which he lives. Failure to see disease in old age in relation to age-related physiological changes, to the immediate and more remote environment, to society and the impact on it of epidemiological and demographic changes prevents us from fully responding to the challenge of old age, sometimes erroneously referred to as the problem of old age.

This book sets out to introduce the medicine of old age in a broad perspective and in a problem-orientated way. It does not attempt to comprehensively cover disease in later life, but rather to deal with some of those aspects of disease which may be of practical everyday use to the practising physician.

The principles of geriatric medicine are relevant to all countries. In that the contents may be of particular use to family doctors preparing for the Diploma in Geriatric Medicine of the Royal College of Physicians in England, it should also be relevant to family doctors in other countries. The sections on demography, the delivery of health care and social services and the legal aspects of medicine of old age aim to fill the gaps left by wholly clinical textbooks.

Acknowledgements

Many people had their lives disrupted while this book was in preparation. In particularly the spouses, families and secretaries of the various contributors had much to endure and deserve our sincere thanks. Editors' prerogative allows us to select three – Norma Pathy, Aileen Finucane and Shirley Green – for special mention.

University of Wales College of Medicine,   M. S. John Pathy
Cardiff, February 1989   Paul Finucane

Contents

Section II. Clinical Problems in the Elderly

Contributors

Delyth Alldrick, MB MRCPsych
Consultant Psychiatrist for the Elderly, Whitchurch Hospital,
Cardiff, UK

June Arnold, MD FRCP
Consultant Physician in Geriatric Medicine (Retired), Clwyd North
Health Authority, Clwyd, UK

A. J. Bayer, MB BCh
Lecturer in Geriatric Medicine, University of Wales College of
Medicine, Cardiff, UK

Lyn Beck, FRCS, DO
Consultant Ophthalmologist, University Hospital of Wales,
Cardiff, UK

G. V. Boswell, MB MRCP (UK)
Consultant Physician in Geriatric Medicine, Dyfed/Powys Health
Authority, Dyfed, UK

Jane Bradshaw, MB MRCP
Consultant Physician in Geriatric Medicine, Nevill Hall Hospital,
Abergavenny, UK

D. Coakley, MD FRCPI
Professor of Geriatric Medicine, St James's Hospital, Dublin, Eire

Carol Comlay, NCLT
Formerly: Hearing Therapist, Welsh Hearing Institute, University
Hospital of Wales, Cardiff, UK

G. Conlon, CQSW RMN
Assistant Director, Services to the Elderly, County of South
Glamorgan, Cardiff, UK

A. B. Davies, MD MRCP
Consultant Physician in Geriatric Medicine, Cymla Hospital,
Neath, UK

G. Davison, MB(Otago) FRACP
Clinical Lecturer, School of Medicine, University of Auckland,
Auckland, New Zealand

R. T. M. Edwards, MB MRCP
Consultant Physician in Geriatric Medicine, Dewi Sant Hospital,
Pontypridd, UK

P. Finucane, MB MRCPI
Senior Lecturer in Geriatric Medicine, University of Wales College
of Medicine, Cardiff, UK

T. E. Finucane, MD
Assistant Professor of Geriatric Medicine, Johns Hopkins
University School of Medicine, Francis Scott Key Medical Centre,
Baltimore, MD 21224, USA

Anne Freeman, MB MRCP
Consultant Physician in Geriatric Medicine, St. Woolos Hospital,
Newport, UK

Deirdre Hine, MB FFCM
Deputy Chief Medical Officer, Welsh Office, Cardiff, UK

R. D. Hutton, MB MRCPath
Senior Lecturer in Haematology, University Hospital of Wales,
Cardiff, UK

D. F. Jessett, MEd, MChS SRCh
Head of School, School of Chiropody, Cardiff, UK

D. Jones, FRCS (Ed)
Consultant Ophthalmic Surgeon, West Wales General Hospital,
Carmarthen, Dyfed, UK

D. W. Molloy, MD FRCP(C)
Assistant Professor of Medicine, Division of Geriatric Medicine,
McMaster University, Hamilton, Ontario, Canada

Rhian E. Owen, MB MRCP
Consultant Physician in Geriatric Medicine, Dewi Sant Hospital,
Pontypridd, UK

M. S. J. Pathy, FRCP
Professor of Geriatric Medicine, University of Wales College of
Medicine, Cardiff, UK

T. Rudra, MB MRCP(UK)
Senior Registrar in Geriatric Medicine, Cardiff Royal Infirmary,
Cardiff, UK

D. G. Seymour, MD MRCP
Senior Lecturer in Geriatric Medicine, University of Wales College
of Medicine, Cardiff, UK

R. M. Seymour, MB MRCP(UK)
Lecturer in Geriatric Medicine, University of Wales College of
Medicine, Cardiff, UK

K. Smith, BA CHE
Administrator, Health Services, Faculty of Health Sciences,
McMaster University, Hamilton, Ontario, Canada

S. D. G. Stephens, MPhil MRCP
Consultant in Audiological Medicine, Welsh Hearing Institute,
University Hospital of Wales, Cardiff, UK

C. G. Swift, PhD FRCP
Professor, Department of Health Care of the Elderly, King's
College School of Medicine & Dentistry, London, UK

T. P. L. Thomas, MB MRCP
Consultant Physician in Geriatric Medicine, Bryntirion Hospital,
Llanelli, UK

Gladys M. Tinker, MB MRCP
Consultant Physician in Geriatric Medicine, Llandough Hospital,
Penarth, UK

C. Twining, MSc PhD
Top Grade Clinical Psychologist, Department of Psychology,
Whitchurch Hospital, Cardiff, UK

Sally Venn, MB DGM
Registrar, Dewi Sant Hospital, Pontypridd, UK

J. B. Walsh, MRCPI
Consultant Physician in Geriatric Medicine, St James's Hospital,
Dublin 8, Eire

W. E. Wilkins, MB MRCP
Consultant Physician in Geriatric Medicine, Princess of Wales
Hospital, Bridgend, UK

M. Woodward, FRACP
Consultant Physician, Repatriation General Hospital, Heidelberg
West, Victoria, Australia

Section I
Ageing: An Overview

Chapter 1

The Physiology of Ageing

D. G. Seymour and R. M. Seymour

As a person grows old, organ function is challenged both by disease and by the physiological processes associated with ageing. In clinical geriatric medicine, it is pathological change rather than decaying physiology which is the major cause of morbidity and mortality. For example, age-related loss in muscle power is dwarfed by the motor disability precipitated by a cerebral infarction, although the former may be of some importance when attempting to rehabilitate the patient. Thus, a full diagnostic functional assessment in an individual elderly patient together with a rational approach to management needs to take account of the physiological backdrop against which the diseases dealt with in this book occur.

This chapter begins with a number of general statements about the physiology of ageing and then touches on some physiological changes of clinical relevance. Space does not permit a more comprehensive review of the extensive literature in this field, particularly of animal models of physiological ageing. Longitudinal studies of human populations are small in number, probably because they are both expensive and demand a life-long commitment from those who embark on them.

General Concepts about Ageing and Physiology

1. The physiological function of most organ systems tends to decline with age, but there is wide individual variability.
2. Age-related changes in physiology are rarely of clinical significance when the system is at rest, but may become important when it is stressed for example by exercise, disease or drug administration.
3. Homeostatic impairment is a key feature of physiological ageing. Elderly people, for example, take longer to excrete an acid load than younger adults and this must be taken into account when treating diabetic ketoacidosis.
4. Physiological changes determine the *maximum* age of a species (around 120 years in humans), whereas the *average* age at death is determined by disease and/or environmental factors.

Clinical Importance of Age-Related Physiological Changes

1. Physiological changes may affect the way in which a disease *presents* in old age. For example, the tachycardia seen in young patients in response to blood loss or pyrexia may not be evident in older subjects.
2. Impaired physiological function may affect the *susceptibility* of an elderly person to disease. A well-recognised example of this would be the changes in the immune response believed to contribute to the increased incidence of tuberculosis in old age.
3. Once a disease or traumatic event has intervened, age-related homeostatic impairment may hamper *recovery*. A common clinical setting in which this occurs is after surgery when fluid depletion or fluid excess place an additional burden on the renal and cardiovascular systems.
4. *Drug handling* tends to alter with age due to a number of factors which include impairment in renal and hepatic clearance and changes in body composition (see Chap. 24).
5. The *reference ranges of laboratory tests* such as spirometry, cardiac indices and several blood tests are affected by age changes which are partly physiological in nature.

Dangers of Over-emphasising Physiological Decline

1. Treatable diseases may be missed by being ascribed simply to "old age". The vague musculo-skeletal symptoms of osteomalacia or polymyalgia rheumatica or the impaired exercise tolerance of late-onset asthma or cardiac failure can be overlooked under these circumstances, to the detriment of the patient.
2. Over-emphasis on age-related physiological decline may lead to attitudes of nihilism among patients and health professionals alike. Each patient deserves precise diagnosis and assessment of function together with individually tailored management.

Cardiovascular Function

Cardiovascular function does tend to decline with age, though the physiological picture is clouded by the presence of heart and arterial disease which are commonplace in the elderly. Table 1.1 lists ten physiological changes in cardiovascular function which appear to be age-related and these are now discussed with particular reference to changes in cardiac output and blood pressure.

Cardiac Output

Community studies of the 1960s indicated that resting cardiac output fell by about 1% per year after the age of 35. While more recent longitudinal investigations have pointed out that such a decline is not universal, the 1% figure remains a useful clinical guide.

In the absence of heart disease, a fall of 1% per year in cardiac output should not result in dyspnoea at rest, even in centenarians. However, symptoms are likely to develop when the heart is stressed by exercise, pyrexia, anaemia or trauma. Estimates vary, but the maximum cardiac output of a man of 65 is typically 20%–30% less than that of a young adult.

Cardiac output is the stroke volume multiplied by the heart rate. The fall in resting cardiac output with age can be attributed to a fall in stroke volume, resting pulse rate remaining constant. The reduced maximum cardiac output with ageing on the other hand is due to a reduction in both maximum stroke volume and maximum heart rate.

Why do the stroke volume and the maximum heart rate fall with age? A number of possible reasons are highlighted in Table 1.1. Heart wall rigidity tends to increase and this both reduces the efficiency of muscle contraction and prolongs the time necessary for each cycle of contraction to be completed. As well as struggling with the effects of its own rigidity the myocardium must overcome the additional strain placed on it by reduced distensibility in the great vessels and the increased peripheral vascular resistance associated with ageing.

Table 1.1.   Age-related changes in cardiovascular function

1. Resting cardiac output and cardiac index[a] fall
2. Resting left ventricular performance declines
3. Cardiac reserve decreases: lesser rise in cardiac output on exercise, maximal heart rate on exercise decreases
4. Rate of myocardial contraction slows, recovery from contraction is delayed, systole is prolonged
5. Heart wall rigidity increases
6. Loss of elasticity in large arteries, systolic blood pressure rises
7. Peripheral vascular resistance rises
8. Maximal coronary artery flow less than in the young
9. Normal vasomotor tone decreases, vagal influence increases
10. Myocardial irritability increases, arrhythmias become more prevalent

[a] Cardiac index is cardiac output expressed relative to a standardised body surface area.

Because of reduced cardiac reserve, the elderly person may be tipped into heart failure by processes which would have been easily coped with in his or her youth. Examples of such processes include anaemia, sepsis, intravenous fluid overload, supraventricular tachycardia, moderate hypertension and small myocardial infarcts.

Blood Pressure

In Western societies a rise in mean systolic pressure between the age of 20 and 70 has been consistently reported, even in fit people. Diastolic pressures rise similarly, but tend to level off ten years earlier. When everyone, including the healthy in the population, is surveyed, the rises in pressure are marked. Thus two-fifths of men between the age of 55 and 65 can be expected to have diastolic blood pressures over 90 mmHg.

The rise in blood pressure with age is usually attributed to the combined effect of increased peripheral resistance and decreased vessel distensibility. The latter is particularly likely to elevate the systolic blood pressure. While it is tempting to regard these changes in blood pressure in Western populations as an inevitable consequence of ageing, environmental factors probably also play a part because in non-Western societies a rise in blood pressure with age is by no means universal. The debate as to what constitutes an appropriate "physiological" blood pressure in an elderly individual illustrates an important general point with respect to ageing. Environmental, social and cultural influences play upon our physiology. By understanding, for example, why certain societies maintain a "youthful" blood pressure we may need to modify our ideas as to what is true, fixed physiological ageing and what is modifiable physiology bordering on pathology.

Respiratory Function

Pure physiological ageing changes in the respiratory system are exceptionally difficult to separate from those due to chronic attrition by micro-organisms, cigarettes and a variety of pollutant smokes and dusts in the environment. In addition, we still know little about the response of ageing respiratory tissue to the stresses of hypoxia, hypercapnia and exercise, which may be more important clinically than simple spirometry and static lung volumes.

Routine Tests of Lung Function

It is widely appreciated that account must be taken of a patient's age and sex when interpreting lung volumes. Tables of age-related predicted values are readily available. There is considerable individual variation, however, and serial measurements may be necessary in any one patient to separate pathological from physiological change.

Peak expiratory flow rates (PEFR), forced expiratory volume in one second (FEV_1) and forced vital capacity (FVC) all decline with age, though the rate of fall is debated. The FEV_1/FVC ratio shows a less clear-cut change. It appears to fall initially, but beyond the age of 70 it may increase.

Total lung capacity appears to change little over the years, but with the gradual loss of elastic tissue that occurs with ageing there is an increase in residual volume and functional residual capacity and a diminution in vital capacity. Transfer factor, for complex reasons, also shows a small decline with age.

Closing Volumes

Chest wall compliance decreases with age as muscle, ligament and bony changes cause the thoracic cage to become less mobile. Within the parenchyma of the lung, elastic tissue is slowly lost and this, together with as yet ill-defined changes in the airways, influences the closing volume of the lung (i.e. the volume at which small airways start to close on expiration). In older individuals, closure occurs at higher lung volumes in the more dependent areas of the lung fields. These observations become clinically important in the immobile elderly patient when atelectasis, sputum retention and superinfection become a threat. Preventive programmes of physiotherapy such as proper positioning of the patient and incentive spirometry have attracted considerable interest, but the benefits remain to be fully proven.

Altered ventilation/perfusion rates in the elderly, together possibly with more complex changes at the alveolar–capillary interface mean that arterial oxygen tensions in older individuals are lower than at a younger age, though values for carbon dioxide appear to remain constant throughout life in the absence of disease.

Defence Mechanisms and the Lung

Several factors combine to render the elderly lung more vulnerable to attack by respiratory pathogens. Changed closing volumes, impaired humoral and cell-mediated immunity, diminished forcefulness of coughing with chest wall "stiffening" and increased neuromuscular incoordination during swallowing (predisposing to aspiration of foodstuffs) all play a part in this increased vulnerability. Experiments have also shown that the tracheobronchial mucus carpet moves more slowly so that expulsion of foreign material is less efficient.

Central Control of Respiration

There is some evidence that the ventilatory response in the elderly to hypoxia and hypercapnia is blunted at rest, but paradoxically it appears to increase with exercise. It is not known where the physiological changes occur which lead to these altered ventilatory responses, nor is their clinical relevance fully understood. Much interest recently has been focused on irregular patterns of ventilation and apnoeic periods during sleep in the elderly and the reader is referred to more specialised texts on this subject.

Renal Function

The classic cross-sectional studies of renal function have led to the concept that glomerular filtration rate (as measured by creatinine clearance) tends to fall with age by about 1% per year after the age of 35 years. While more recent longitudinal studies have shown that such renal decline does not occur in every individual, it is a reasonable first assumption in clinical practice that a patient of 75 will possess only about 60% of the creatinine clearance of a patient of 35. Such falls in creatinine clearance with ageing may be accompanied by only a minor rise in serum creatinine as muscle mass (and hence the rate of creatinine production) tends to decrease in the elderly.

A 50% fall of creatinine clearance does not of itself produce symptoms and common adverse effects in clinical practice are usually confined to the accumulation of renally excreted drugs such as digoxin. On average the maintenance dose of digoxin required in the elderly tends to be half that needed in younger adults and this may be a useful concept when therapy is initiated in the older patient. However, thereafter, dosage in individual elderly patients needs to be adjusted using clinical criteria (such as the heart rate in atrial fibrillation) not by reference to books of physiology. The dangers of overdosage of digoxin in the elderly have been so well publicised that it is becoming increasingly common to encounter elderly patients who are under-digitalised.

For selected renally excreted drugs, such as gentamicin and (to a lesser extent) digoxin, the measurement of blood levels is of value in defining dosage regimens.

Compared with the creatinine clearance rate the effect of ageing on other aspects of renal function has been relatively little explored. However, it has been established that the ability to concentrate and dilute urine and the ability to excrete an acid or alkaline load falls with age. Ability to concentrate or dilute urine is an important means of maintaining salt and water balance, and its reduction in old age makes the elderly patient vulnerable to the effects of inadequate fluid intake or excessive loss on the one hand or fluid overload on the other. The unthinking prescription of "two litres of dextrose and one of saline" per day in the elderly post-operative patient may lead to disaster. Difficulties in handling acid loads may lead to delayed recovery from diabetic ketoacidosis in the elderly.

It is not clear whether the commonly observed decline in renal function which occurs with age is primarily due to ageing or the effects of subclinical disease over the years. For clinical purposes the distinction is probably unimportant; what matters is the recognition that such a decline is likely to have occurred in an elderly patient.

Gastrointestinal Function

Motility

Some authors describe a condition of "presbyoesophagus" in many elderly people which is composed of delayed oesophageal emptying, dilatation and an increased incidence of ineffective peristalsis with so-called tertiary contractions. The physical basis of these changes is unclear, but they may lead to an increased incidence of reflux oesophagitis and aspiration of gastric contents. Elsewhere in the gastrointestinal tract, motility measurements are more difficult, although delayed gastric emptying with age has been described. In the lower bowel, transit time is often increased and it is tempting to attribute this to an age-related decline in colonic smooth muscle power, often aggravated by years of laxative abuse. However, studies of the sigmoid colon have more often encountered *over-active* rather than hypotonic muscle, although this often leads to hypersegmentation and associated *slowing* of transit time. Again, it is not clear whether such changes are physiological or secondary to a lifetime of purgation and low fibre diets.

It must be stressed that a *change* in bowel habit in an elderly person must never be attributed to "old age" and must always be investigated.

Absorption

Atrophy of the gastric mucosa is common in old age, even in the absence of pernicious anaemia. While this may increase the chances of peptic ulceration, it is difficult to prove that absorption of drugs and nutrients is significantly affected. Similarly, in the small intestine, while the absorptive surface area is decreased in old age, it has yet to be established that this has a major effect on absorption.

Liver

Liver size and blood flow falls with age, but the considerable reserve capacity of this organ enables it to cope with normal body requirements even in extreme old age. Many of the liver enzyme systems become less efficient with age, however, and this may affect the metabolism of certain drugs (see Chap. 24).

Exocrine Pancreatic Function

The amount of exocrine tissue in the pancreas falls with age, but the loss falls far short of the 90% reduction that would be required to produce steatorrhoea.

Glucose Tolerance

It has long been recognised that the incidence of glucose intolerance increases with age. The rise in fasting plasma glucose is small (of the order of 0.05 mmol/l per decade), but there is an impaired ability to handle a glucose load. In 1980, the World Health Organization proposed new criteria for frank "diabetes mellitus" and recognised an intermediate state of "impaired glucose tolerance" (Table 1.2). The majority of elderly people who develop glucose intolerance with age fall into the "impaired glucose tolerance" rather than into the true "diabetes mellitus" group.

The reason for impaired glucose tolerance with age is probably multifactorial. Some research studies have pointed to altered patterns of insulin release while others have stressed alterations in peripheral insulin receptors.

Table 1.2. Diagnostic values on glucose tolerance tests[a] (WHO recommendations 1980)

	Venous plasma glucose (mmol/l)[b]		
	Fasting		2 hours post-glucose
Normal	<8	and	<8
Impaired glucose tolerance	<8	and	≥8 but <11
Diabetes mellitus	≥8	and/or	≥11

[a] After a 75-g oral glucose load in 250–350 ml water.
[b] Capillary whole blood samples or venous whole blood samples give values which are up to 15% lower.

The Nervous System and Ageing

Physiological changes occurring in the nervous system are those most associated in the lay mind with "senescence" and although they do not often threaten life they may certainly diminish its quality. To illustrate this point a few of these changes are discussed here and the reader is referred to more detailed texts for further information.

The Special Senses

With regard to *vision*, physiological changes occur in both the optical apparatus and the central visual pathway. These result in a diminution in corneal sensitivity, a small pupil which reacts less briskly to light, and impaired accommodation and long-sightedness (due to increased lens stiffness). Yellowing of the lens leads to poor blue–green colour discrimination and less efficient adaptation to the dark leads to reduced visual acuity in low lighting and at night. Some upward gaze and ocular movements become progressively impaired. Visual evoked responses are diminished, suggesting a central ageing effect, and perception of visual stimuli is altered causing difficulty in picking out embedded figures from a confusing background.

Two lessons can be drawn from these observations. Firstly, physiological changes must be taken into account when examining elderly cranial nerves II, III, IV and VI. Secondly, efforts need to be made to help older eyes function at their physiological best by providing well-lit, unambiguous environments for old people and immediate referral to an ophthalmologist once failing vision is complained of.

With regard to *hearing*, age-related changes in inner ear structure lead to progressive bilateral sensorineural hearing loss at high frequencies. High-pitched consonants such as "p", "t" and "c" are lost while low-pitched vowels are preserved. In addition, central ageing processes which are not understood lead to difficulties in comprehending speech, particularly against a background of confusing noise. A hearing aid is not the automatic answer to this problem. Slowly spoken, clear speech (not necessarily louder) should be adopted when communicating with older patients with possible hearing loss. Physical examination of every older patient should include as complete an assessment of hearing as possible.

Both *taste* and *smell* appear to decline with age possibly related to a loss of taste buds and olfactory neurons. Because of these dulled sensations, food may lose its flavour making it difficult to persuade elderly people to eat adequately.

Cerebral Function

Changes in the cellular structure and neurochemistry of the brain are a major preoccupation of groups seeking to understand the pathogenesis of dementias. In "normal" elderly brains there appears to be a loss of neurons in certain areas, a decrease in brain weight, mild ventricular dilatation, gyral atrophy and a small accumulation of amyloid-like material, senile plaques, lipofuscin and neurofibrillary tangles. Small changes in the cholinergic, catecholamine and gamma-aminobutyric acid (GABA) neurotransmitter systems have been described by some groups, though these changes are not as consistent or as marked as those noted in dementias.

Despite the growth of neurophysiological information about the elderly brain we do not yet know which, if any, of these changes underline the impairments of cognitive function frequently associated with ageing such as diminished ability to solve new problems and failure of storage of recent information. Slow mentation and apparently poor memory may, however, be the presenting feature of a wide variety of physical diseases, reactions to drugs or mental disorders so should never be dismissed as "old age" or, even worse, "hardening of the arteries".

Sleep

Elderly people frequently complain of disturbed sleep, but studies have suggested that frequent arousals from sleep are probably part of a normal pattern of ageing, although if excessive this can lead to daytime somnolence and napping. Less time appears to be spent in Stage 4, deep sleep. A switch to an interrupted pattern of sleep tends to disturb certain physiological diurnal rhythms such as cortisol production, although the effect that this disturbance has on other physiological processes and the well-being of elderly individuals is not known.

Peripheral Nervous System

With regard to sensory changes, clinicians are well aware of the fact that vibration sense diminishes in older people and may be absent in the distal lower limbs in a third or more "normal" people aged over 75 years. More sensitive techniques show that fine touch may also be diminished. Loss of the ankle jerk is often described as a "normal" finding in patients over 70. Once again, we know almost nothing about the cellular and biochemical changes which are responsible for these observations. Moreover, questions have recently been raised by those interested in the neurology of the elderly as to whether the above findings are truly physiological or may represent a sub-group with minor pathological conditions.

The fall in muscle power observed in old age is probably due to a mixture of myopathic and neuropathic change. Muscle bulk diminishes and histological studies incriminate loss of Type II fast twitch fibres. The number of motor units may also decline, although this is debated. Muscles appear to take longer to relax and contract and the strength of the hand grip and quadriceps strength diminish by about 40% between the ages of 30 and 70. Both motor and sensory changes, though part of normal ageing, may play a part in the aetiology of falls (see Chap. 17) and also need to be considered in programmes of physiotherapy and occupational therapy. Changes in muscle power must also have an effect on the ease with which patients can climb stairs, cross roads and rise from the toilet.

Bone Mass

Total bone mass increases up to the age of about 35 years and thereafter decreases, even in fit people. The rate of decline in women is greater than that of men, particularly in the decade after the menopause when the protective effect of oestrogens is removed. There is, however, considerable variation from person to person. Cortical bone mass tends to decrease steadily with age so that, by the age of 80, around 50% of men and 75% of women have cortical bone densities below the "normal" range for young adults. Trabecular bone mass declines with age, but the rate of loss slows in the seventh and eighth decades. According to some studies, about 25% of men and 50% of women at the age of 70 have trabecular bone densities below the "normal" range for young adults.

The bone mass of an individual is determined by a number of genetic, environmental, endocrinological and pathological factors and it is difficult to be dogmatic about whether loss of bone mass is a true physiological process. Factors known to favour a low bone mass are a low body weight, lack of activity, poor calcium intake before the age of 35, excessive tobacco, alcohol and caffeine, early menopause, chronic malabsorption, corticosteroids, thyrotoxicosis and possibly any long-term debilitating disease.

Body Temperature Control

The maintenance of body temperature is one of the homeostatic mechanisms which can become impaired in old age. At rest, in comfortable surroundings, the body temperature of a fit old person is no different from that of a young adult. Problems may arise, however, when the elderly are exposed to temperature extremes.

As the external temperature falls, the onset of shivering may be delayed in the old as compared with the young, placing them at greater risk from hypothermia. In addition, the lower basal metabolic activity of the elderly (due to lower muscle mass) places them at an extra disadvantage in the cold. Some elderly people also appear to be less aware of the coldness of their surroundings than are young people, which may result in delays in putting on extra clothing or turning up the heating. Matters may be made worse by factors which are more to do with finance and social tradition than physiology. The British practice of sleeping in a cold bedroom with a window open to let in "fresh air" may be particularly hazardous. Once clinical hypothermia has developed in the elderly, the mortality rate tends to be higher than in the young, possibly because of impaired homeostatic function in renal and cardiovascular systems.

At the other extreme, old people are particularly susceptible to hyperthermia during heatwaves and are more likely to die when hyperthermia has developed. Identifiable problems here include a reduced renal ability to conserve salt and water, a thirst mechanism which may be less keen and a delay in the onset of sweating when the body temperature rises.

Combating Physiological Decline

While physiological decline is the rule with old age, this should not result in undue pessimism in doctors dealing with the elderly. The reserve capacity of most organs is considerable, and in any case the quality of life of a person living in the controlled environment of a modern society is largely unaffected by the physiological changes of ageing. There is also the exciting possibility that we may be able to halt some of those declines in physiological function that have been attributed to the "inevitable" effects of ageing by encouraging "healthier" life styles in early life. Diet and exercise are important variables open to modification. Details of exercise prescription in the elderly are beyond the scope of this chapter, but the reader is directed to the important work of Shephard and his colleagues in Canada. The benefits of exercise therapy can be demonstrated even in the very elderly. They include increased cardiac efficiency, possibly increased vital capacity, weight reduction, better joint flexibility and an increased sense of well-being. A maintenance of muscle strength and bone mass may also be possible as the result of longer term programmes of exercise.

Finally, despite the growth of geriatric medicine, the general public still seem to see ageing as an inexorable symptomatic physiological decline involving diminishing vision, hearing, memory and sexuality, aches and pains, breathlessness and a host of other "failing" organ systems. It is important that health professionals take active steps to educate patients positively about ageing. "It's just your age" should be a diagnosis of last resort, if indeed it is supportable as a diagnosis at all.

Further Reading

Albert ML (ed) (1984) Clinical neurology of ageing. Oxford University Press, Oxford

Avioli LV (ed) (1987) The osteoporotic syndrome: detection, prevention and treatment, 2nd edn. Grune and Stratton, New York

Geokas MC (ed) (1985) Symposium on the aging process. Clin Geriatr Med 1:1–309

Goldman R, Rockstein M (eds) (1975) The physiology and pathology of human aging. Academic Press, New York

Rowe JW, Andres R, Tobin JD, Norris AH, Shock NW (1976) The effect of age on creatinine clearance in men: a cross-sectional and longitudinal study. J Gerontol 31:155–163

Seymour DG (1986) Medical assessment of the elderly surgical patient. Croom Helm, London, pp 27–29, 82–89, 189–194

Shephard RJ (1985) Physical fitness: exercise and ageing. In: Pathy MSJ (ed) Principles and practice of geriatric medicine. Wiley, Chichester, pp 163–177

Shephard RJ (1987) Physical activity and aging, 2nd edn. Croom Helm, London

Tallis RC, Caird FI (eds) (1986) Hypertension in the elderly. Churchill Livingstone, Edinburgh, pp 79–106. (Advanced geriatric medicine 5)

Chapter 2

Demography and Epidemiology of Old Age

Deirdre Hine

Demography

Few well-informed adults, let alone those working in health or social care services, can be unaware that one of the most striking and well-documented demographic trends of this century has been the increase, in both relative and absolute numbers, of elderly people in the population. Though most evident in the developed industrialised countries, this is a world-wide phenomenon with the numbers of old people in developing countries also increasing. Brazil, Mexico and Nigeria, for example, will experience a more than tenfold increase in the number of people aged 60 and over between the years 1950 and 2025.

The description of these changes as "the greying of nations" is a reminder that the absolute number of old people (the white hairs in the greying head), together with their frequency in relation to the young (the black hairs), determine the characteristics of the total population. This is well illustrated for the population of Great Britain by Fig. 2.1. The study of this phenomenon and the analysis of the factors which have led to it are important for all those working with the elderly and in planning services for them. Perhaps more importantly, however, misconceived ideas about the cause of this phenomenon can play a potent part in generating those hostile attitudes to old people known collectively as "ageism". Such attitudes are unfortunately not uncommon in both professional and lay people who come into contact with the elderly or have influence over the provision of resources to meet their needs.

The Current Population Structure and Its Determinants

The number of elderly people in Great Britain, defined for the purposes of the census carried out by the Office of Population Censuses and Surveys (OPCS) as women over 60 and men over 65, has been increasing for many years. These mem-

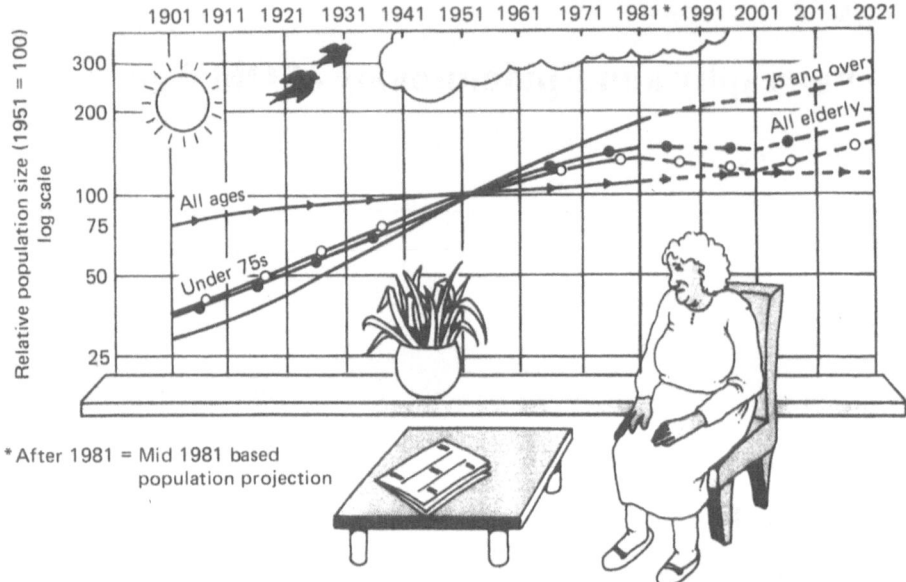

Fig. 2.1. Relative size of the elderly population of Great Britain 1901–2021 (1951=100). (From Office of Population Censuses and Surveys Census Guide 1: Britain's elderly population 1984.)

bers of the population are by reason of their age eligible for a State pension and are thus referred to as the population of pensionable age. Their numbers have risen from less than 3 million in 1911 to almost 10 million in 1981 (Table 2.1). This trebling in absolute numbers has been accompanied by a similar rise in the proportion of the population made up of elderly people which increased from 6% in 1911 to 18% in 1981. This phenomenon of an increasingly aged population is worldwide. In the United States, for example, the number of persons aged 65 and over has risen more than eightfold from 3.1 million in 1900 to over 25 million today. This compares with a threefold increase in the total US population during the same period.

Popular opinion usually ascribes these increases to the success of medical science in keeping elderly people alive for longer and longer, often unfortunately with the tacit implication that the old have outstayed their time and have no right to continued care and support. Rather it is an increase in life expectancy which has resulted in the increasing numbers of old people and medicine and health care services have played a comparatively small role in this improvement. This increase in life expectancy took place not at the end of the life span of today's old people, but in their earliest years.

The number of old people alive today is the product of the number of births occurring at or around the turn of the last century and the mortality experience of that cohort of people over the total period since then. An examination of the data shows that the annual number of live births in Great Britain reached its peak at approximately 900 000 per annum during the decade 1900–1910 and has declined rapidly ever since. The infant mortality rate (deaths under 1 year per 1000 live

Table 2.1. The elderly population of Great Britain by broad age groups: 1851–2001 census data[a]

	1851	1871	1891	1911	1931	1951	1961	1971	1981	1991[b]	2001[b]
Number by age (millions)											
60–64 women	0.3	0.4	0.5	0.6	1.0	1.3	1.5	1.7	1.5	1.5	1.4
65–74 women	0.4	0.5	0.6	0.9	1.4	2.1	2.3	2.7	2.8	2.8	2.5
men	0.3	0.4	0.5	0.7	1.1	1.5	1.6	1.9	2.2	2.2	2.1
persons	0.7	0.9	1.1	1.5	2.4	3.6	3.9	4.6	5.0	5.0	4.6
75–84 women	0.1	0.2	0.2	0.3	0.5	0.9	1.2	1.4	1.7	1.9	1.9
men	0.1	0.1	0.2	0.2	0.3	0.6	0.7	0.7	0.9	1.1	1.1
persons	0.3	0.3	0.4	0.5	0.8	1.5	1.8	2.1	2.6	3.0	3.0
85 and over women	–	–	–	–	0.1	0.2	0.2	0.3	0.4	0.6	0.8
men	–	–	–	–	–	0.1	0.1	0.1	0.1	0.2	0.3
persons	–	–	0.1	0.1	0.1	0.2	0.3	0.5	0.6	0.8	1.0
Total numbers (millions)											
60–65 and over[c]	1.3	1.6	2.1	2.7	4.3	6.7	7.6	8.8	9.7	10.3	10.1
75 and over	0.3	0.4	0.4	0.6	0.9	1.7	2.3	2.5	3.1	3.8	4.1
85 and over	–	–	0.1	0.1	0.1	0.2	0.3	0.5	0.6	0.8	1.0
Population: all ages (millions)	20.8	26.1	33.0	40.8	44.8	48.9	51.3	54.0	54.3	55.4	56.4

(Taken from OPCS (1984) Census guide 1: Britain's elderly population.)
[a] 1851–1981 give census counts (no census taken in 1941).
[b] 1991 and 2001 show projections of the provisional mid 1981 estimates of the usually resident population.
[c] 60–65 and over means women aged 60 and over plus men aged 65 and over.

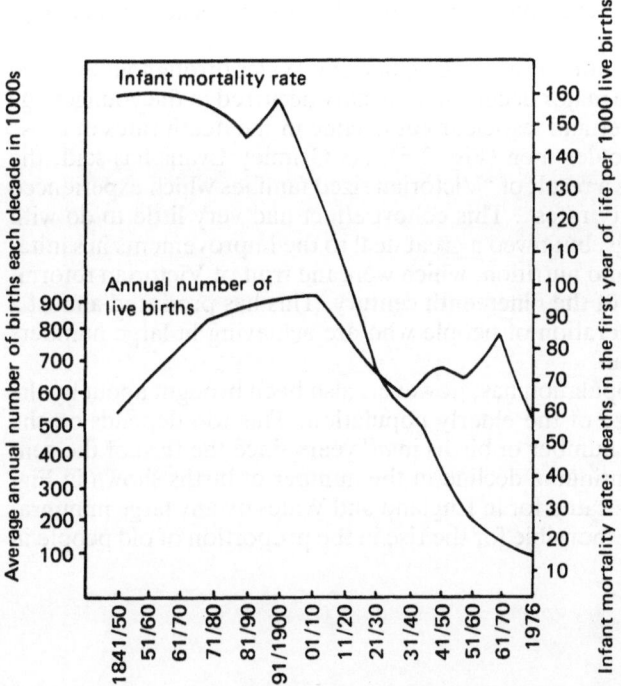

Fig. 2.2. Number of live births and infant mortality rate in Great Britain. (From Muir Gray 1985.)

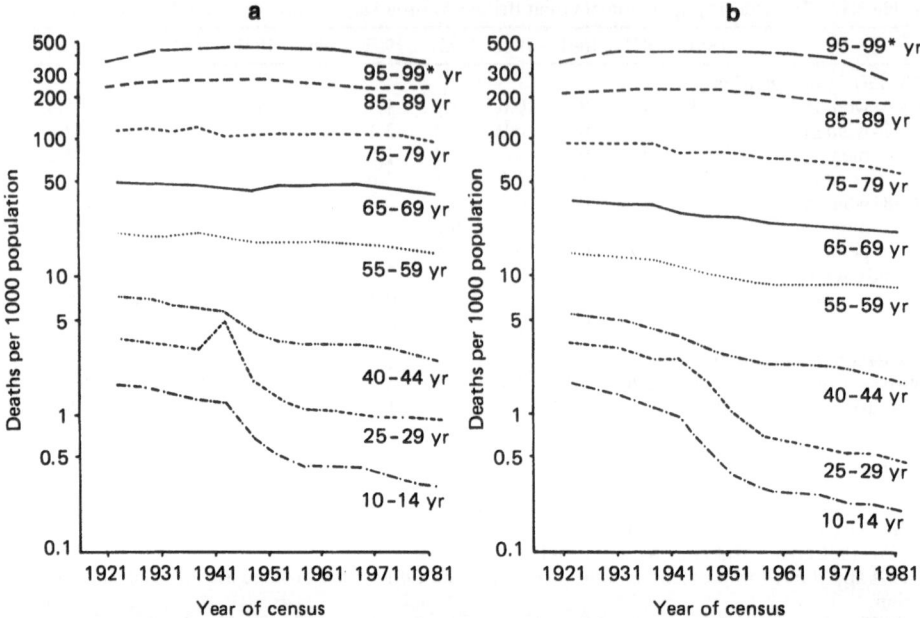

Fig. 2.3. Mortality rates in males (**a**) and in females (**b**), England and Wales 1921–1984. *Ninety-five years and over in 1981. (From Alderson 1986.)

births) began a similar and even more dramatic fall about a decade earlier (Fig. 2.2).

If we examine mortality rates by age in England and Wales throughout this century it is very clear that the major decline in mortality occurred in the younger age groups, with a much slower and less clear-cut decline in the death rates of those over 60, especially so in older men (Fig. 2.3). As Grimley Evans has said, the number of elderly today is a result of "Victorian sized families which experienced Edwardian infant mortality rates". This cohort effect had very little to do with medical treatment or drugs, but owed a great deal to the improvements in sanitation, housing, education and nutrition, which were the fruit of Victorian reforming zeal in the later years of the nineteenth century. This has produced almost a century later the first generation of people who are achieving in large numbers their full biological life span.

The "greying" of the population has, however, also been brought about by the increase in the *relative* size of the elderly population. This too depends on the number of births, but the number of births in *all* years since the turn of the century. The marked and continuing decline in the number of births shown in Fig. 2.2, which was not compensated for in England and Wales by any large immigration of young people, is responsible for the rise in the proportion of old people in the population.

Future Trends

Looking forward to the end of this century the trend of increasing numbers of elderly people is set to continue (Table 2.1). The mid-1981 population projections show an increase in the total number of pensioners from 9.7 million in 1981 to 10.3 million in 1991. By the year 2001, however, the increase will have ceased and there will be a slight reduction to 10.1 million. Thus the total number of elderly people looks likely to reach a plateau at about 10 million. Within these figures, however, the more important trend is that of the numbers in the oldest age groups. A reduction from 5 million to 4.6 million persons aged 65–74 years between 1951 and 2001 is balanced by an increase from 3.1 million to 4.1 million people aged over 75 years, and by 2001, one million of these will be over 85 years (Fig. 2.4). Although in absolute terms these numbers are not great in relation to the projected total population of 56 million people in 2001, the knowledge that these age groups make the heaviest demand for health and social services (because of age-related diseases and disability) gives a substantial significance to these projections and indicates a serious challenge to the planners of such services.

The lack of homogeneity in the elderly population, a matter which is all too frequently forgotten when we refer to "the elderly", has other facets and implications in addition to stratification by age. There is a notable lack of balance in the proportion of the two sexes, with only one-third being men. This is produced to some extent artificially by the inclusion of women of 60–64 in the pensionable age group while men are not included until 65. The greater longevity of women is also responsible, however, as evidenced by the ratio of two women to every man in the

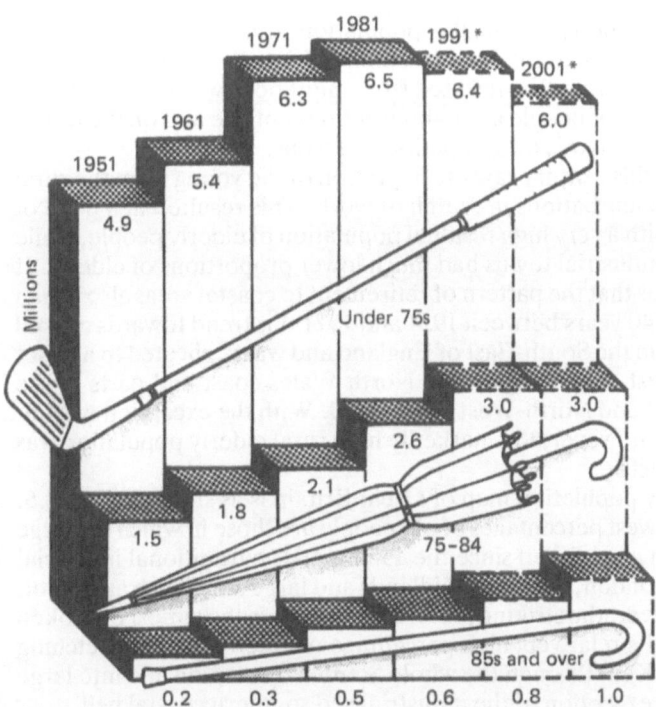

Fig. 2.4. Numbers of the elderly by broad sub-groups, Great Britain 1951–2001. *Mid-1981 based population projection. (From Office of Population Censuses and Surveys and the Central Office of Information 1984.)

75–84 age group, and even more dramatically by four women to every man in the over-85 age group.

Further differences in the characteristics of the age/sex groups also result from this greater longevity of women. Nearly three-quarters of elderly men are married with a wife still living, while less than half of the elderly women have a living spouse. Of these about 11% were never married and in the over-85 age group this rises to 16% reflecting partly the enormous loss of marriage opportunity resulting from the large loss of young men in the First World War. The number of women who never marry is now very much less, but the likelihood that an elderly "ever married" woman will be widowed will remain high while the life expectancy of women continues to outstrip that of men. The data for 1981–1983 suggest that women, with a life expectancy of 77.4 years, still have a 6-year advantage over men, who have a life expectancy of 71.3 years. The increasing trend towards divorce and remarriage will also affect the chances that elderly men and women of the future have of the support of a spouse in coping with the health and social problems of old age. Since the spouse is by far the most frequent and in most cases the most acceptable "carer" of old people, these data also have considerable significance for health services.

The Distribution of Old People

The distribution of the elderly within the population also lacks homogeneity, either in broad geographical terms, within communities, or within household types. Geographical distribution has resulted from migrations within the country; on the one hand migration of people at or about retirement age and on the other, of the young for social, economic or occupational reasons.

The early decades of this century saw the migration of the young from the rural areas to the industrial conurbations in search of work. This resulted in a band of central rural counties with a very high residual population of elderly people, while the rapidly expanding industrial towns had much lower proportions of elderly. It was during these decades that the pattern of retirement to coastal areas also began to develop. During the 40 years between 1931 and 1971 this trend towards coastal retirement accelerated in the South-East of England and was replicated to a lesser extent in the South-West, East Anglia, the North Wales coast and parts of the coasts of the North-East and North-West of England. With the exception of Mid-Wales and the Borders, however, the markedly high rural elderly population was much reduced by the 1980s.

Currently, the elderly population map of Great Britain is as shown in Fig. 2.5. The districts with the lowest percentages of old people are those in which the large "new towns" have been established since the 1950s and the traditional industrial development areas of London, the West Midlands and large cities such as Bristol, Cardiff and Hull. However, the striking feature of the map is the almost unbroken band of authorities with a relatively high percentage of elderly people stretching from the south coast of Kent through the whole South-West region and into large areas of Wales with the exception of the industrialised southern coastal belt.

Variations in the proportion of elderly people between different local authority districts are not very extreme in numerical terms. Rotherham with 35%, Worth-

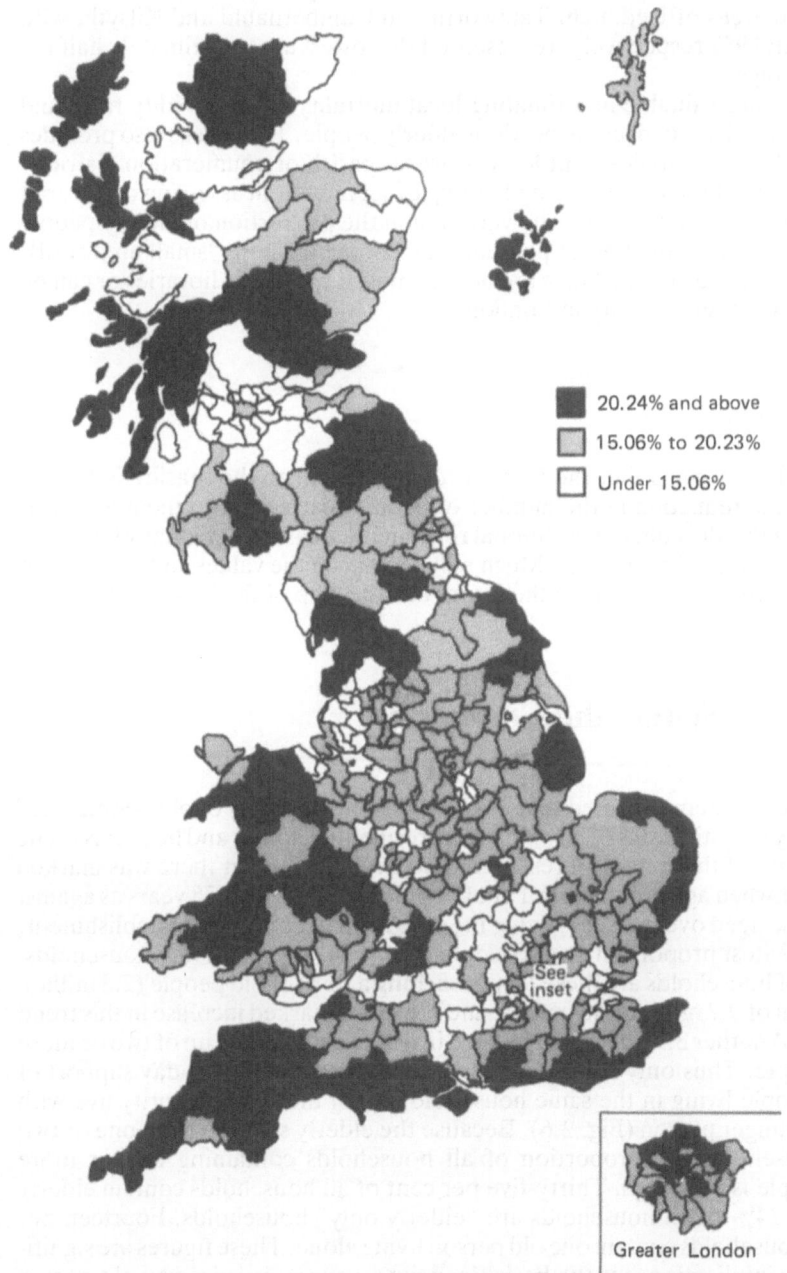

Fig. 2.5.   The proportion of elderly people in each local authority district of Great Britain 1981. (From Office of Population Censuses and Surveys and the Central Office of Information 1984.)

ing with 35% and Eastbourne with 34% were the "top three" in 1981, while the rapid growth areas of Redditch, Tamworth and Cumbernauld and Kilsyth, with 11%, 10% and 9% respectively, represented the lowest at approximately half the national average.

These data are valuable in estimating local mortality and morbidity rates and for planning services to meet the needs of elderly people. The census also provides data at smaller geographical unit levels – ward, parish or enumeration district – which can be invaluable in detailed planning of services or in assessing the overall health needs of the population. The variation in the proportion of elderly people is greater the smaller the unit of population examined. These "small area statistics" are published as tables which are held at most large public libraries or can be consulted at the OPCS library in London.

Future Trends

There are already signs that the fashion for retirement to the seaside is past its peak. With the reduction in the number of people reaching retirement age after the middle of this decade, the traditional retirement areas may gradually lose their record proportions of old people. Much will depend on the values and attitudes of the "new elderly" in determining the future old age map of the United Kingdom.

The Elderly Within the Community

The 1981 Census demonstrated that only a tiny minority (3%) of old people were permanently in institutions of any kind (e.g. residential homes and hospitals). The great majority of these were in residential homes. Here again there was marked variation between age groups with 1% of people aged less than 75 years as against 19% of those aged over 85 years living in some form of communal establishment.

So the greatest proportion of old people (i.e. 97%) live in private households. What sort of households are these? Approaching a third of old people (2.8 million out of a total of 9.7 million), live alone and there is a marked increase in this trend since 1961. Another 3.9 million (43%) live in a household made up of two or more elderly people. Thus only 2.4 million old people have the day-to-day support of younger people living in the same household and of these the majority live with only one younger person (Fig. 2.6). Because the elderly so often form one or two person households the proportion of all households containing one or more elderly people is very high. Thirty-five per cent of all households contain elderly people and 24% of all households are "elderly only" households. Fourteen per cent of all households contain one old person living alone. These figures are significant in their implications for the basic financial resources required by old people for rent, rates, fuel costs, repair and maintenance and for the proportion of individual income which may have to be spent on them. This in turn affects the availability of money for old people's nutritional and social necessities, which have such a marked influence on their physical and mental health. These observations provide a natural introduction to the epidemiology of old age.

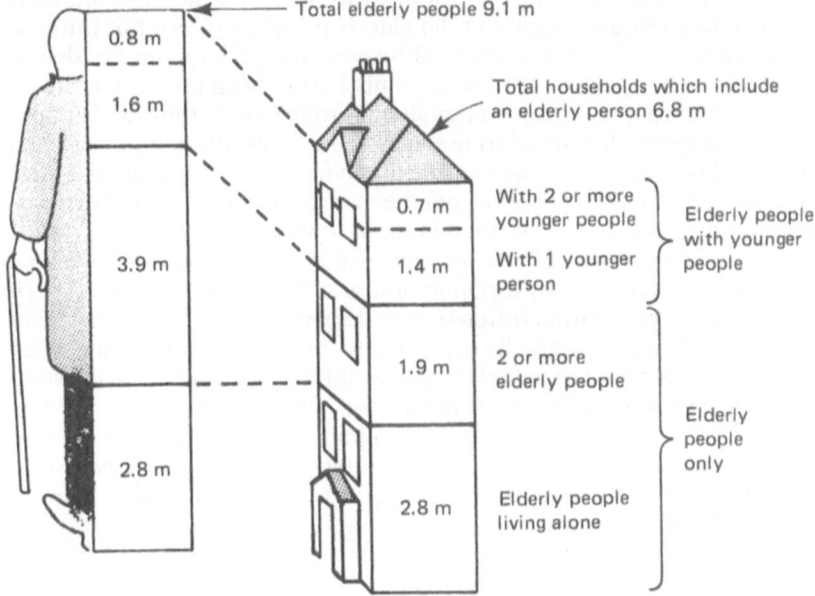

Fig. 2.6. Composition of households containing elderly people: Great Britain 1981. (From OPCS Guide 1: Britain's elderly population 1984.)

Epidemiology

Epidemiology is the study of the distribution and determinants of health and ill health in populations and the application of the results of these investigations to the control of disease and the provision of health services.

Information required for such study is principally obtained from routinely collected data, mainly population data, mortality data and morbidity data. These may be supplemented by information obtained from research and from ad hoc surveys. The epidemiology of old age is compiled from these same sources, all of which are to some degree unreliable or incomplete and, as we shall see, there are reasons why this may be particularly so for the elderly population.

The basic unit of measurement of disease in populations is the "rate". This is calculated from the number of people in whom the disease is present (the numerator), the total number in the population (the denominator) and the time period over which the measurement is being made. Such a rate calculated for the whole population of a defined geographical area is called a "crude" rate. The annual crude death rate, for example, is expressed as the number of deaths in the year divided by the number of people in the total population. It is usual to express this as the death rate per thousand by multiplying the resulting figure by 1000.

It has been shown in the previous section that old people differ in many ways from the general population and that the elderly population itself is far from homogeneous in its characteristics. Quite clearly these differences are likely to result in mortality and morbidity experience of old people being substantially different from that of the rest of the population. Crude rates are therefore unlikely to give an accurate picture of disease in the elderly population. For this purpose we require specific rates, i.e. rates obtained by measuring the number of deaths (though it could be the episodes of illness, admissions to hospital, etc) in the elderly sub-group of the population and in small sub-groups within the elderly population. For such purposes it is usual to use age- and sex-specific sub-groups, and the need to examine carefully the age- and sex-specific rates for each decade after the age of 60 will be easily understood from the marked difference in characteristics of these sub-groups already described in the section on demography.

Death rates can be further refined by standardisation: comparing the actual number of deaths experienced by a population or a sub-group to those experienced by a "standard" population (often the whole population is used as the standard). The ratio of the deaths actually occurring to those which would have been expected had the study population had the same mortality experience as the standard population is expressed as a percentage and called the Standardised Mortality Ratio (SMR). The SMR is the ratio of the number of observed deaths to the number of expected deaths expressed as a percentage. SMR values above 100% represent unfavourable mortality experience and values below 100% indicate favourable mortality experience.

Population Data

Attention has been drawn to the deficiencies of routinely collected data used in epidemiological studies. The population data required are obtained in Great Britain from the Census carried out by OPCS and repeated every 10 years. The last Census was undertaken in April 1981 and the next will be due in 1991. The Census is carried out by means of a questionnaire filled in by the head of each household, assisted if necessary by a trained enumerator responsible for about 200 households. The questionnaire requires the names, dates of birth, marital status and other information to be provided for each member of the household. The forms are processed centrally with strict confidentiality being observed. The results, as we have seen in the section on demography, give valuable information. The major deficiencies of the census as a data source relate to occupational and social class data and fortunately have little impact on its accuracy as a tool for studying the epidemiology of old age. Even the 10-year interval between censuses, which is compensated for by calculating projections on the census population for each intervening year taking into account births, deaths and migrations, is of lesser importance in studying the elderly than in studies relating to, for example, the first 5 or 10 years of life.

Mortality Data

The source of mortality data is the certification by doctors and the registration by a responsible relative or other person of all deaths. This information is collected locally by local authorities in a system administered by Superintendent Registrars and coordinated centrally by OPCS. The main advantage of mortality data is that the events which make them up are dramatic and unlikely to be missed, and have been required to be registered by law for more than 100 years. The data are thus comprehensive and easily available.

The reliability of the information given on death certificates should not be overestimated; the certified cause of death is in most cases based on clinical opinion and not supported by post-mortem examination. It has been shown that certification of death in old people is less accurate than for younger people. Death is common in old people, is often not unexpected, causes less concern than deaths at younger ages and is thus unlikely to be fully investigated. Multiple pathology is the rule in the elderly as is atypical presentation of well-recognised conditions such as myocardial infarction. It may well be that the idea of a single cause of death is inappropriate in this age group and that death certification as currently practised conceals more than it reveals.

Morbidity Data

Data on illness, whether or not resulting in death, are important in obtaining a picture of disease prevalence in a population. Morbidity data are collected in a number of different ways, with four main sources of statistics on hospital patients:

1. Hospital Activity Analysis (HAA) provides an abstract of case notes on all people admitted to hospital other than to maternity and psychiatric beds.
2. Hospital In-patient Enquiry (HIPE). This analyses a 10% sample of deaths and discharges from HAA data.
3. Annual returns are made by hospitals in England and Wales to the Department of Health and the Welsh Office for both in-patients and out-patients, giving administrative but no clinical information.
4. The Mental Health Enquiry (MHE) collects data on psychiatric patients from all National Health Service (NHS) psychiatric units and hospitals in England and Wales.

The limitations of information from these sources as a contribution to the overall picture of disease in the elderly relate to their accuracy and their limited coverage since they give information only on conditions for which hospital care is given. There is evidence that referral rates to hospital are lower for many conditions in elderly people than for younger age groups. Neither HAA nor HIPE distinguish between episodes of disease and individual patients experiencing them, the system being designed to count events and not people. Thus morbidity rates for different age cohorts cannot be calculated.

Morbidity data from primary health care sources are not routinely collected either locally or nationally. However, the Royal College of General Practitioners, in collaboration with OPCS and the former Department of Health and Social Security (DHSS), has undertaken three National Studies of Morbidity Statistics from General Practice in 1956–1957, 1970–1972 and 1981–1982. The most recent study covered 330 000 people on the lists of 48 practices selected from practices who volunteered for the study. It is not therefore a random sample of the population, though efforts were made to provide a balance of types of practice. In the absence of any routinely collected national data from primary care these studies are valuable as they deal with a wide range of chronic diseases which are unlikely to present to hospital for treatment. They give more information about both the early stages of the more serious conditions and, in some cases, the terminal stages.

The morbidity statistics from general practice do not, of course, give any information on illnesses not recognised as such by the patient or those for which the patient does not seek medical help, both of which are circumstances known to be common in the elderly population. The General Household Survey (GHS) collects information, including some limited information on health, by questioning a representative sample of 15 000 private households annually. The health-related information collected includes questions about episodes of acute illness, the presence of chronic illness and disability, taking of medicines, use of health and local authority services, smoking habits and the consumption of alcohol. In spite of the obvious inaccuracies inherent in a system which relies on the ability of respondents to remember and accurately report their own health and illness experience, the GHS collects useful information on both declared and undeclared illness and a range of variables which may be associated with illness and disability.

Perhaps the only other national source of useful epidemiological data on the elderly is the National Cancer Registry. This is maintained by OPCS and holds registration cards giving the identity and type of neoplasm for all cases of cancer diagnosed. Some information on the stage of the tumour and the treatment given is also entered, and the date of death and duration of survival are obtained by linkage to the national mortality information. Failure of registration of cases resulting in unsatisfactory coverage is a problem, as it is with all registration systems. Other registers from which some information on the elderly may be obtained include psychiatric case registers, local authority registers of handicapped people (including the blind register) and registers which may be maintained locally by clinicians interested in the epidemiology of particular disease processes, for example, thyroid disease registers.

These sources can be supplemented by the findings of ad hoc surveys of the elderly of which that undertaken by Hunt (1978) and reported as *The elderly at home* is a particularly useful example, though it is now becoming somewhat out of date. With all these problems in collection and in the limitations in quality of information, however, some definite patterns of disease and disability specific to old age emerge.

The level of disability in the elderly population was reported by a survey of all age groups undertaken in 1968–1969. This showed that at age over 75 years, 11% of males and 15% of females reported that they were severely handicapped and an additional 7% of males and 10% of females reported very severe handicap. The GHS of 1983 reported that over two-thirds of men and women over the age of 75 considered that they had some form of limiting long-standing illness.

Mortality

The very high rates of death in the newborn period drop rapidly over the first few years of life, reaching their lowest point at around 10 years of age. They then begin to rise, and rise very steeply from the age of 45, reaching and passing the newborn mortality rates in the late fifties for men and at around 60 years for women and continuing to increase very markedly with age from that point. From the very earliest years the rates for males are higher than for females and this gap is maintained until the very oldest age groups (Fig. 2.7).

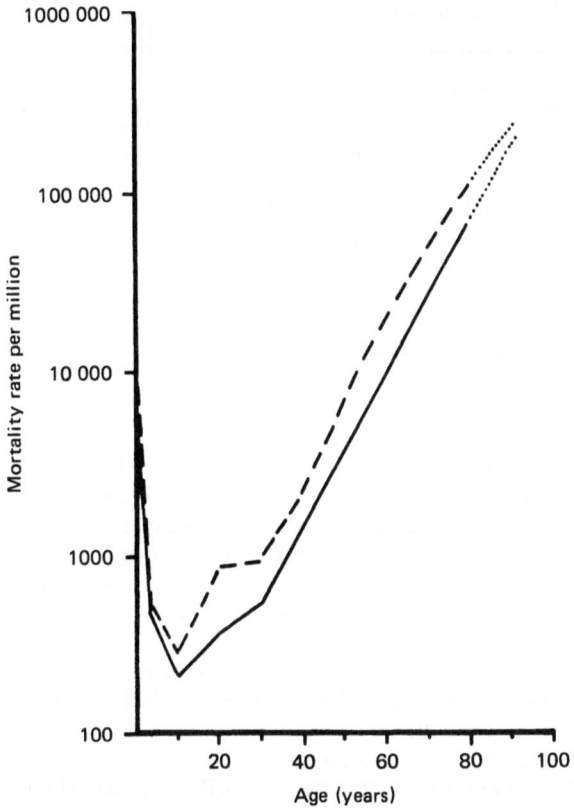

Fig. 2.7. Mortality rates per million for males (------) and females (————) by age in England and Wales. (From Alderson 1986.)

The five main causes of death in the age range 60–84 years are shown in Table 2.2 together with the percentage of all deaths which they represent for this age range. Ischaemic heart disease, accounting for one-third of all deaths in males and over a quarter of deaths in females, has remained level throughout the last two decades.

Lung cancer is the second commonest cause of death in men and the fifth in women. Its frequency as a cause of death for those aged over 85 years is still rising, though the over-75 age group has shown a static picture. For women an increase in death from lung cancer is noted in all the elderly age groups.

Cerebrovascular disease, the third commonest cause of death in men and the second in women, has shown a steady decline in mortality from 1950, which is reflected in the age-specific rates. This may be due to improving control of hypertension at all ages.

Cancer of the digestive organs, which includes several forms of cancer commonest in the older age groups, i.e. stomach, colorectal and biliary system cancers, is the fourth ranking cause of death in men and the third in women. Cancer of the stomach is declining in incidence throughout the world, though oesophageal cancer has shown a recent increase.

Table 2.2. Main cause of death in British people aged 60–84 years

Sex	Rank	Cause	%
Male	1	Ischaemic heart disease	33
	2	Lung cancer	11
	3	Cerebrovascular disease	10
	4	Digestive organ cancer	8
	5	Chronic obstructive airways disease	8
Female	1	Ischaemic heart disease	27
	2	Cerebrovascular disease	16
	3	Digestive organ cancer	8
	4	Breast cancer	5
	5	Lung cancer	4

From Alderson (1986).

Breast cancer in women, the commonest cancer for this sex in all 10-year age groups from the age of 50, is the fourth commonest cause of female deaths in the elderly and shows no change in its age-specific mortality during the last 50 years. The prospect of more comprehensive early detection offered by the recent UK Government decision to implement a breast cancer screening programme aimed at all women over 50 years of age may displace this in future years as a main cause of death.

Death rates from chronic obstructive pulmonary disease, the fifth ranking cause of death in older men have shown some fall in the elderly as in the whole population from the beginning of the 1960s. This contrasts vividly with the absence of a fall to date in the rates for lung cancer and for pneumonia.

Conditions which cause death in old people may not necessarily be those which cause the major burden of morbidity or disability. Chronically disabling but non-fatal conditions such as the arthropathies are understandably under-represented in the mortality figures. However, for most health care purposes it is precisely these chronically disabling conditions which are of greatest interest, since they are the conditions which require long-term treatment and support and are thus associated with major consumption of resources.

Future Trends

Some of the factors known to be related to disease, for example, cigarette smoking, diet, alcohol and lack of exercise, can give some clue as to the likely future pattern of morbidity and mortality in old people. Results from several different sources have indicated that successive male cohorts coming into the elderly age range show decreasing cumulative cigarette consumption, while the data for females show a steady increase in cigarette consumption. Thus we may expect a decrease in cigarette-associated diseases in the "new elderly" males, but an increase in these diseases among elderly women.

Reported alcohol consumption, as obtained by the GHS, indicates a lower proportion of moderate and heavy drinkers in the over-65 age group than in the general population and a higher proportion of complete abstainers (11% of males and 22% of females compared with 5% males and 12% females aged 45–64 years).

Thus we may expect an increase in alcohol-related disease as this younger age group becomes elderly.

Information on the adequacy and quality of diet in old people today and in those who will become elderly over the next two decades is difficult to obtain. The National Food Survey provides data on food expenditure by category of food and the age of the housewife. There is a lower expenditure per person per week in households where the housewife is 65–74 years than in a household where the housewife is younger. The lowest expenditure occurs where the housewife is 75 years and over. This gives some indication that nutrient intake in the elderly is poor compared with that of younger age groups. The lower expenditure is more marked for protein than for all other foods. The current emphasis on "healthy eating" is already affecting the diet of much of the younger population. Elderly people, however, are likely to be much more resistant to advice on changes in dietary habit and it remains to be seen whether the change in diet in those aged 45–65 years will have a beneficial effect on their health as they enter old age.

The current increase in interest in physical exercise as an aid to healthy living may similarly bear fruit in reducing the physical infirmity of tomorrow's elderly. The acquisition at a younger age of the habit of taking exercise may prove to be extremely valuable. It has been estimated that only 9% of those aged 70 years and over walk 2 miles (3 km) at least once in 4 weeks and that less than 0.5% go swimming. It has recently been argued that regular exercise can help to maintain physical ability with advancing age. The attainment of physical fitness is feasible in people irrespective of their age. A 10%–20% improvement in the strength of the quadriceps muscles of 70-year-old men can readily be produced, and a 10%–25% improvement in maximum oxygen uptake can be induced by several weeks of endurance training. Measures to increase the habitual physical activity of the elderly population are an urgent public health priority in order to reduce the functional consequences of the age-associated decline in physical ability. There is need for a change in professional and lay attitudes to exercise, the expectations of elderly people should be increased and appropriate recreational facilities should be provided.

These trends in health-associated behaviours may be crucial in deciding whether the improvement in mortality projected by demographic and epidemiological forecasts is associated with an increasing number of "full timers" who are healthy or an increasing number of "survivors" with chronic disease. It is vitally important that every opportunity be taken to ensure that those whose potentially fatal disease is postponed remain, as far as possible, mobile, independent and enjoying a good quality of life.

Further Reading

Alderson M (1986) An ageing population: some demographic and health trends. Public Health 100:263–277

Butler RN (1979) The greying of nations: creative responses. Age Concern, London

Donaldson RJ, Donaldson LJ (1983) Essential community medicine. MTP Press, Lancaster

General Household Survey Annual Reports 1971–84 (1973–1985) Office of the Population Censuses and Surveys, HMSO, London

Hunt A (1978) The elderly at home. HMSO, London

Kalache A, Muir Gray JA (1985) Health problems of older people in the developing world. In: Pathy
    MS (ed) Principles and practice of geriatric medicine. Wiley, Chichester, pp 1279–1283
Muir Gray JA (1985) Social and community aspects of ageing. In: Pathy MS (ed) Principles and prac-
    tice of geriatric medicine. Wiley, Chichester, pp 17–55
Office of Population Censuses and Surveys and the Central Office of Information (1984) Census guide
    1: Britain's elderly population. HMSO, London
Office of Population Censuses and Surveys (1985) Mortality statistics: cause. England and Wales
    series DH2 no. 11. HMSO, London

Section II
Clinical Problems in the Elderly

Chapter 3

Headache and Facial Pain

T. P. L. Thomas

The main pain-sensitive structures in the head are the blood vessels, sensory nerves and nerve roots. Pain is appreciated when these are irritated, or in the case of blood vessels, when they are displaced or dilated. Pain can also arise from organs and tissues such as the skin, eye, nasal sinuses, temporomandibular joint, teeth and bone. It follows, then, that the cause of headache and facial pain is varied, though in practice the number of conditions responsible for the problem is finite and diagnosis and management is usually straightforward.

The natural history of headache and of the disorders causing it are altered in old age. The ageing brain occupies less volume so that the cranium can accommodate large masses without producing symptoms. Thus headache is seen in fewer than half of patients with intracranial tumours. As a rule migraine becomes less frequent and individual attacks become less severe. Headache of recent onset is unlikely to be due to migraine, which seldom presents in old age.

Though headache becomes increasingly uncommon with advancing age, when it does occur it should be regarded as an indicator of underlying disease and the search for the cause must be as diligent as it would be in younger subjects.

Headache

The causes of headache are listed in Table 3.1. As with many problems in the elderly, two or more disorders may combine to cause symptoms.

Tension Headache

Tension headache or "muscle-contraction" headache is the commonest type in people of all ages. Muscular spasm in the scalp and neck from emotional tension are most often implicated, though cervical osteoarthritis may also play a part. Such headache often begins insidiously in the late afternoon or early evening. It is

Table 3.1.   Cause of headache in old people

Tension headache

Vascular headache (migraine; giant cell arteritis; hypertension; arterio-venous malformation; aneurysm)

Meningeal irritation (meningitis; sub-arachnoid haemorrhage)

Raised intracranial pressure (neoplasm; abscess; hydrocephalus; subdural haematoma)

Metabolic vasodilation (febrile illness; CO_2 retention; anaemia; hypoxia; uraemia)

Drugs and toxins (vasodilators; NSAIDs; dipyridamole; CO)

Other causes (cough headache; post lumbar puncture; Paget's disease)

Referred pain (disorders of the eye; teeth; nasal sinuses; cervical spine; ear etc.)

---

usually bilateral, involving part of the temporal, frontal or occipital regions and is often described as a band-like pressure or constant ache with superimposed short episodes of stabbing pain. Not uncommonly, patients describe ill-defined discomfort in the neck region, radiating anteriorly to the temples and forehead.

Tension headache can be episodic or continuous for months or years. It does not interfere with sleep as a rule and associated vomiting is not a feature. The most important differential diagnosis in old people is from the headache associated with raised intracranial pressure.

Reassurance of the patient is the most important aspect of management. Often the knowledge that headache is not due to a brain tumour will alleviate symptoms. Should the headache persist a short course of simple analgesics, taken regularly rather than on an "as required" basis, may break the continuing pain–tension–pain cycle. If it is felt that the pain is exacerbated by cervical osteoarthritis, anxiety or depression, however, appropriate management will be required.

"Vascular" Headaches

True *migraine* headaches are uncommon in the elderly, perhaps because the cerebral blood vessels can no longer dilate enough to stimulate the nerve endings surrounding the major blood vessels and in the dura. A diagnosis of migrainous headaches is usually untenable in an elderly patient without a long-standing history.

Giant cell arteritis (temporal arteritis) is a chronic inflammatory disease of medium-sized arteries which contain elastic tissue. Prompt and accurate diagnosis of this cause of headache is extremely important in elderly patients in order to minimise the risk of permanent blindness. While it is very rare before the age of 55 years, its incidence rises sharply thereafter, with a tenfold increase between the sixth and ninth decade. Women are more often affected than men.

The headache is severe and constant. It may last for many hours or even days and may be resistant to any form of analgesia except opiate therapy. Characteristically the temporal arteries are involved while the external carotid, ophthalmic, posterior ciliary and vertebral arteries and their branches are also commonly affected (Fig. 3.1). Inflamed vessels are swollen, tender and painful. Overlying skin may be red, the scalp is often tender and large irregular arteries may be visible and palpable.

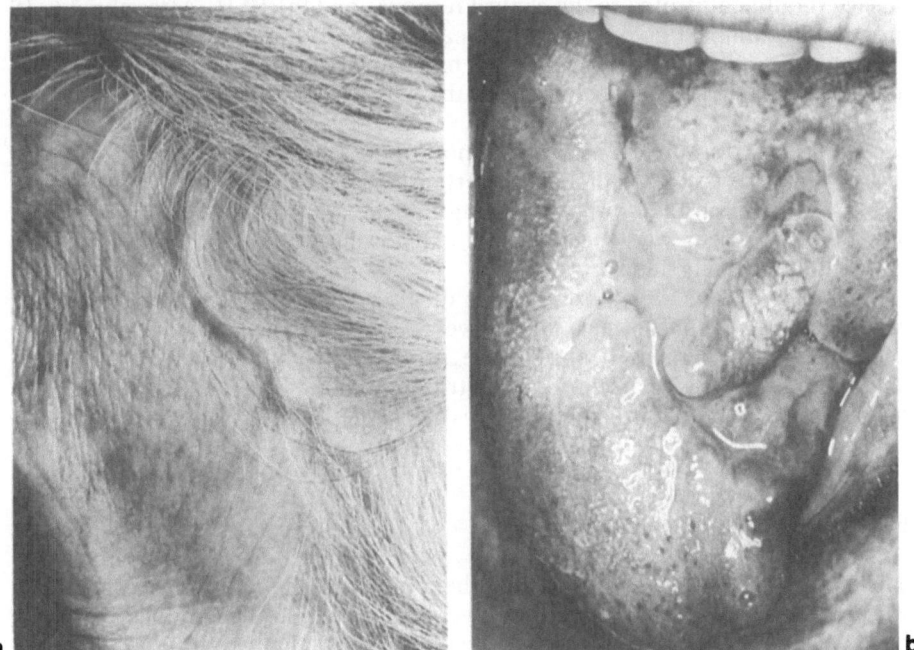
a
b

Fig. 3.1. Cranial arteritis with **a** a tortuous swollen temporal artery and **b** necrosis of the tongue from involvement of the lingual artery.

Sudden blindness may occur when occlusion of the posterior ciliary artery results in an ischaemic optic neuritis (see Chap. 13). Oculomotor palsies can be produced by involvement of other arteries supplying the orbit. Myalgia occurs in 25% of patients and other symptoms such as shoulder pain, anaemia, weight loss and fever reflect the widespread involvement found in some patients. Jaw claudication is considered to be pathognomonic.

All elderly patients with headache of recent onset should have an erythrocyte sedimentation rate (ESR) estimation. In giant cell arteritis, it is usually elevated to greater than 50 mm/h. This test, however, is neither specific nor sensitive; the ESR rises with age in the absence of disease and rarely it may be normal in the presence of arteritis. The diagnosis is confirmed by the histological appearance of a temporal artery biopsy, although 10%–15% of people with arteritis will have normal biopsy findings. It is best to biopsy a pulsatile vessel and the diagnostic yield will be increased if a large sample is taken. The typical histological features include loss of the internal elastic lamina and infiltration of the vascular wall by a chronic inflammatory process with giant cells. A therapeutic trial of steroids may obviate the need for cranial artery biopsy as a rapid resolution in symptoms (within 48 hours) and a falling ESR would be accepted by many as being of diagnostic significance.

Prednisolone in high dosage (up to 80 mg/day) should be started immediately. This will reduce the risk of blindness but will not alter the natural course of the disease. The disease is self-limiting so that approximately one-third of people no longer need steroids after between 6 months and a year of treatment. The steroid dosage should be titrated to the clinical response and the ESR. After about 6–18 months an attempt should be made to wean patients off treatment.

In elderly patients, giant cell arteritis must always be borne in mind even if an alternative diagnosis seems obvious, as the penalty for a mis-diagnosis can be so great.

Mild to moderate *hypertension* does not produce headache, though it is a feature of severe or accelerated phase hypertension (see Chap. 8).

An *arterio-venous malformation*, being congenital, is unlikely to present in old age. It may present with focal seizures. Headache when it occurs tends to be unilateral, throbbing and recurrent.

Small *berry aneurysms* (up to 2 cm in diameter) are not a cause of headaches which are recurrent or chronic. However, posterior communicating artery aneurysms may compress the third nerve, producing a painful palsy with pupillary dilatation. Pain can also occur in the distribution of the first and occasionally the second divisions of the fifth nerve due to direct compression by an aneurysm.

Meningeal Irritation

The meninges are irritated by blood or the products of inflammation. All patients whose headache is accompanied by fever, neck stiffness or Kernig's sign must have *meningitis* excluded. The headache may be frontal or generalised, or it may radiate into the neck and back. It is progressive in severity and is often associated with vomiting. It should be remembered that nuchal rigidity may not be present in elderly patients and a high index of suspicion is important. Delay in diagnosis severely affects outcome, pneumococcal meningitis having a mortality of greater than 50% in elderly patients. Those who are ill with vague symptoms should be considered for lumbar puncture, even in the absence of neurological signs. This may reveal a chronic pyogenic meningitis, most often due to the pneumococcus, though tuberculosis is another important cause.

The clinical diagnosis of *sub-arachnoid haemorrhage* (SAH) is usually straight-forward, though a quarter of patients are not diagnosed when first seen.

It is important to remember that an unconscious patient may have a space-occupying lesion. This is more likely if there are focal neurological signs. Inappropriate lumbar puncture may cause coning of the mid-brain, although this risk is obviated by performing a computed tomography (CT) brain scan. This can show blood in the sub-arachnoid space or ventricles as well as sometimes revealing unexpected findings such as an extracerebral or intracerebral haematoma and, uncommonly, a cerebral abscess.

Raised Intracranial Pressure

Raised intracranial pressure can be due to a tumour, obstructive hydrocephalus or a brain abscess. The headache is usually progressive and bursting, though initially it may be episodic. Characteristically it wakes the patient from sleep and disappears after rising. It is exacerbated by manoeuvres which raise intracranial pressure further, such as stooping or coughing. Headache is seen in fewer than half of old people with intracranial tumours and associated papilloedema is seen in only 5%–30%.

The incidence of *intracerebral tumours* has been estimated at 60 per 100 000 at the age of 70. Information on tumours in older people is less certain as a histological diagnosis is less frequently obtained. Metastatic tumours are known to be twice as common as primary tumours. Those causing obstruction to the flow of CSF can produce obstructive hydrocephalus; this produces a rise in intracranial pressure with headache as a prominent feature, as is vomiting and ataxia.

While age itself is not a contraindication to surgery, few tumours are amenable to such intervention. Hydrocephalus can be treated with a shunt and thereby relieve headache. The use of high-dose steroids (e.g. dexamethasone 5 mg t.d.s.) often causes a dramatic reduction in cerebral oedema surrounding the tumour. It may also lower intracranial pressure and result in rapid and prolonged relief of symptoms. Other drugs may shrink specific tumours. Dopamine agonists (e.g. bromocriptine) can often successfully reduce the size of a prolactin or growth hormone secreting pituitary tumour. Radiotherapy may be effective in the palliation of cerebral metastases (e.g. from bronchogenic carcinoma) and can be combined with steroid therapy.

A *chronic subdural haematoma* (CSH) may occur following trivial trauma which is not remembered by half of patients, even with the benefit of hindsight. Chronic alcoholism and anticoagulant therapy are underlying risk factors. Associated headache may have no characteristic pattern. Apathy, confusion and drowsiness are other features. A progressive neurological deficit should alert one to the possibility of a CSH, while the absence of a fluctuating level of consciousness cannot reliably exclude the condition.

An *extradural haematoma*, unlike a CSH, occurs swiftly following minor head trauma and is more amenable to surgery than CSH.

Metabolic Vasodilation

Most *febrile conditions* (e.g. influenza) can be associated with headache. However, in the elderly febrile patient with headache, one should always consider diseases of the ears, nasal sinuses and especially meningitis.

In a minority of elderly patients with chronic pulmonary disease, *carbon dioxide retention* produces headache not unlike that of raised intracranial pressure. *Anaemia* and *hypoxaemia* can also produce vascular distension and headache. Chronic *uraemia* can cause generalised headache, possibly related to a low-grade cerebral oedema.

Drugs and Toxins

A generalised throbbing headache of a variable degree can be generated by *drugs and toxins* causing vasodilatation. Such agents include short- and long-acting nitrates, hydralazine and other vasodilators. Non-steroidal anti-inflammatory drugs (NSAIDs) and dipyridamole are also implicated. Elderly patients are susceptible to the toxic effects of carbon monoxide at low concentrations. Coal-burning stoves occasionally produce enough CO to produce headache but no other symptom.

Other Causes

Cough headaches are brief, immediate, severe pains in the head precipitated by coughing. They usually occur in middle-aged and elderly men. The condition is generally benign and resolves spontaneously, though if it occurs for the first time in old age, a CT scan may be necessary to exclude a posterior fossa lesion.

Lumbar puncture headache is attributed to a sudden lowering of CSF pressure by needle puncture of the dura mater. It is exacerbated by standing, relieved by lying down and eventually resolves spontaneously.

Paget's disease commonly produces a deep-seated pain, most often in the occiput. It is discussed in more detail in Chap. 6.

Facial Pain

The causes of facial pain are summarised in Table 3.2.

Table 3.2. Cause of facial pain in old people

Herpes zoster
Post-herpetic neuralgia
Trigeminal neuralgia
Glossopharyngeal neuralgia
Atypical facial neuralgia
Cluster headache
Tumours
Referred pain

Herpes Zoster

Herpes zoster is due to reactivation of the varicella-zoster virus lying dormant in the posterior root ganglion. In the cranial nerves it mainly involves the Gasserian ganglion, involvement of the geniculate ganglion being rare. With Gasserian ganglion involvement the ophthalmic division of the trigeminal nerve is most often affected, so that two-thirds of all people with zoster of the cranial nerves will have herpes zoster ophthalmicus. A vesicular rash resembling chicken-pox is seen (Fig. 3.2). This may involve the cornea, causing ulceration and scarring. Pain often precedes the rash and indeed may be the only manifestation, although occasionally there is sensory loss in the area affected. Motor cranial nerves can (rarely) be affected due to inflammation of the anterior horn cell or of the peripheral nerve. This can result in oculomotor palsy and ptosis.

Geniculate herpes zoster (Ramsay Hunt syndrome) accounts for only 5% of cranial nerve zoster. The pain and rash is localised to the external auditory meatus and pinna of the ear. Loss of taste sensation is found on the anterior two-thirds of the tongue. Paralysis of the nerve to the stapedius causes hyperacusis and a lower motor neurone facial palsy can occur.

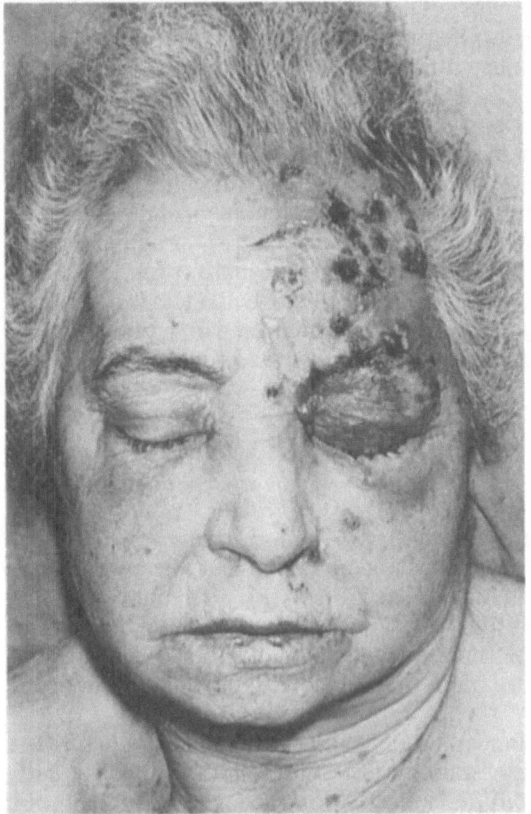

Fig. 3.2. Herpes zoster ophthalmicus (by permission of Dr B. S. D. Sastry).

Antiviral therapy with vidarabine or acyclovir should be given for zoster of the cranial nerves, especially if eye-sight is threatened by corneal ulceration. This will shorten the attack and may lessen the risk of post-herpetic neuralgia.

Post-herpetic Neuralgia

Most episodes of zoster resolve with few sequelae apart from possible scarring of the skin. The most difficult residual problem is persistent intractable pain (post-herpetic neuralgia), which is particularly troublesome in elderly patients. In one series 43% of patients aged over 50 years with zoster subsequently developed this complication. It is thought to be due to fibrosis of peripheral nerves or to an inability to block painful afferent stimuli in the dorsal root ganglion.

Post-herpetic neuralgia is characterised by chronic persistent deep-seated pain and hyperaesthesia to sensory stimuli. Descriptions of the discomfort include "burning", "prickly" and "itchy". Lancinating pains are elicited by sensory stimuli. The pain may persist for years and drive the patient to distraction.

Physical examination may reveal a loss of sensation in the painful area. Typical scarring of the skin or cornea may also be present and residual motor nerve dysfunction may be found. The facial palsy, for example, is less likely to resolve than is that of an idiopathic Bell's palsy.

There is some evidence that corticosteroids given at the time of the rash may reduce the risk of post-herpetic neuralgia and anti-viral therapy may have the same effect. Once established, however, neuralgia is very difficult to treat. Carbamazepine and phenytoin are only rarely helpful. Non-opiate analgesics seldom control pain and opiates are contraindicated because of the risk of addiction that comes with prolonged therapy. Antidepressants occasionally produce relief. Sometimes electrical cutaneous stimulation can be effective and local application of ethyl chloride spray is worth trying. Surgical intervention with a phenol block of the Gasserian ganglion is unhelpful and even total surgical denervation seldom produces lasting relief.

Trigeminal Neuralgia

The aetiology of trigeminal neuralgia is unknown in most cases. It usually develops after the age of 50 and is by no means uncommon in patients over 70; it is slightly commoner in females than in males. The pain occurs with equal incidence over the territory of the second and third divisions of the fifth cranial nerve. The first division is involved in about 5% of cases, but almost never in isolation. The right side of the face is affected more often than the left, while bilateral involvement rarely occurs.

The pain can be very intense, is lancinating in character and may be described by the patient as an "electric shock", "stabbing" or "shooting". The onset is sudden and the paroxysms may occur in quick succession throughout the day (but usually not at night) and lead to a more continuous pain.

The majority of patients will have a "trigger-zone": an area of mucous membrane or skin in the trigeminal area, which when stimulated induces a bout of pain. Various activities and stimuli (e.g. eating, shaving, washing or a cold wind) can trigger a paroxysm. This can be severely incapacitating and is a recognised cause of significant weight loss in elderly patients. The neurological examination is normal.

Carbamazepine is the mainstay of treatment which, if given continuously, reduces the frequency and severity of attacks. The starting dose is 100 mg daily, increasing as necessary to a daily dose of 600–800 mg in divided doses. Side effects include leucopenia, skin rashes, drowsiness and ataxia. Other effective drugs include phenytoin, baclofen and clonazepam. If medical treatment fails then phenol infiltration of the peripheral branches of the fifth nerve, either in the supraorbital notch or in the distribution of the lingual territory, is sometimes successful. The degree of anaesthesia left following such a procedure is usually quite acceptable. Other therapeutic manoeuvres include thermocoagulation of the sensory root and destruction of nerve fibres with radio-frequency waves.

Glossopharyngeal Neuralgia

Glossopharyngeal neuralgia occurs approximately a hundred times less often than trigeminal neuralgia. The pain is similar in type and quality producing paroxysms of lancinating pain in the territory of the ninth cranial nerve at the back of the mouth and the ear. Trigger-zones are present and often stimulated by swallowing, thereby causing reluctance to eat and weight loss. Sensory or motor signs produced in this or adjacent nerves suggest an underlying cause requiring further investigation.

Atypical Facial Neuralgia

Atypical facial neuralgia occurs mainly in women and is described as a "boring" or "burning" pain in one cheek which is often continuous, but may be episodic. It is not strictly localised to the distribution of any cranial nerve. Attacks are usually unilateral and trigger-zones are almost never found. The majority of patients will have some underlying psychological problem and symptoms may respond to antidepressant therapy. Other forms of therapy are ineffective.

Cluster Headache

Cluster headache (periodic migrainous neuralgia) is extremely rare in elderly patients but can produce facial pain. It predominantly affects males. Attacks occur mainly at night, the patient waking from sleep with severe boring pain in one eye, radiating to the forehead and temple. The affected eye is injected and lacrimates. Attacks occur in clusters, occurring regularly for weeks or months, then remitting for similar periods.

   If cluster headache occurs for the first time in old age, a CT brain scan is indicated since the presentation may be indistinguishable from the pain produced by a retro-orbital tumour or a sphenoidal ring meningioma.

Tumours

Pain can be caused by tumours when the nerve itself is the primary site (e.g. schwannoma) or when the nerve is compressed by an extrinsic tumour (e.g. meningioma). Metastases and infiltrating carcinomas may compress various cranial nerves and cause facial pain. Tumours of the nasopharynx, for instance, can track along the base of the skull and involve the cranial nerves at the foramina, producing a sixth nerve palsy and pain in the temple. Tumours invading the deep soft tissues may produce a dull ache which can be referred to the vertex, the frontal region or to the back of the ear.

Referred Pain

Disorders of the *temporomandibular joint* may produce an aching pain, often unilateral, which involves the area of the joint and radiates around the ear. Pain is often aggravated by chewing. Tenderness over the mandibular condyle is a useful sign.

Frontal headache can be produced by *eye disorders* such as errors of refraction, glaucoma and uveitis. Painful proptosis and ophthalmoplegia caused by the Tolosa–Hunt syndrome can sometimes be treated effectively with steroids.

Other sources of referred facial pain and headache are the *teeth* and *nasal sinuses*.

Clinical Evaluation

There is no substitute for a careful history coupled with an adequate physical examination. This is almost always more informative than the specialist investigations which are increasingly available. A detailed description of the pain is the first requirement. Note whether it is constant or intermittent, its character, its onset and duration, its distribution, and the presence of precipitating or relieving factors and associated symptoms. Both the past history and drug history are important. Note specifically the presence of diabetes mellitus, herpes zoster and weight loss.

The history alone often allows one to make a confident diagnosis. Trigeminal neuralgia, for instance, is characterised by its paroxysmal nature, the absence of pain between attacks and the presence of precipitating factors and trigger-zones. It is localised to the distribution of all or part of the trigeminal nerve. The pain of post-herpetic neuralgia on the other hand is constant and localised to the distribution of the nerve affected. Atypical facial pain is dull and constant in nature and is not localised to the distribution of any particular nerve.

The physical examination obviously concentrates on the central nervous system though other systems must not be neglected. The level of consciousness and the mental state should be assessed, followed by examination of the cranial nerves. Findings may alter the likely diagnosis so, for example, when the history is suggestive of trigeminal neuralgia, the presence of sensory loss or wasting of facial muscles would suggest instead a compressive lesion such as a posterior fossa tumour.

Examine the neck for stiffness. The temporal arteries should be inspected and palpated; they may be tender though not necessarily palpable in patients with temporal arteritis. The temporomandibular joint may be tender if arthritis is present. Evidence of sinusitis is present if there is localised swelling or oedema; there may also be localised tenderness. The teeth and eyes must also be examined systematically. Look for scarring from old zoster infection on the skin of the face.

Investigation

The ability to accurately diagnose the cause of headache and facial pain has recently improved, particularly due to advances in the field of diagnostic radiology. Neurosurgical techniques have also improved considerably.

It should be noted that a gamma radionuclide scan is a sensitive investigation for chronic subdural haematoma and has the advantage of a shorter "filming" time in agitated patients. Skull radiographs may show a shifted pineal gland, although EEG is seldom helpful. Skull X-rays (including views of the temporomandibular joint) and X-rays of the teeth and nasal sinuses are sometimes helpful.

It is important that older patients share in the resulting benefits of these improved techniques and have access to appropriate facilities. Problems can arise when large numbers of elderly people (who are prone to head injury and neurological disorders) make demands on services that cannot readily be met. This problem is well described and beautifully articulated in the article by Kalbag and every physician responsible for geriatric patients would do well to read it.

Further Reading

Kalbag RM (1984) Geriatric medicine and the neurosurgeon in the era of the CT scan. In: Evans JG, Caird FI (eds) Advanced geriatric medicine 4. Pitman, London, pp 162–172

Chapter 4

Chest Pain

M. S. J. Pathy

Pain in the chest is one of the most frequent presenting symptoms in old age and commonly gives rise to considerable concern as the patient rightly or wrongly believes it to represent serious heart disease. A methodological approach to the problem might be by systems, but it is often simpler to use a clinico-anatomical strategy to arrive at a differential diagnosis. Such an approach allows one to classify chest pain as either central or lateral.

Central Chest Pain

It is at this site that pain causes the greatest diagnostic difficulties (see Table 4.1).

Table 4.1. Causes of central chest pain

Cardiac pain (myocardial ischaemia and infarction, pericarditis, mitral
  valve prolapse)
Aortic disease (acute dissection, thoracic aneurysm)
Pulmonary embolus
Oesophageal disease (oesophagitis, oesophageal spasm, achalasia,
  carcinoma)
Mediastinal lesions (tumours, mediastinitis)
Musculo-skeletal disorders
Manubriosternal and xiphoid syndromes
Psychogenic causes
Abdominal disorders

Myocardial Ischaemia

Myocardial ischaemia is undoubtedly the most important cause of retrosternal pain. In the overwhelming majority of patients coronary atherosclerosis is the cause of angina pectoris but, exceptionally, giant cell arteritis or polyarteritis nodosa affect the coronary arterial vasculature and the ostia of the coronary arteries may be stenosed in syphilitic aortitis.

Retrosternal pain which is recurrent and clearly precipitated by exertion and relieved by rest and glyceryl tinitrin (GTN) is angina pectoris. The pain is typically retrosternal but may be more marked slightly to the right or, more often, the left of the mid-line. If the pain radiates it may be to the jaw or down the inner aspect of one or both arms. Occasionally it may be confined to a peripheral site, e.g. jaw, elbow or wrist and may be attributed to local pathology. The site of radiation is often characteristic for a given individual and pain does not, for example, tend to radiate to the jaw on one occasion and the wrist at another time.

Ischaemic heart pain is typically described as gripping, constricting or as a tightness or dull pressure under the sternum. Descriptions such as sharp, stabbing and a series of jabs of pain that last for a few seconds do not represent angina pectoris. Anginal pain normally lasts for a few minutes and only rarely for more than half an hour. Factors which may prolong its duration include a persistent tachyarrhythmia, concomitant anaemia, persistence of severe stress or aortic valve disease. Commonly pain follows an established pattern or quantum of activity, but exertion after meals or during exposure to cold may induce angina after less than customary exercise. Where coronary vasoconstriction significantly contributes to ischaemic symptoms, the relationship to exercise may be less predictable and chest pain may occur at rest on some occasions and only after considerable exertion at other times in the same patient. Increased cardiac output in the recumbent position is probably responsible for decubitus angina which may be a feature of aortic valve disease, though it also occurs in severe triple coronary artery disease.

Clinical examination most often demonstrates no abnormal physical signs. Cardiomegaly may be due to associated conditions such as hypertension, aortic valve disease or syphilitic aortitis, or it may result from ischaemic heart disease per se. A third or loud fourth heart sound are common in subjects with angina, though a fourth heart sound is not uncommon in apparently fit old people. Early, late or pan-systolic murmurs may be present particularly where there has been a previous myocardial infarction.

The resting ECG is normal in about a third of patients. Abnormalities are often non-specific and include conduction disturbances, particularly left bundle branch block and ventricular premature beats or other rhythm changes. More specific features include ST–T changes or Q waves. Exercise stress electrocardiography provides useful positive evidence of relevant ischaemic heart disease, but many elderly patients are unable to undertake the amount of exercise required to produce 85% or more of maximum predicted heart rate. Stress radionuclide imaging tests may be also precluded for similar reasons.

Episodes of angina are treated by GTN. The drug is administered sublingually to discourage premature swallowing before it is absorbed from the buccal mucosa. GTN is destroyed during its passage through the liver. The drug is absorbed most rapidly by chewing it and keeping the contents in the mouth for 30 seconds after which it can be spat out. Alternatively, it can be given sublingually in an aerosol spray. For patients who have more than occasional attacks of angina pectoris, prophylactic treatment with longer acting nitrate preparations or with calcium antagonists are warranted. Beta-blockers have a lesser role in the management of angina in old people than in a younger population as they have a greater tendency to cause heart failure, bronchospasm and exacerbate peripheral vascular disease.

Myocardial Infarction

Central chest pain is the commonest single presenting feature of infarction of the myocardium occurring at any age, but its incidence is decidedly less in the very old. Other presenting symptoms such as breathlessness, confusion and syncope are prominent in advanced age and may give rise to diagnostic uncertainties where chest pain is absent or indefinite. Pain is retrosternal, gripping, pressing or heavy like a stone under the breast bone; it is often intense, requiring opiates for its relief. In the absence of treatment, the duration of pain is measured in hours, rather than in minutes. Nausea or vomiting, breathlessness, feeling of faintness or intense weakness may be accompanying symptoms or may dominate the clinical scene. Presentation may be with acute left ventricular failure or with a stroke and the underlying cardiac infarction may go undetected.

A modest fall of blood pressure is often found on physical examination, but severe hypotension is an ominous complication. An atrial gallop rhythm is common and a variety of dysrhythmias are frequently identified in the early hours following infarction. The old are particularly likely to have evidence of left ventricular failure, though congestive heart failure is less common. An evanescent pericardial rub may be detected after a day or two.

Serial electrocardiography is the single most useful diagnostic test, though pre-existing abnormalities such as left bundle branch block may make diagnostic interpretation uncertain or impossible. Pathological Q waves, S–T segment elevation with its convexity upwards and T wave inversion are the most useful diagnostic features. Characteristically the creatine phosphokinase (CPK) rises to a peak and then falls within 2–3 days. This is not specific as muscle disease and trauma, including that sustained by prolonged lying on the floor, injections and strokes also give rise to elevated CPK. The rise of the aspartate transaminase and lactate dehydrogenase may persist for several days after the peak CPK.

Pericarditis

Myocardial infarction is the commonest cause of pericarditis in old people, but any chest pain from the pericarditis is usually masked by ischaemic pain. In the days following an acute infarct, a Dressler's syndrome develops in a minority of elderly patients and may give rise to pericardial pain. A large effusion must raise the possibility of hypothyroidism. The fibrinous pericarditis associated with uraemia is more often noted as an autopsy finding than as a clinical phenomenon in old people. Rheumatic, tuberculous or bacterial causes are usually identified by the association of evidence of the underlying disease. Coxsackie B virus infection is uncommon in old age.

The pain of pericarditis is usually sudden in onset and substernal, but it may also be felt in the left precordium. The supine position intensifies the pain and leaning forwards lessens it. Swallowing and coughing may aggravate the discomfort and, if the adjacent pleura is involved, deep breathing may produce sharp stabs of left chest pain. Hyperpnoea and dyspnoea may be accompanying symptoms.

The diagnostic finding is the pericardial friction rub which is frequently evanescent. It has a high-pitched grating or squeaking sound, frequently with a to-and-fro quality. Sometimes three components to the friction rub can be clearly identified, less commonly only one component. Firm pressure with the diaphragm of the stethoscope intensifies the auscultatory sound of the rub.

Serial electrocardiography may show the typical S–T segment elevation in all leads with preservation of the normal upward concavity. T wave inversion develops usually after several days. Echocardiography is useful in diagnosing the presence of an effusion.

Treatment will depend on the underlying cause and this may need to be controlled before the pericarditis resolves. With Dressler's syndrome, there is usually rapid pain relief with non-steroidal anti-inflammatory drugs. Very large effusions will need to be drained if there is evidence of cardiac tamponade.

Mitral Valve Prolapse

Mitral valve prolapse is often asymptomatic, though it may be associated with central chest pain. Such pain is intermittent and may resemble angina in quality but has little or no temporal relationship to exertion and lasts from minutes to hours on different occasions. The cardinal physical signs are an apical mid-systolic click and late systolic murmur on auscultation. If the degree of mitral regurgitation is severe, the murmur may be prolonged and occupy the whole of systole. Diagnostic support is provided by echocardiography.

Acute Aortic Dissection

In this disorder pain is intense, often appropriately described as tearing in character and develops acutely in the retrosternal region or back. Pain may later progress down into the abdomen, but rarely into the arms. Syncope may be a presenting feature. The patient may appear pale, cold and sweating but blood pressure tends to be maintained or elevated, particularly in peripheral dissection which is more common in old people. Aortic regurgitation may result from proximal dissection involving the aortic valve and can precipitate acute heart failure.

The dominant physical findings are absent pulses on one or both sides in the subclavian arteries or its branches or in the femoral artery. Clinical evidence may suggest involvement of mesenteric or renal arteries. Rarely a paraplegia or hemiplegia may develop. In proximal dissection signs of free aortic regurgitation may be apparent. The electrocardiograph is usually normal and chest radiographs show widening of the aorta, but this is often difficult to distinguish from an unfolded aorta which is so common in old people. Diagnosis may be supported by echocardiography and the CT scan may provide additional diagnostic information (Fig. 4.1). The most precise information is derived from retrograde aortic angiography.

The primary objective in acute dissection is to prevent the tear from extending. Intravenous sodium nitroprusside should be given so as to rapidly reduce systolic blood pressure to about 100 mm Hg together with beta-adrenergic blockade to reduce the velocity of left ventricular ejection. Management should be undertaken in an intensive care setting where the blood pressure, pulse, central venous pressure and urine output can be adequately monitored. Continued medical management is the policy of choice for distal aortic dissection, whereas for proximal dissection surgical intervention is preferable except when the patient is very frail.

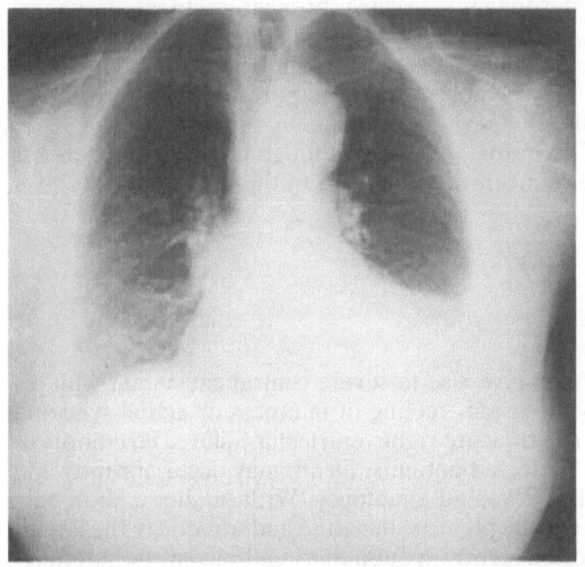

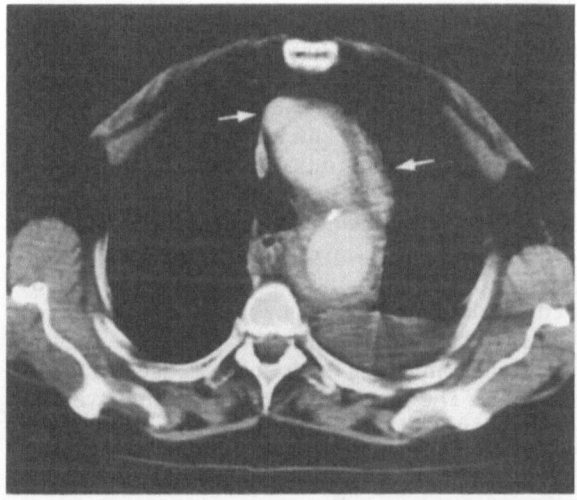

Fig. 4.1a, b. Dissecting thoracic aortic aneurysm. **a** The chest radiograph shows a widened aortic arch and fluid in the left pleural cavity compatible with but not specific for aortic aneurysm. **b** The contrasted CT scan shows contrast material outside the aortic lumen (arrowed) which is pathognomonic of dissection. (By permission of Dr. D. Cochlin.)

Aneurysm of the Thoracic Aorta

Aneurysms in this site are now uncommon, being due to syphilis, cystic medial necrosis or trauma. Most often pain is absent or a deep-seated ache, aggravated by exertion, insidiously develops. Where there is erosion of ribs, sternum or spine, intense boring pain may dominate the clinical picture. Compression of neighbouring structures, e.g. oesophagus, trachea, bronchi, recurrent laryngeal nerve and superior vena cava, together with free aortic regurgitation and abnormal chest wall pulsation renders clinical diagnosis abundantly clear. However, many or all of these findings may be absent and it requires radiography and/or echocardiography for diagnosis.

Surgery is the only form of definitive treatment, though the potential benefits must be weighed against the not inconsiderable risks of this course of action for the individual patient.

Pulmonary Embolus

Massive pulmonary embolus may give rise to severe central chest pain with associated dyspnoea, cough, hypotension, feeling of faintness or actual syncope, peripheral cyanosis and evidence of acute right ventricular failure. Haemoptysis occurs in less than a quarter of affected patients. Death may occur abruptly and without warning; the diagnosis is revealed at autopsy. With smaller emboli pain may be absent or if it occurs it may be pleuritic in nature and situated in the lateral chest. Symptoms of small and often recurrent pulmonary emboli may be indefinite or misleading and it is only the presence of immobility, recent surgery, lower limb fracture or intractable heart failure that heightens the index of suspicion. Overt deep vein thrombosis will suggest the diagnosis in the presence of new cardio-respiratory symptoms but not infrequently evidence of a pulmonary embolus may precede the clinical picture of deep vein thrombosis. The combination of cough, dyspnoea, pyrexia and crackles at one lung base on auscultation may be misdiagnosed as a chest infection. Sputum, if any, is usually mucoid or occasionally blood streaked but not purulent.

ECG changes are variable and only rarely provide diagnostic certitude. Conduction disturbances, S–T changes and T wave inversion are most commonly seen. A P pulmonale with a deep S, prominent Q and inverted T waves in lead 3 indicate acute cor pulmonale. This is diagnostically valuable though an uncommon finding, being only seen in massive pulmonary infarction. A chest radiograph is often normal though it may show oligaemic lung fields and a wedge-shaped infarct may indicate a previous embolus. The diagnosis is confirmed by a ventilation/perfusion scan which demonstrates non-perfusion of a ventilated area of lung (Fig. 4.2). Pulmonary angiography is an alternative though more invasive diagnostic tool. However, it is of little value in detecting small emboli.

Anticoagulation may prevent the disorder from progressing. Associated symptoms such as chest pain and hypoxia will need appropriate therapy. In the face of massive pulmonary embolism, thrombolytic therapy may be considered.

Oesophageal Disorders

Oesophageal disorders are discussed in Chap. 21. Gastro-oesophageal reflux is the single most likely condition to be mistaken for ischaemic heart pain in old people. The two disorders may co-exist and oesophageal pain may be relieved by glyceryl trinitrate and so compound the diagnostic difficulties. If pain is extant at

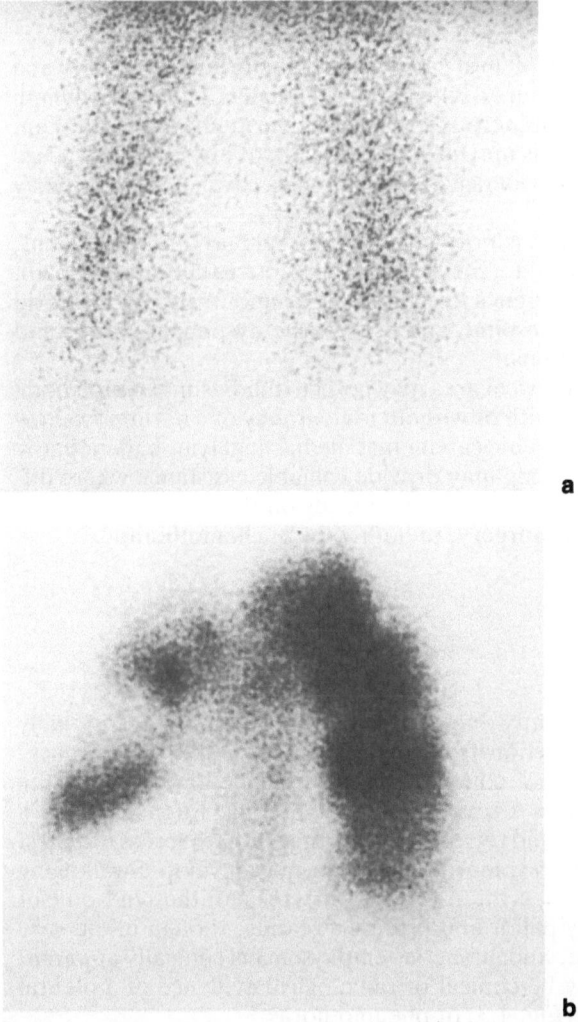

Fig. 4.2. Ventilation scan (**a**) and perfusion scan (**b**) showing multiple perfusion defects without corresponding ventilation defects and indicating multiple pulmonary emboli. (By permission of Dr. D. Cochlin.)

the time of examination, rapid relief following an adequate dose of a liquid antacid may assist in the differential diagnosis. Diffuse oesophageal spasm gives rise to bouts of retrosternal pain which may simulate ischaemic heart pain, but commonly symptoms are induced by swallowing. Beta-blocking agents may induce oesophageal spasm and give rise to retrosternal chest pain. Where the drug is administered for angina, misdiagnosis is common.

Mediastinal Tumours

The restricted space between the pleural cavities and the sternum anteriorly and spine posteriorly may house tumours of the lung, oesophagus, thymus or lymph nodes or aortic aneurysms. The numerous structures in the mediastinal space are vulnerable to compression and this may produce a wealth of physical signs. Dysphagia, Horner's syndrome and evidence of superior vena caval obstruction may be prominent.

The pain of mediastinal disease is normally retrosternal and often persistent, but malignant involvement of the intercostal nerves gives rise to lateral chest pain. Pain may be absent or a late occurrence even with large tumours producing florid signs. A cough, often loud and rasping, and progressive dyspnoea, stridor and hoarseness are suggestive symptoms.

Palpable lymph nodes in the cervical area may point to mediastinal lymph node involvement. Chest radiographs with or without tomography or a barium swallow examination may define bronchogenic carcinoma, mediastinal lymphadenopathy or oesophageal disease. CT scanning may provide valuable assistance where differential diagnosis is problematic. Treatment depends on the underlying cause, some tumours being amenable to surgery, radiotherapy or chemotherapy.

Acute Mediastinitis

Acute mediastinitis is predominantly due to oesophageal tears, but occasionally it is secondary to spread of infection from the superficial tissues of the neck. Oesophageal perforation may be a complication of instrumentation or, in the Mallory–Weiss syndrome, follows a severe bout of vomiting. Intense pain is a characteristic feature; it is severe and retrosternal and may radiate across the chest or through to the back. Later lateral pleuritic chest pain may develop. Swallowing is particularly painful. The patient is intensely ill with pyrexia or the syndrome of shock with hypotension, a grey pallor and profuse sweating, though in the very aged sweating is less prominent. Subcutaneous emphysema is clinically apparent in most patients and there may be clinical or radiological evidence of a pleural effusion, pneumomediastinum (Fig. 4.3) or pneumothorax.

Musculo-skeletal Disorders

Local and referred pain of musculo-skeletal derivation is common in adult life and is often diagnostically misinterpreted in old people. Injury may have been causal but forgotten by the patient. Local tenderness may indicate injury or inflammation. Pain from nerve root compression at the level of the lower cervical and upper dorsal spine may be referred to the anterior chest wall. Cervical spondylosis associated with severe disc degeneration is a common cause of root compression in the old, but it may also be due to myeloma or to metastatic bone disease. Osteoporosis is the commonest cause of vertebral crush fractures, but the lower thoracic vertebrae are usually affected and nerve root compression is rare.

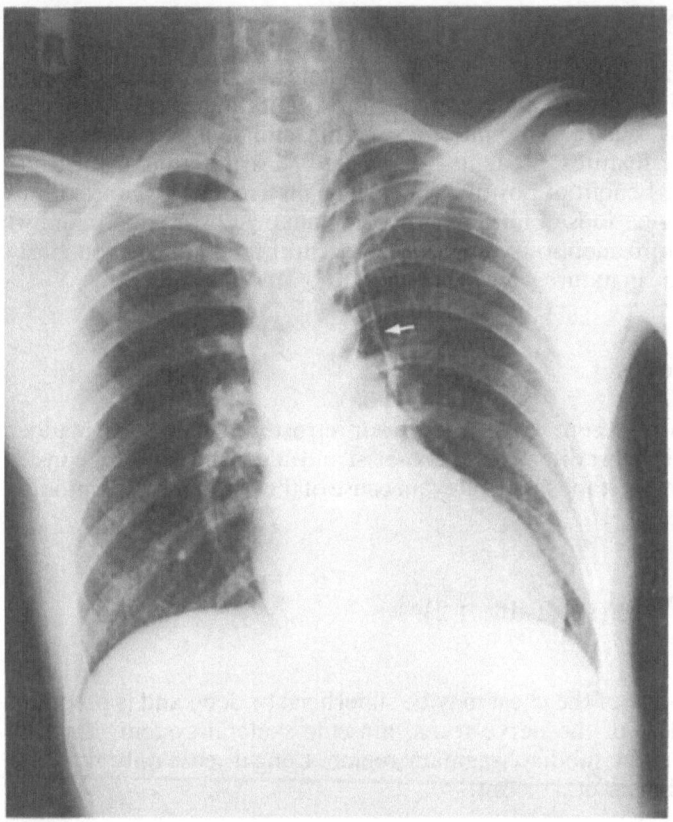

Fig. 4.3. Mediastinitis, showing displacement of the mediastinal pleura (arrowed) due to the presence of air. (By permission of Dr. D. Cochlin.)

Manubriosternal and Xiphoid Process Syndromes

Pain due to the manubriosternal syndrome is sharp and localised to the affected area and is brought on or accentuated by flexion, extension or twisting of the trunk or by coughing or sneezing. The pain may at times be a constant dull ache. Local tenderness with occasional swelling and increased warmth in the region of the manubriosternal junction is of diagnostic import. Rheumatoid arthritis may be present.

The xiphoid syndrome is characterised by symptoms comparable with the manubriosternal syndrome, but pain and tenderness is experienced over the lower central chest. Exercise, particularly walking, may precipitate attacks of pain and be mistaken for angina. However the pain is typically sharp and stitch-like.

Psychogenic Causes

Functional chest pain is often a feature of anxiety states. Typically it is localised to the left precordial or inframammary area and precipitating events are either non-specific or stress-related. Palpitation, sweating and hyperventilation are commonly associated features. Patients who have had a previous myocardial infarction without the benefit of positive counselling are frequently conscious of their heart and during periods of tension may complain of substernal discomfort and a disastrous reinforcement of symptoms can occur if the pain is erroneously diagnosed as ischaemic in nature.

Abdominal Disorders

Acute cholecystitis may present with severe lower retrosternal pain. Gall bladder disorder and ischaemic heart disease often co-exist and at times it requires considerable clinical acumen to establish the relevant cause of the presenting symptoms.

Lateral Chest Pain (see Table 4.2)

Pain outside the mid-line of the chest may be superficial or deep and is predominantly due to disorders of the nerve roots, musculo-skeletal system, lungs or pleura or referred from the subdiaphragmatic region. Lung disease only gives rise to pain by involving the parietal pleura.

Table 4.2. Causes of lateral chest pain

Herpes zoster
Cervical spondylosis
Costrochondritis
Trauma
Disorders of lung and pleura
Spontaneous pneumothorax

Herpes Zoster

Herpes zoster is predominantly a disease of old age, the attack rate increasing from 3.5 per 1000 under the age of 50 to 10.1 per 1000 in the eighth decade. The disorder is precipitated by reactivation of the varicella-zoster virus. The virus has a predilection for the posterior root ganglion. There is often a prodromal period of up to four days characterised by intense burning pain in the distribution of the dermatome of the affected nerve root.

The chest is the site of involvement in over 50% of cases. The unilateral segmental rash is initially erythematous, but within hours becomes vesicular. The clear vesicular fluid becomes turbid if secondary infection develops. The lesions shrivel and scab over in less than a week. After separation pink scars remain which eventually turn white to provide lasting evidence of the disorder. Additional to this segmental rash, a scattered eruption of variable intensity and characteristic of chickenpox may occur. The rash is particularly intense in patients who are immunocompromised due to underlying leukaemia, multiple myeloma, reticuloses or cortico-steroid administration. Post-herpetic neuralgia is a painful complication, often intensely so, and may persist for months or years. Occasionally, there is no skin eruption with an acute attack of zoster.

Treatment with acyclovir in the early stages may abort or significantly modify an acute attack. The pain of post-herpetic neuralgia is often responsive to anti-convulsant or anti-depressant medication. The use of transcutaneous nerve stimulating devices may also be beneficial.

Cervical Spondylosis

Cervical spondylosis refers to the degenerative changes in the intervertebral discs and associated osteoarthritic changes in the diarthrodial neurocentral and apophyseal joints. Bony spurs resulting from these changes cause cervical myelopathy (see Chap. 15) by compressing the spinal nerve roots. If the lowest cervical vertebrae are involved, central or lateral chest pain may develop. Pain may be episodic or a constant dull ache and may radiate down the ulnar border of the arm and inner two fingers with associated parasthesia. Cervical movement may precipitate or exacerbate episodes of pain. Sensory impairment to light touch and pin-prick may be detected over the C7, T1 dermatomes.

Costochondritis

Costochondritis is not an uncommon cause of chest pain which is sometimes prolonged and gnawing in character. It is readily identified by local tenderness on direct pressure over the affected costal cartilages or by indirect pressure over the sternum. In the localised and severe form of chondritis – Tietze's syndrome – the second costochondral junction is commonly involved with swelling and marked tenderness being evident. The condition is self-limiting though analgesia will be required, sometimes for prolonged periods.

Trauma

Chest pain may result from direct or indirect trauma. Direct trauma usually results from a blow to or a knock on the chest wall. Most commonly a clear history of injury is available, but disturbed levels of consciousness due to disease, drugs or alcohol or due to a seizure may necessitate a clinical or radiological search for evidence of trauma. Painful injury may result from cardio-pulmonary resuscitation. Indirect trauma may be a sequence of severe bouts of coughing or vomiting and chest pain may be mistakenly attributed to underlying respiratory or abdominal pathology. Rib fractures following direct or indirect trauma are surprisingly common in old people and often overlooked. Local tenderness is always to be found in patients with traumatic chest pain if diligently sought and local infiltration with 1% lignocaine hydrochloride usually produces prompt symptom relief.

Disorders of Lungs and Pleura

Disease of the lung parenchyma and visceral pleura does not produce pain. It is only when the disease process extends to involve parietal pleura, the chest wall and the structures in the mediastinum that pain is experienced. The parietal pleura is richly supplied with pain nerve fibres from the intercostal nerves. As these nerves originate from the thoracic segments of the spinal cord, pain from parietal pleural disease is located in the appropriate dermatomes of the chest wall. The central portion of the diaphragmatic pleura is supplied by the phrenic nerve which originates from the 3rd, 4th and 5th cervical nerve roots. Inflammatory involvement in this area of pleura may produce pain referred to the neck and shoulder.

Pleurisy is most often due to disease of the underlying lung, though chest wall trauma is an important cause. Bacterial pneumonia, pulmonary infarction, bronchiectasis, pulmonary tuberculosis, lung abscess or bronchogenic carcinoma may be the primary underlying disorder. Mesotheliomas may widely infiltrate the pleural surfaces producing severe chest pain, cough and dyspnoea. The collagen disorders such as systemic lupus erythematosus and rheumatoid arthritis may be associated with pleurisy.

Pleuritic pain is typically sharp, stabbing or tearing in quality, but may be no more than a dull ache. It is aggravated by or may only occur on deep breathing or coughing. Patients will often try to limit pain by shallow breathing or hold the sides of their chest when coughing. A pleural friction rub is the characteristic physical sign. It is accentuated by deep breathing and disappears if the patient holds his breath. Depending on the underlying pathology a pleural effusion may develop with the associated physical signs of dullness to percussion, diminished vocal fremitus and diminished or absent breath sounds over the affected area.

Spontaneous Pneumothorax

Spontaneous pneumothorax occurs most frequently as a consequence of rupture of a small visceral subpleural bleb in a radiologically normal lung, but emphysematous changes may be apparent (Fig. 4.4). Air may enter the pleural space from outside the body by penetrating traumatic injury to the chest wall or following diagnostic intervention such as a pleural biopsy. In the past therapeutic pneumothorax was induced in an effort to control cavitating tuberculosis.

Spontaneous pneumothorax may present with acute lateral chest pain and breathlessness. A slowly enlarging pneumothorax may be pain free and only associated with breathlessness on exertion. Some small pneumothoraces are symptom free. At the other extreme a positive pressure tension pneumothorax may result in dramatic signs of circulatory collapse which may be relieved equally dramatically by a needle in the chest wall as a temporary emergency procedure.

A chest radiograph in both inspiration and expiration will confirm the diagnosis and define the extent of the pneumothorax, the presence of adhesions and

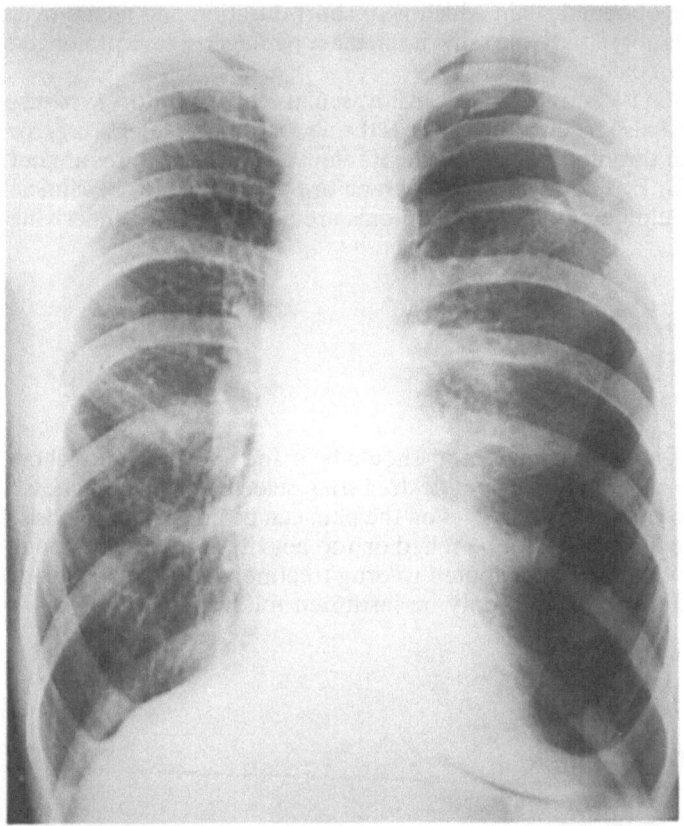

Fig. 4.4. Left sided pneumothorax due to spontaneous rupture of an emphysematous bulla in a patient with chronic obstructive airways disease. (By permission of Dr. D. Cochlin.)

mediastinal shift. With small pneumothoraces air will usually be resorbed spontaneously, whereas intercostal drainage will be required for large lesions; this is especially so if respiratory function is compromised.

Clinical Evaluation

A meticulous history is of cardinal importance. False economy of time in history taking is the commonest cause of diagnostic error and leads to inappropriate and unrewarding investigation. The clinical presentation and circumstances are crucial diagnostic signposts.

Symptoms in the aged may be influenced by the vagaries of the memory, contamination by multiple disease and the side effects of polypharmacy; yet it is vital to characterise each symptom from the not infrequent clinical pot-pourri. The onset and duration of the pain, its site and radiation together with a description of its character must be obtained. Pain which is of short duration and recurs over weeks or months does not require the same immediacy of diagnosis as a prolonged and isolated episode of pain.

Physical examination is centred on the cardiovascular and respiratory systems, though attention must also be directed towards the abdomen, neck, legs (e.g. for evidence of deep vein thrombosis) and psyche if relevant clinical features are not to be overlooked. An ECG and chest radiograph are extensions to the clinical examination and should be obtained if symptoms are acute or if the underlying cause is not apparent.

Management

While investigation is in progress, attempts should be made to control such chest pain as distresses the patient. A therapeutic drug trial, selected on a "best guess" basis is sometimes necessary and its effect on the pain can be an aid to diagnosis. However, such strategies should not be relied on too heavily as the spontaneous resolution of pain can be falsely attributed to drug treatment and a wrong diagnosis made. Specific treatment can only be instituted following accurate diagnosis.

Further Reading

Constant J (ed) (1985) Bedside cardiology, 3rd edn. Little, Brown and Company, Boston
Hamdy RC (1984) Chest pain. In: Hamdy RC Geriatric medicine; a problem-solving approach. Ballière Tindall, London pp 41–51
Timmis GC, Westveer DC, Hauser AM, Stewart JR, Dressendorfer RH, O'Neill WW (1985) Cardiovascular review, 6th edn. Grune and Stratton, Orlando

Chapter 5

Abdominal Pain

W. E. Wilkins

Abdominal pain is common in the general population. In only a minority does the symptom reflect serious disease. This probably explains the paucity of published information on its incidence. Data based on consecutive admissions to the Emergency Room at the University of Virginia Medical Center suggest that 1 in 100 adults per year develop abdominal pain of sufficient magnitude to seek medical advice. Abdominal pain was a significant factor in 1 out of 10 presentations at the centre (Brewer et al. 1976).

There is a particular absence of published data on the incidence of abdominal pain in old people. Anecdotal evidence with some support from the literature indicates that presentation with abdominal pain in old age is far more likely to reflect serious illness than in the younger patient. The study of Brewer et al. quoted above showed that 33% of patients aged over 65 years required urgent surgical treatment as opposed to 16% of those aged under 65. The mortality rate among the older group was 8.4% as compared with 0.9% in the younger group. Bolt's study based on emergency referrals to the West Middlesex Hospital quoted a mortality rate of 25% in patients over the age of 70 years with abdominal pain (Bolt 1960).

Perception of Abdominal Pain

Two neuronal pathways are involved in the perception of abdominal pain.

Visceral Pain

Visceral (organ) pain results from the stimulation of "pain" nerve endings located in the smooth muscle of the arterial and bowel wall. Certain organs such as the liver are devoid of pain receptors and pain is perceived when receptors in the organ capsule are stimulated by stretching. Visceral pain fibres are unmyelinated and travel via the sympathetic nerves to the spinal cord at the level of T6 to L2. After entering the spinal cord the fibres synapse and travel to the cerebral cortex via the lateral spinothalamic tract.

Visceral pain tends to be dull and poorly localised. There are exceptions to this, as in the case of peptic ulcer pain which localises well and can be severe even though a small area of pain receptors are involved. Perhaps the presence of gastric disease sensitises the receptors or co-existent muscle spasm augments pain symptoms.

Visceral pain is perceived to originate from the embryological rather than the anatomical site of the diseased organ. Thus in the early stages of acute appendicitis, visceral pain is perceived to originate from the centre of the abdomen. Sometimes visceral pain is felt on the surface of the body in an area removed from the diseased organ – a phenomenon known as *referred pain*. This can occur when those sensory neurones supplying the organ and those supplying the area of the body surface enter the spinal cord at the same level. For example, visceral pain originating from the kidney, may be perceived in the groin.

Parietal Pain

Parietal (body surface) pain occurs as a result of spread of disease from the viscus to the overlying parietal peritoneum. In contrast to the visceral peritoneum, the parietal peritoneum is very well endowed with pain receptors. The nerve supply results from nerve fibres which "penetrate" inwards from the skin and indeed parietal nerve receptors are similar to those found in the skin. Parietal pain can be localised accurately and its description is much more precise than that of visceral pain. The only exception to this rule of localisation is the pain resulting from the diaphragmatic peritoneum which may be localised to the shoulder.

Irritation of the parietal peritoneum invokes reflex responses (the peritocutaneous and peritoneomuscular reflex of Morley) resulting in hyperaesthesia and muscular guarding. It is possible that as an associated phenomenon of ageing these neuronal mechanisms may degenerate and that this may explain the paucity of clinical signs seen occasionally in elderly people with peritonitis. The role of prostaglandin synthesis in mediating these mechanisms remains to be determined.

The causes of abdominal pain can be usefully divided in those conditions causing acute pain and chronic pain.

Acute Abdominal Pain

A useful classification of the causes of acute abdominal pain in old people has been suggested by Bolt and Table 5.1 lists the commoner causes. There are four main aetiological groups:

distension of a viscus
intra-abdominal sepsis
vascular disease
miscellaneous

Table 5.1. Causes of acute abdominal pain

Distension of a viscus (urinary retention, intestinal obstruction)
Intra-abdominal sepsis (acute cholecystitis, appendicitis, acute
  pancreatitis)
Vascular disease (aortic dissection, vascular occlusion)
Miscellaneous (extra-abdominal disorders, diabetes mellitus, adrenal
  insufficiency, retroperitoneal haemorrhage)

Distension of a Viscus

Urinary retention is a common cause of abdominal pain and seldom poses a problem in diagnosis. The history is usually suggestive and patients are almost always male, prostatic hypertrophy being the commonest cause. In the female presenting with acute retention, a vaginal examination to exclude a gynaecological tumour is essential.

Intestinal obstruction is an important cause of acute pain in old people, its incidence being second only to urinary retention in the male and gallbladder disease in the female.

When the small bowel is obstructed, the causes include an incarcerated hernia, adhesions due to previous surgery and gallstone ileus. Small bowel malignancy is very rare. Gallstone ileus, although rare in young people occurs not uncommonly in old age. This relates directly to the increased prevalence of gallstones with increasing age. When assessing a patient with small bowel obstruction, the history can be insidious and the clinical signs atypical. Examination of the hernial orifices is essential. Particular care should be taken with obese females since an incarcerated femoral hernia can easily go unnoticed. Evidence of an obstructing gallstone

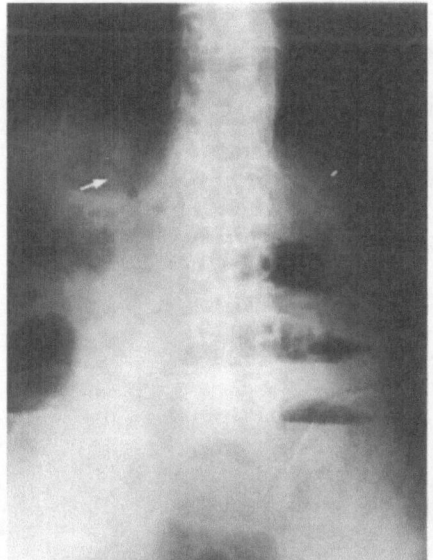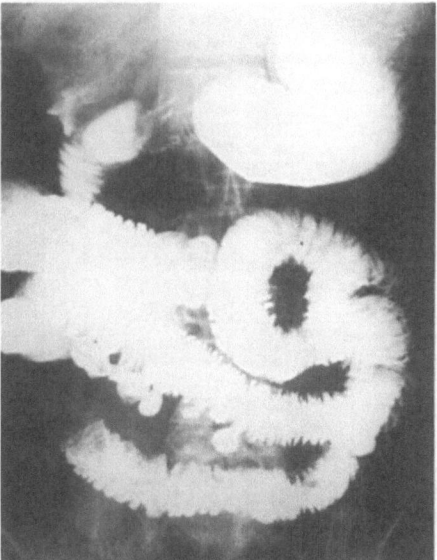

a   b

Fig. 5.1. Gallstone ileus. **a** Plain abdominal film shows gas in the biliary tree (arrowed) and fluid levels. **b** Subsequent barium follow through examination shows obstruction at the terminal ileum.

at the terminal ileum and gas shadowing within the biliary tree are useful radiographic signs of gallstone ileus (Fig. 5.1). Small bowel obstruction usually presents late and the mortality rate varies between 25% and 50%.

Large bowel obstruction is almost always due to colorectal carcinoma (see Chap. 11). Early symptoms such as rectal bleeding may be absent, unnoticed or ignored by the patient who then presents late with abdominal pain due to obstruction. This is particularly frustrating since elderly patients fare well after colonic surgery (as compared with gallbladder surgery, for example) and "short" colonoscopy provides an excellent and well-tolerated method of investigation.

People with chronic constipation and atonic bowels are at particular risk of volvulus of the colon. The large bowel is on a pedicle at the caecum, transverse colon and the sigmoid. Volvulus can occur at caecal and sigmoid levels. The former presents acutely with pain, nausea and abdominal distension. Volvulus of the sigmoid can be much more insidious. An awareness of the "at risk" group is important. A plain abdominal radiograph will show marked dilatation of the sigmoid loop; sigmoidoscopy may be therapeutic (Fig. 5.2).

Intra-abdominal Sepsis

The commonest source of intra-abdominal sepsis is disease in the biliary tract. The prevalence of gallstones increases with advancing age and post mortem studies show the presence of gallstones in 40% of people over the age of 80 years. The natural history of gallstones is unknown but in the majority of patients they are asymptomatic. Impaction of a gallstone in the cystic duct is the usual cause of *acute cholecystitis* and overall this is the commonest cause of acute abdominal pain in old people.

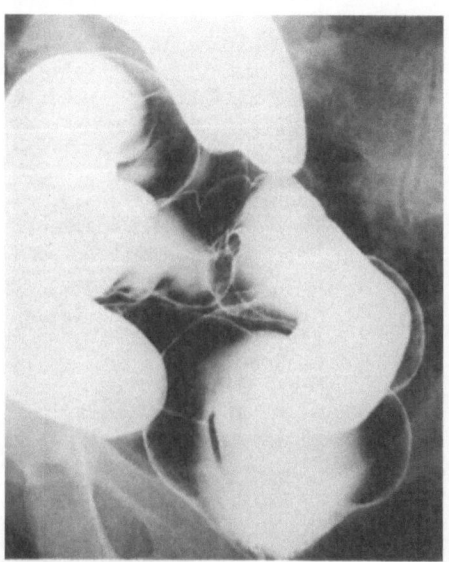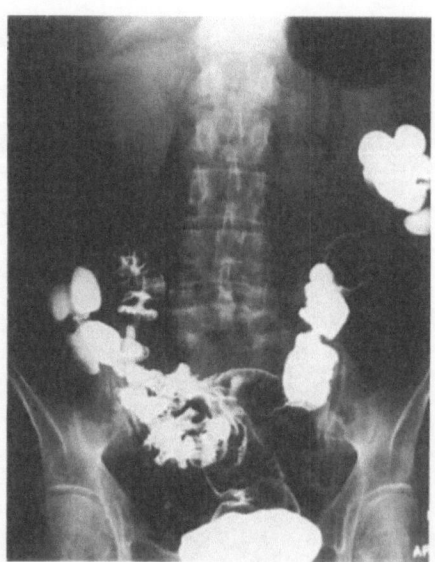

a   b

Fig. 5.2.   Sigmoid volvulus immediately before (a) and following (b) decompensation. Note the twist in the sigmoid loop.

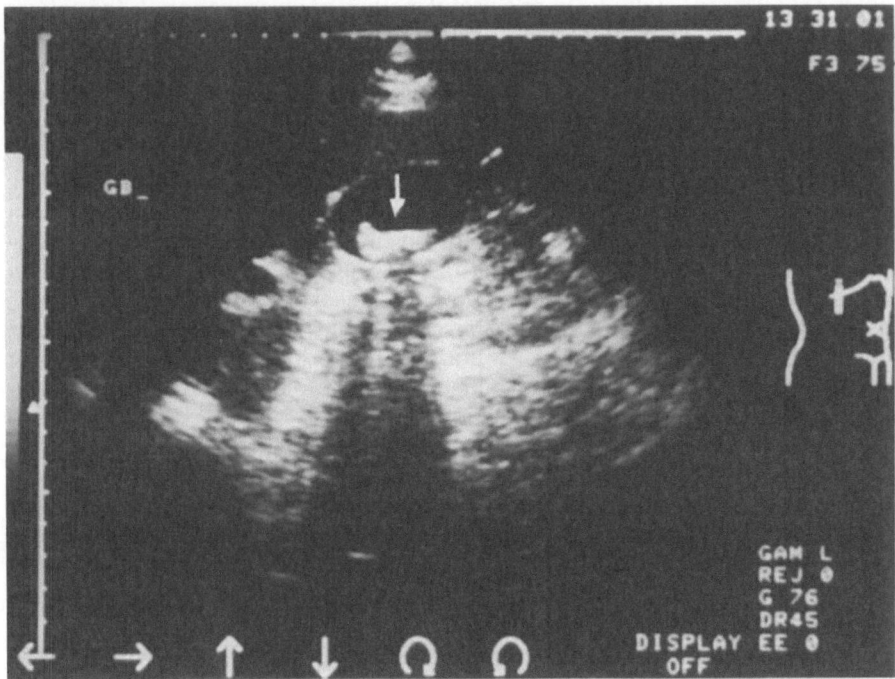

Fig. 5.3. Ultrasound examination of the abdomen showing stones in the gallbladder (arrowed).

The majority of biliary duct stones either pass spontaneously or fall back into the gallbladder. Stones traversing the cystic duct cause pain resulting principally from the gallbladder spasm; the term biliary colic is a misnomer. The pain is constant, severe and localised to the epigastrium or right hypochondrium and accompanied by a positive Murphy's sign. Occasionally the pain is reported as pleuritic in type. It is usually associated with nausea and vomiting. In an uncomplicated attack the pain begins to resolve within 24 hours of onset. There may be a neutrophil response and a transient rise in liver enzymes. Sometimes, however, the impaction of a biliary stone is painless and may mimic the presentation of a malignant obstruction.

Passage of a biliary stone may result in damage to the common bile duct and this in turn may lead to chronic stasis and infection, leading to ascending cholangitis and even bacterial hepatitis. Signs of sepsis may be apparent at this stage, though a quarter of elderly people remain apyrexial and non-specific signs such as mental confusion may predominate. Septicaemia is usual and blood cultures are often positive. If impaction persists a gallbladder empyema may develop. The appearance of a mass in the right hypochondrium signifies an omental response or the development of an empyema. The gallbladder may become gangrenous and subsequently perforate.

Abdominal ultrasound is a particularly good method of investigating such patients. The presence of stones is characterised by the "comet's tail" sign (Fig. 5.3). The absence of gallbladder concentrating function is a good marker of disease and contrast cholecystography remains a useful method of investigation. If the patient remains jaundiced, percutaneous transhepatic cholangiography or endoscopic retrograde choledochopancreatography (ERCP) may be required. It must not be assumed that abdominal pain in the presence of gallstones signifies cholecystitis. Other conditions (e.g. myocardial infarction and pneumonia) can present with similar pain.

Intra-abdominal sepsis secondary to gallbladder disease carries a high mortality unless treatment is prompt. The bowel should be rested, so naso-gastric suction should be applied and intravenous fluids given. Parenteral analgesia and antibiotics will be required. Care must be taken to use an antibiotic regime which covers anaerobic organisms. Once the patient recovers from the acute attack, an elective cholecystectomy should be carried out promptly. As a rule, old people tolerate biliary tract surgery poorly, the perioperative mortality being much greater than that found with younger patients. In particular, there is a high incidence of post-operative chest infection.

Acute appendicitis is often erroneously assumed to be rare in old age. As in younger people, the presentation is usually with central abdominal pain which later localises to the right iliac fossa with associated pyrexia and constitutional upset. In common with other acute abdominal conditions in old age, the presentation may be atypical and diagnosis consequently delayed. The appendix is often gangrenous or even perforated at laparotomy and the perioperative mortality is then high.

Acute pancreatitis in old people is probably under-diagnosed. It is usually due to gallstone impaction, although alcohol is an increasingly important cause. It can complicate recovery from hypothermia (see Chap. 22) and is occasionally seen in hypercalcaemic states and with pancreatic carcinoma. Abdominal pain is accompanied by vomiting and there is epigastric tenderness. Once it is considered, the diagnosis is easily established, since estimation of serum amylase is a simple and accurate test. Sometimes the rise in serum amylase may be missed since levels can peak and return to normal within 24 hours after the onset of symptoms. Measurement of urinary amylase can be useful since abnormal "lag" excretion of amylase may persist for 48 hours after the onset of acute symptoms. Persistent elevation of serum amylase and persisting abdominal pain should question the possibility of a pancreatic pseudocyst. Blood calcium usually falls with pancreatitis. Abdominal ultrasound or CT scanning can be useful in showing pancreatic necrosis with secondary sepsis. This may require surgical treatment.

Vascular Disease

Vascular disease in the form of dissection or occlusion of a major vessel causes acute and severe abdominal pain.

With abdominal *aortic dissection* the vessel is invariably atherosclerotic and the patient is usually hypertensive. The severe pain is followed by symptoms referable to acute blood loss and ischaemia of the intra-abdominal organs. Resuscitation and an emergency surgical repair of the dissecting vessel offers the only hope of survival. Perioperative mortality rates are very high.

There are two main syndromes of *vascular occlusion* seen in elderly patients. Acute massive necrosis results from occlusion of the superior mesenteric artery which alone supplies the small intestine and the large intestine as far as the splenic flexure. The presentation is usually explosive with rapid progression to gangrene and perforation. Occasionally the clinical features are less marked and abdominal pain may be entirely absent. Rarely, this syndrome is due to vasculitis and the initial investigations should include an estimation of erythrocyte sedimentation rate or blood viscosity. Early laparotomy and resection offers the only hope of survival. The mortality rate approximates 75%.

The second syndrome is that of ischaemic colitis due to inferior mesenteric artery hypoperfusion. This has a very characteristic presentation of sudden onset bloody diarrhoea associated with left iliac fossa colicky abdominal pain. Plain abdominal radiography can be useful since it often shows the characteristic "thumb printing" appearance due to oedema of the bowel wall. The majority of cases recover with conservative treatment, though the bowel may perforate and some patients develop a stricture at the site of ischaemia. Anticoagulation is of no proven value.

Miscellaneous Causes

The importance of *extra-abdominal disorders* such as pneumonia and myocardial infarction in producing pain referred to the abdomen has already been mentioned. The assessment of all patients presenting with acute abdominal pain should include a chest radiograph and serial ECGs.

With *diabetic ketoacidosis* abdominal pain is often due to a paralytic ileus with gross gastric distension. *Adrenal insufficiency* can also present with acute abdominal pain. The patient is usually very ill with hypovolaemia and an elevated blood urea. Serum potassium is usually elevated and sodium and glucose levels are low. If biochemical and clinical features support the diagnosis then a random blood sample should be taken for cortisol levels and corticosteroids given immediately. To confirm the diagnosis, a Synacthen test with dexamethasone cover can be carried out when the patient's condition has improved. *Hypercalcaemic states* can present with acute abdominal pain secondary to pancreatitis, duodenal ulceration, renal stones or constipation. Primary hyperparathyroidism is relatively common in old age, especially in females.

Other causes include *retroperitoneal haemorrhage* in elderly patients on anticoagulants. Abdominal pain associated with a sudden drop in haemoglobin concentration without evidence of haematemesis or melaena are suggestive features.

Chronic Abdominal Pain

The causes of chronic abdominal pain are summarised in Table 5.2.

Table 5.2.   Causes of chronic abdominal pain

Upper gastrointestinal tract disorders (peptic ulceration, chronic calculous cholecystitis, chronic pancreatitis)
Mesenteric ischaemia
Lower gastrointestinal tract disorders (diverticular disease, irritable bowel syndrome)
Neuromuscular disorders (post-herpetic neuralgia, irritation of nerve root and peripheral nerves)
Miscellaneous disorders (hypercalcaemia, Addison's disease)

Upper Gastrointestinal Tract Disorders

The majority of patients will have disease in the upper gastrointestinal tract either in the stomach, duodenum, biliary tract or pancreas.

Peptic Ulcer

Peptic ulceration is discussed in Chap. 21. While abdominal pain is a common symptom, it is often non-specific and may be entirely absent. This is particularly the case in patients who take non-steroidal anti-inflammatory drugs.

Chronic Cholecystitis

The continued presence of stones in the gallbladder results in chronic inflammation, usually with superimposed episodes of acute cholecystitis. The gallbladder becomes shrunken and fibrosed. It can be the source of pain or discomfort in the right hypochondrium, shoulder or scapular region. Fatty food intolerance is a common associated symptom.

Chronic Pancreatitis

Chronic pancreatitis predominantly presents with central abdominal pain which tends to be recurrent and relieved by adopting a forward crouching posture. Features of pancreatic insufficiency (see Chap. 10) are usually found in association.

Mesenteric Ischaemia

Chronic abdominal pain due to vascular insufficiency (intestinal angina) is rare but its incidence increases with age. Typically the patient presents with upper abdominal cramp-like pain 10 to 20 minutes after eating. There is significant weight loss as a result of food avoidance and malabsorption (see Chap. 10). The diagnosis is confirmed by mesenteric angiography. Surgery offers the only hope of correction.

Lower Gastrointestinal Disorders

The role of the lower gastrointestinal tract in the aetiology of chronic abdominal pain is difficult to determine. Some 50% of old people in Western societies have diverticular disease, so that when this is found, it must not automatically be assumed to be the cause of chronic abdominal pain. Likewise one should be cautious in attributing symptoms to the irritable bowel syndrome without first undertaking appropriate investigations. There is, however, a small group of patients whose pain is undoubtedly due to colonic spasm.

An adequate barium examination or colonoscopy is essential for assessment of the colon. In the irritable bowel syndrome, colonoscopic examination will often reveal a "spastic" appearance of the lower bowel, and during the procedure, the patient may perceive the pain with which he has presented.

Neuromuscular Disorders

Post-herpetic neuralgia can cause severe and prolonged abdominal pain in the distribution of the affected dermatome. Occasionally, no skin eruption accompanies the acute attack of herpes zoster and this can cause diagnostic confusion among the uninitiated.

A vague, band-like ache across the abdomen occurs as a consequence of *nerve root or peripheral nerve irritation*. Nerve root compression can follow an osteoporotic vertebral collapse or be due to diabetic radiculopathy, malignant infiltration and intervertebral disc prolapse. Peripheral neuropathy (see Chap. 15) occasionally causes chronic abdominal pain. Often the precise cause of referred abdominal pain remains obscure despite intensive investigation. In such patients a block of the intercostal nerve in the relevant dermatome with local anaesthetic will relieve the pain if it is due to benign spinal root disease. This helps to clarify the diagnosis.

Miscellaneous Causes

Other and more unusual causes of chronic abdominal pain include hypercalcaemic states and adrenal insufficiency. These have already been mentioned in the context of acute abdominal pain.

Clinical Evaluation

The evaluation of abdominal pain in old people is often difficult. Patients may be confused and the clinical features may be altered or clouded by the presence of coincidental disease. Accurate diagnosis depends on an awareness of the atypical presentation of illnesses, the development and application of intuitive clinical skills and in informed use of modern investigative techniques. In the younger patient clinical skills alone should lead to an accurate diagnosis in 80% of patients. With old people, however, the diagnostic yield based on the history and clinical examination falls to well below 50%.

The clinical history is fundamental to diagnosis and it should attempt to define the site, onset and duration, intensity, type and periodicity of the pain, aggravating and relieving factors, together with associated symptoms. The site of the pain can indicate its likely source, though the perception of pain in areas removed from the site of disease can cause diagnostic confusion. The mode of onset of the pain is important; an explosive onset suggests vascular occlusion for example. The severity of the pain can be useful in diagnosis; this is illustrated by renal colic which is agonising and is associated with pallor and profuse sweating. When the pain of obstruction becomes established, its periodicity may suggest the underlying cause. Thus the pain of small bowel obstruction has a periodicity of a few minutes while that of biliary obstruction can vary between 15 minutes and 2 hours. In elderly patients and particularly in the very old, this periodicity may not become established. It is important to recognise that very serious acute intra-abdominal disease can develop in old people in the absence of significant abdominal pain. This phenomenon is increasingly recognised in patients who regularly ingest non-steroidal anti-inflammatory drugs and it is suggested that these agents interfere with pain perception by their effect on prostaglandin synthesis.

As in young children, signs of intra-abdominal disease can be surprisingly sparse in the elderly patient. Taking intra-abdominal sepsis as an example, body temperature can be normal or low, there may be no abdominal tenderness and signs of peritonitis may be absent even in advanced disease. The white cell count can be normal.

While examination of the abdomen itself is of prime importance, the examination of the heart, chest, spine and other organs must not be neglected in view of their possible contribution to abdominal pain. Evidence of weight loss is an important marker of serious disease (see Chap. 10).

Further Investigation

Recent technological advances have revolutionised the assessment of abdominal pain and have benefited old people as well as other age groups. The role of endoscopy and abdominal ultrasonography, for example, is now well established. These facilities should be easily accessible to old people and the threshold for their use should be low as they are well-tolerated and have a high diagnostic yield. However, their use should not be viewed as a substitute for a good clinical assessment. All patients with abdominal pain should have a baseline series of blood investigations.

Blood Count and Blood Viscosity

A microcytic hypochromic anaemia suggests gastrointestinal blood loss and should be viewed with great suspicion. Poor dietary intake should never be accepted as a cause of iron deficiency in old people until gastrointestinal disease has been excluded. Investigations should be initially directed towards the upper gastrointestinal tract. Common sources of blood loss include oesophagitis, gastric and duodenal ulceration, gastric and pancreatic malignancy. If upper gastro-intestinal endoscopy is normal, attention should then be directed towards the lower intestine. Carcinoma of the large bowel is the commonest malignancy in old age, although abdominal pain is not usually a prominent feature.

Raised blood viscosity is a non-specific finding but marked elevation should suggest a hyperviscosity syndrome (e.g. multiple myeloma) or autoimmune disease with vasculitis.

Blood Biochemistry

The blood sugar should always be estimated as diabetic ketoacidosis can present with abdominal pain. Abnormalities in blood urea and electrolytes can provide useful diagnostic clues. The electrolyte disturbance of renal failure can cause a paralytic ileus. Gastrin excretion depends on reasonable renal function and in renal failure raised levels will increase the risk of peptic ulceration. If the patient is dehydrated then there is an increased risk of mesenteric thrombosis.

Abnormal liver function tests are also of diagnostic use. Conjugated hyperbilirubinaemia with significant elevation of alkaline phosphatase suggests biliary obstruction. It is important to remember that other intra-abdominal organs (e.g. kidney, pancreas) can produce alkaline phosphatase, especially when they are cancerous. Referred pain from metastatic involvement of the dorsal spine should also be considered in patients with a raised alkaline phosphatase. When aspartate transaminase levels are elevated to above ten times normal then this is more suggestive of hepatitis than biliary obstruction.

There is a significant association between hypercalcaemia and intra-abdominal disease so that serum calcium should be routinely measured.

Radiology

A chest radiograph (and an ECG) should be routinely obtained to exclude cardiac and pulmonary disease. There has been much debate about the need for routine, plain abdominal radiography. In the general population there is low diagnostic yield so that this examination is wasteful. In elderly patients, however, the insidious nature of peritonitis due to a perforated viscus should lead to a more liberal use of this investigation, particularly in the very old.

CT scanning will allow visualisation of many abdominal organs. It is of particular value in patients who develop abdominal pain while on anticoagulants since it accurately defines haemorrhage. Abscess cavities containing air will also be seen well.

Biliary scintigraphy using ^{99}Tcm-labelled radiopharmaceuticals can be of considerable use in suspected gallbladder disease. In addition to documenting non-function of the gallbladder, it also supplies information on gallbladder emptying. Modern radiopharmaceuticals concentrate well in the gallbladder with minimal renal excretion.

Ultrasonography and Endoscopy

Abdominal ultrasonography is an extremely valuable diagnostic tool particularly in the investigation of biliary duct obstruction. In the majority of cases it will obviate the need for the more invasive tests such as percutaneous intrahepatic cholangiography or ERCP. It is also of value in the diagnosis of metastatic liver disease and in obstructive and malignant renal disease. It has advantages over CT scanning in that it is easier to use and does not expose the patient to radiation.

Both CT scanning and ultrasound examination compare very unfavourably with endoscopy and barium examination in the assessment of bowel disorders;

both also frequently fail to show small pancreatic tumours. Clinical discretion is essential to the appropriate use of CT scanning and ultrasonography. The diagnostic yield from both is extremely poor when abdominal pain is the only symptom and when other pointers towards intra-abdominal pathology are absent.

Fibre optic endoscopy is an exciting development in the investigation of bowel disease. Upper gastrointestinal endoscopy is valuable in the investigation of pain in the upper abdomen. The technique is technically easy, safe and well tolerated by old people and has a high diagnostic yield. It is of therapeutic benefit with stenosing lesions of the oesophagus and in the management of impacted gallstones.

Lower gastrointestinal endoscopy is also very useful. Short colonoscopy with a 60 cm long flexible endoscope can be carried out with ease to the splenic flexure. However, the diagnostic yield in patients with abdominal pain but no other symptom is low.

Management

The management of abdominal pain is dictated by the diagnosis. It is beyond the confines of this chapter to discuss the management of individual causes. It is, however, important to recognise that a small but significant number of patients will remain without a diagnosis in spite of intensive investigation. It is important to adopt a positive approach with such patients. This should include an explanation of the situation and a message of positive reassurance. If the pain is severe, advice should be sought on anaesthetic and psychotherapeutic methods of relief.

Further Reading

Benson M, Bree RC, Schwab RE et al. (1985) Computed tomographic studies of the painful abdomen. Radiology 155:1443–1444

Bolt DE (1960) Geriatric surgical emergency. Br Med J i:832–836

Brewer RJ, Golden GT, Hitch DC et al. (1976) Abdominal pain: an analysis of 1000 cases in a university hospital emergency room. Am J Surg 131:219–233

Clinch D, Banerjee AR, Ostick G (1984) Absence of abdominal pain in elderly patients with peptic ulcer. Age Ageing 13:120–123

De Dombal FT (1985) Analysis of symptoms in the acute abdomen. Clin Gastroenterol 14(3):531–543

Ponka JL, Welborn JK, Brush BE (1963) Acute abdominal pain in aged patients: an analysis of 200 cases. J Am Geriatr Soc 11:993–1007

Steinheber FU (1976) Interpretation of gastrointestinal symptoms in the elderly. Med Clin North Am 60(6):1151–1154

Chapter 6

Musculo-skeletal Pain

June Arnold

Musculo-skeletal pain accounts for much of the morbidity and half of the disability suffered by pensioners in the United Kingdom. It can be attributed to pain in muscles, tendons, ligaments, entheses (insertions), bursae, joints or bone. While pain itself impairs the quality of life for many people, it is also often accompanied by loss of function in an affected muscle or joint. The resulting immobility and its accompanying problems are discussed in more detail in Chapter 15.

Joint Disorders (Table 6.1)

Osteoarthritis

Osteoarthritis (OA) affects some 5–6 million people in the United Kingdom and its prevalence increases dramatically with age. The causes are unknown and its relationship to the ageing process is uncertain, age perhaps merely allowing time for the disease to develop. Previous trauma to a joint, anatomical joint abnormalities and hereditary factors (possibly related to the structure of cartilage) are important aetiological factors. There is also an association with diseases such as diabetes mellitus, haemochromatosis, rheumatoid disease and other inflammatory arthroses.

Table 6.1. Articular causes of musculo-skeletal pain

Osteoarthritis
Rheumatoid disease
Gout
Pseudogout
Seronegative spondyloarthritides
Infective arthritis
Haemarthrosis
Hypertrophic pulmonary osteoarthropathy

With regard to pathogenesis a suggested sequence is stiffening of the adjacent bone followed by alteration in the structure of the cartilage which then retains water and becomes less resilient. Later the cartilage is destroyed. There is an overgrowth of bone resulting in nodes or osteophytes which can break off and form loose bodies in the joints. The synovial fluid is less viscous and may be increased in amount. Ultimately joint space is lost and the joint fuses. Concomitantly the central joints in the spine, which have no synovial membrane, show disc degeneration. The central nucleus may prolapse vertically into the vertebral body, backwards into the spinal canal compressing the spinal cord, or sideways compressing nerve roots. The combination of disc degeneration and osteoarthritic changes in the apophyseal joints is called spondylosis.

There is a worldwide geographical variation in the joints commonly affected. Those most frequently involved are those that move most, take the heaviest weight or are most readily injured. The condition can be asymptomatic, being an incidental radiological finding. When symptoms are present, pain is the predominant feature. This typically occurs asymmetrically in one or more joints; hips, knees, hands, spine and feet are the most commonly affected. Stiffness occurs after quite short periods of rest making it difficult to get out of a chair or bed, but it is not prolonged for hours at a time as in the inflammatory arthroses. Progression is variable beginning with pain present only on exercise. Later the pain becomes more persistent and takes longer and longer to ease with rest. Finally, it can be continuous, deep-seated and boring, interfering with sleep. Some patients experience sudden lancinating pains and episodes of swelling and redness in individual joints. Disability can be severe, with joints fixed and the patient confined to bed or chair, though progression to such a stage can and should be prevented. As the disorder is confined to joints general health is unimpaired. Patients are, however, frequently overweight.

With hip involvement, pain is usually felt in the groin and inner thigh, but may be in the knee, acetabular area or buttock. There is limitation of movement, especially rotation, and the leg may be shortened. The patient will then swing to the side of the lesion on walking and may keep the opposite knee flexed, thereby increasing the stress and the likelihood of osteoarthritis in that knee.

In the knee, both patello-femoral and tibio-femoral joints can be affected. Lax ligaments, previous injury and obesity are important predisposing factors. The onset is often acute with pain and swelling due to a large effusion. Other patients have a more chronic course and may develop flexion or valgus deformities. Sometimes a joint effusion may extend into the popliteal area (Baker's cyst). Should the joint capsule rupture, a sudden pain is felt at the back of the knee followed by swelling of the calf and lower leg, a condition that can be confused with a deep vein thrombosis. The correct diagnosis is established by ultrasound or the injection of radio opaque dye into the joint. Treatment is a few days rest, with local steroid if the pain is severe.

The hands are affected early and, though there may be some deformity, pain is usually mild and loss of function minimal. The thickening of the bones at the joint margins results in Heberden's nodes at the distal interphalangeal joints and Bouchard's nodes at the less often involved proximal interphalangeal joints. Pain at the base of the thumb may be troublesome due to involvement of the first carpometacarpal joint (Fig. 6.1).

In the feet the commonly involved joints are the first metatarso-phalangeal, resulting in hallux valgus or hallux rigidus. Bunions develop over the joint, and

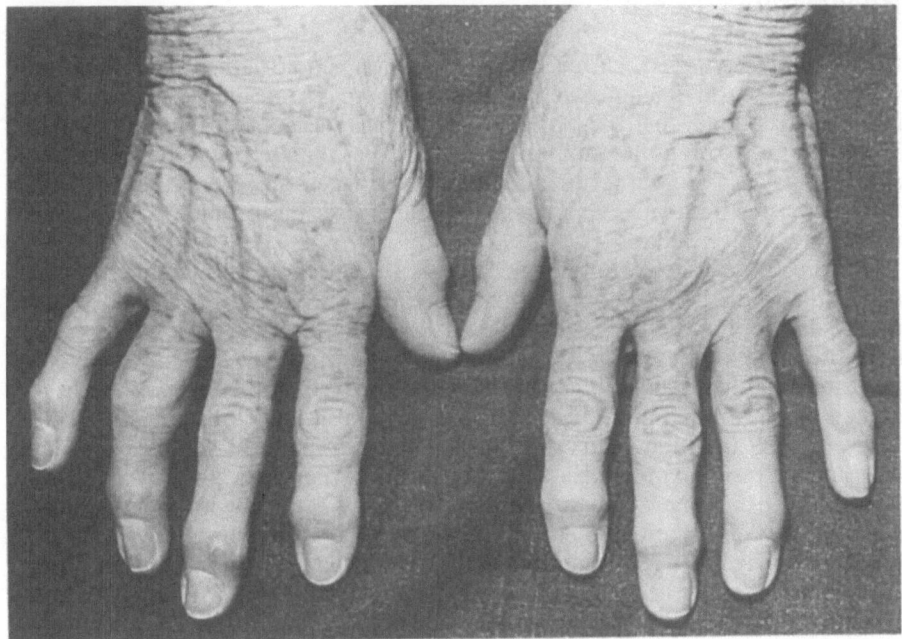

Fig. 6.1. The hand in osteoarthritis, showing Heberden's nodes, Bouchard node and "squaring" of the hands from involvement of the carpo-metacarpal joint of the thumb.

can become infected and lead to infection of the bone and joint. This is particularly likely to occur in patients with diabetes mellitus.

Changes in the spine may be widespread and are most often associated with symptoms in the cervical and lumbar regions. Recent pain is unlikely to be related to long standing abnormalities seen on X-ray. Neck pain may radiate to the shoulders or over the vertex to the forehead and, typically, is worse at night. Pain from disc protrusion is aggravated by coughing and is worse on flexion, whilst osteoarthritis in the apophyseal joints is aggravated by extension. Often multiple joints are involved at multiple levels. Movement may be limited and muscle spasm palpable. Neurological signs can be due to nerve compression or interference with local blood supply to nerves. Sudden neck movements such as looking upwards or sideways can cause ischaemia of the hind brain by compressing the vertebral arteries.

Attacks of low back pain tend to be recurring. There may be a definite relationship to injury or a certain movement. Typically there is mild pain for a day or two, which suddenly becomes severe and radiates into the leg. As with cervical spine lesions movement is limited, spasm present and more than one joint tends to be affected.

The diagnosis of osteoarthritis is made on clinical grounds, radiological examination showing classical changes only when the disease is well advanced.

Rheumatoid Disease

Rheumatoid disease (RD) affects some 1½ million people in the United Kingdom. It is more common in temperate climates and there is some evidence to suggest an increased frequency in urban populations. It presents in early or middle adult life, in women more often than in men, and only occasionally for the first time in old age. As it is disabling rather than fatal, many sufferers survive into old age when their increasing frailty and dependence produces a serious problem for the patient and caring services alike.

The cause or causes are unknown. There is a disorder of immune function which affects the whole body. People with haplotype HLA DR4 or D4 are at increased risk of developing the disease. While 70% of patients with rheumatoid disease have these haplotypes, only 5% with these haplotypes develop rheumatoid disease. It is postulated that this gene or a nearby one is so similar to a possible trigger organism that the patient in combating the organism develops auto-antibodies. Some of these antibodies can be measured by the differential sheep cell and latex tests and the result expressed as a titre; collectively they are known as rheumatoid factor (RF). Rheumatoid factor is not present in all patients with rheumatoid disease, and 10% of unaffected elderly people have a positive test. Levels can vary considerably over the years and reflect the activity and severity of the disease.

The joint changes are characterised by synovial thickening, alterations in the synovial fluid, loss of joint space with erosion of the underlying bone and followed by fibrous ankylosis and osteoarthritis. Nearly every joint in the body may be affected, though the first carpo-metacarpal joint at the base of the thumb is often spared. As this joint is commonly involved in osteoarthritis, this feature is sometimes of value in the differential diagnosis.

The usual presentation is insidious, with pain, stiffness and swelling affecting joints in a symmetrical manner. Non-specific disease symptoms are the rule and patients may feel vaguely unwell, tire easily and lose weight. Initially, there is involvement of the metacarpo-phalangeal joints and interphalangeal joints, giving the fingers a spindle-like appearance. Later, with joint destruction, swan-neck or boutonnière finger deformities result (Fig. 6.2). Synovial tendon sheaths may be involved leading to swelling and sometimes tendon rupture. A carpal tunnel syndrome may be an early feature due to median nerve compression from synovial hypertrophy. The tendency of the hands to ulnar deviation also increases the likelihood of tendon rupture. Painful wrists can interfere with lifting even light objects such as a cup. Involvement of the cervical spine may cause subluxation of the atlanto-axial joint compressing nearby nerve roots and the cervical cord, resulting in loss of power in the legs and, rarely, in sudden death.

Extra-articular manifestations of the disease are legion. Rheumatoid nodules may develop on extensor surfaces and indicate active disease. These occasionally ulcerate and can be troublesome, especially if over pressure areas such as the sacrum. Treatment should be protective, removal being unsuccessful as the wound fails to heal. Other complications include dry eyes (a fairly common finding in the elderly without rheumatoid disease), which is treated by frequent instillation of methylcellulose eye-drops, and dry mouth which is much more difficult to help. This combination of atrophy of the lacrimal and salivary glands is known as Sjogren's syndrome.

The disease follows an intermittent course of attacks and remissions. Intercurrent illness, stress, bereavement or too much exercise may all make the patient worse, but equally the patient may relapse in the absence of any of these factors.

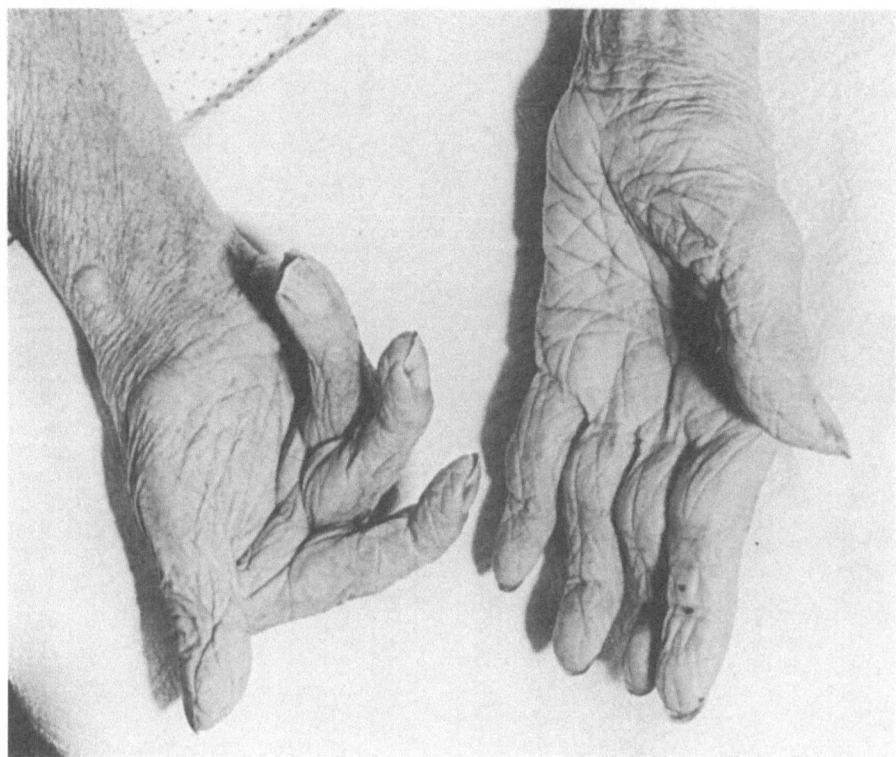

Fig. 6.2. Rheumatoid disease with "swan-neck" deformity of the fingers of the left hand and "Z-shaped" deformity of the left thumb.

Many patients remain in good health for years with the disease apparently controlled. A few others deteriorate steadily and rapidly, while the majority get slowly worse. The inflammatory features may become less prominent with time, the condition coming to resemble osteoarthritis; by this stage, however, the damage may be widespread.

As for osteoarthritis diagnosis is made on clinical grounds, with typical radiological features confirming the diagnosis only in long-standing disease. A high titre of rheumatoid factor is highly suggestive of the diagnosis in the early stages, but this test is neither fully sensitive nor specific.

Drug treatment in the initial stages consists of non-steroidal anti-inflammatory drugs (NSAIDs), which generally control symptoms but do not influence the progression of the disease. Agents which do modify the course of rheumatoid disease, at least in some patients, include gold, penicillamine, antimalarial agents and cytotoxic drugs (e.g. azathioprine and cyclophosphamide). They should only be used when the disease is severe and progressive and has failed to respond to simpler measures. Such agents are seldom required in old age. Only 40% of patients can continue on treatment because of side effects, and of these only two-thirds will benefit. A few that improve will later relapse. One of the other preparations may be tolerated if the first choice has to be abandoned. If the patient responds, the treatment should be continued indefinitely.

Gold and penicillamine can cause rashes, oral ulceration, bone marrow depres-

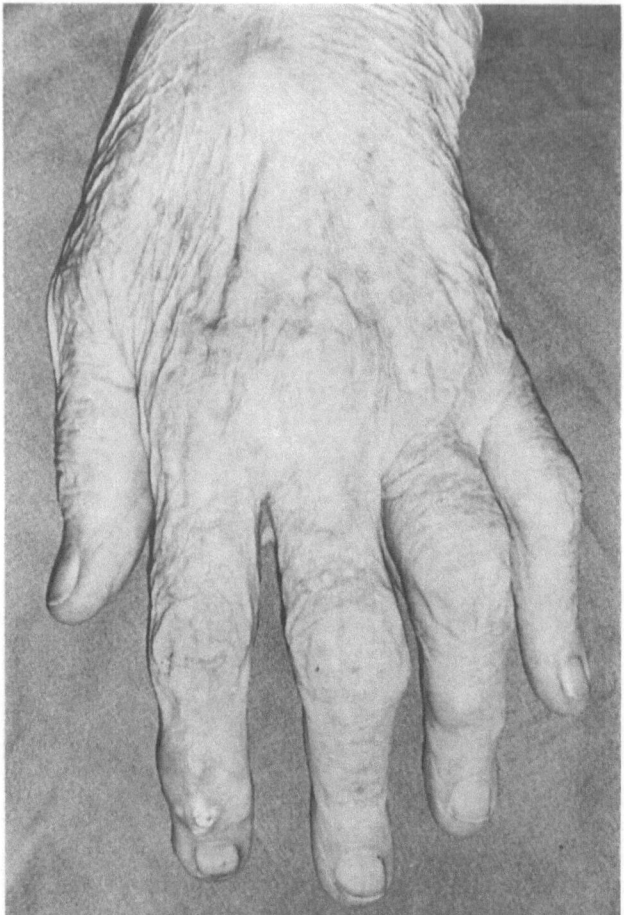

Fig. 6.3.   Chronic tophacious gout with tophi on the index finger. The patient also had rheumatoid disease.

sion and renal failure. A test dose must be given before starting gold as hypersensitivity reactions can occur. Penicillamine may cause a drug-induced lupus syndrome, Goodpasture's syndrome or myasthenia gravis. Skin, blood counts and urine must be examined monthly whilst patients are on either of these preparations. Antimalarials may cause blindness, so regular ophthalmoscopic examinations are necessary.

Gout

Like osteoarthritis gout has been known since early times. The incidence has increased in recent years, particularly in women, though the disease remains more common in men. There is a hereditary predisposition and in some individuals alcohol and purine-rich foods may precipitate attacks. Most cases have no family history and attacks follow diuretic or cytotoxic therapy or are associated with a myelo-proliferative disorder. The pain is very severe, the slightest vibration in the vicinity being viewed with anxiety. The first metatarso-phalangeal joint is most frequently affected, but the knee, ankle or wrist may also be involved. During acute attacks the joint is red, shiny and swollen. Blood urate is raised, though levels are variable and high levels may occur in the absence of joint involvement. The definitive diagnosis is made by finding crystals of sodium monourate in the synovial fluid. The joint recovers completely following an acute attack.

While single attacks do occur, often the disorder is recurring or chronic, with many joints involved and pain less severe. Extra-articular deposits of sodium monourate form gouty tophi in soft tissues, most notably on the ears and fingertips (Fig. 6.3).

The diagnosis is suspected on clinical grounds and confirmed by finding uric acid crystals on joint aspiration. Treatment of the acute attack is with an NSAID (such as indomethacin) in full doses until the pain and swelling subsides. Colchicine is a useful alternative, especially if there is a contraindication to the use of NSAIDs. Symptoms are usually controlled within a few days of commencing therapy. Prophylactic therapy may be required in the face of very high blood urate levels, recurring attacks or absence of avoidable precipitating factors. Allopurinol, which inhibits xanthine oxidase and prevents the formation of uric acid, is the drug of choice. Initially blood urate may be increased because of mobilisation from the tissues and a further attack of gout experienced. For this reason indomethacin or a similar preparation is given for the first 4–8 weeks of allopurinol therapy. Once started allopurinol should be continued indefinitely; fortunately, side effects are rare.

Pseudogout

Pseudogout causes less acute symptoms than gout. Large joints, especially the knees, are affected. The clinical features may be similar to osteoarthritis, though episodes of acute arthritis are more commonly found. The diagnosis is often made unexpectedly by finding typical calcification on X-ray of the joint and is confirmed by finding crystals of calcium pyrophosphate in the synovial fluid.

Other crystals may cause arthritis. Calcium hydroxyapatite is found in bone and has been demonstrated in soft tissues surrounding joints. More recently it has been found in joints, particularly the shoulder. In the past such patients were thought to have osteoarthritis.

Seronegative Spondyloarthritides

Seronegative spondyloarthritides comprise a group of nine or more inflammatory arthritides in which rheumatoid factor is absent. They are much less common than osteo- and rheumatoid arthritis and include ankylosing spondylitis, psoriatic arthritis and arthritis associated with inflammatory bowel disease. An asymmetrical polyarthritis, sacroileitis and spondylitis are common to all forms of seronegative spondyloarthritis. There is an association with haplotype HLA B27.

Ankylosing spondylitis first affects the axial skeleton, starting with the sacroiliac joints. It is more common in men, starts early in life and presents in the second

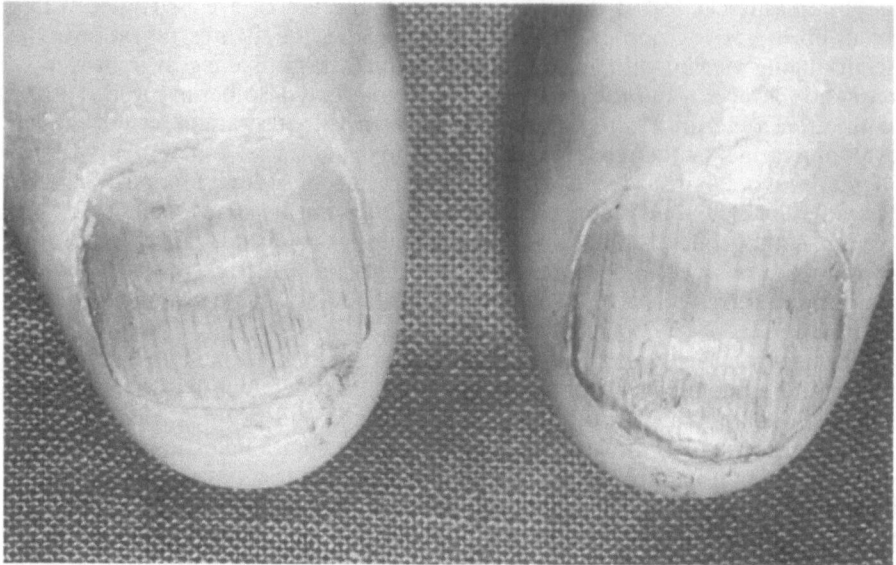

Fig. 6.4.   Pitting of the fingernails in psoriasis.

or third decade with stiffness in the back. Without vigorous treatment about 20% of cases may progress to ankylosis of the spine and sacroiliac joints, the contour of the spine coming to resemble a question mark. Treatment has little to offer in the late stages though exercises, especially in extension, are important to maintain mobility. The patient should be prone for some hours each day and swimming in particular is of therapeutic benefit.

Psoriatic arthritis is an asymmetrical general arthritis frequently involving the interphalangeal joints but has many variations and may be clinically indistinguishable from rheumatoid disease. The lesions can be mild, moderately severe or, occasionally, very destructive. There is often associated pitting of the fingernails (Fig. 6.4).

Inflammatory bowel disease such as ulcerative colitis and Crohn's disease are associated with ankylosing spondylitis and a peripheral non-destructive polyarthritis. Amelioration of the bowel disease may help the peripheral arthritis, though spinal involvement tends to get progressively worse.

Infective Arthritis

Infective arthritis presents with pain in one joint, usually accompanied by redness and swelling, pyrexia and leucocytosis, but swelling may be less obvious in the hip or spine. Systemic signs are not always pronounced, especially in elderly people. Sepsis may complicate long-standing arthritis, especially if there has been joint surgery. With tuberculosis infection, signs of inflammation are less marked than with other bacterial organisms. Large joints or the spine are usually affected and a spinal lesion may give rise to a psoas abscess. The diagnosis is made by joint aspiration and joint and blood cultures. Prolonged courses of antibiotics are necessary.

Haemarthrosis

Haemarthrosis in the older person suggests either trauma to the joint or blood dyscrasia, though injury may be slight or forgotten. There is a sudden onset of pain or swelling of a joint, the knee being most frequently affected. The diagnosis is made by aspiration. The blood should be removed and, as with any acute arthritis, the joint rested in optimum position during the acute phase and then exercised later.

Hypertrophic Pulmonary Osteoarthropathy

Hypertrophic pulmonary osteoarthropathy is an inflammatory polyarthritis affecting the distal joints of the arms and legs with associated finger clubbing and tenderness of the long bones. Radiographs of affected joints show periostitis. The condition is usually associated with lung carcinoma and improves if the carcinoma is successfully treated.

Soft Tissue Pain (Table 6.2)

Polymyalgia Rheumatica

Polymyalgia rheumatica is a fairly common condition, involving only older people, and is closely related to cranial (temporal) arteritis. It may precede the arteritis, more rarely succeed it, or both may occur together. Typically the patient is unwell for a few weeks with aches and pains in the shoulder and to a lesser extent the pelvic girdle. Stiffness occurs particularly in the morning and becomes increasingly severe. Tenderness is confined to the muscles, there is no loss of power and joint movements are full. Peripheral arteries should be examined for tenderness and absence of pulsation. The patient is often mildly anaemic and the ESR is raised to levels of 50 mm/h or more. The response to steroids is dramatic, all symptoms clearing within 2 to 3 days. Prednisolone is given in doses of 10–20 mg/day until the ESR falls to normal levels. The dose is then tapered to around 5 mg daily with further reductions of 1 mg a month depending on the ESR and recur-

Table 6.2. Non-articular causes of musculo-skeletal pain

Muscular pain (polymyalgia rheumatica; frozen shoulder)
Bone pain (Paget's disease; osteopenia; osteomalacia; tumour)
Ligament injury
Bursitis

rence of symptoms. Treatment may need to be continued for several years. Cranial arteritis requires a higher initial dose of steroids.

Frozen Shoulder

Frozen shoulder is common at all ages, but is much less likely to improve spontaneously in the elderly. The causes are various and include trauma, myocardial infarction and hemiplegia. The site of the original lesion may be in the muscles, tendons, entheses, bursae, bones or joint. The treatment is exercise, though this will have to be delayed for a few days if there is a dislocation, or confined to twice-daily gentle passive movement for 2–3 weeks when the humeral neck is fractured. Otherwise the joint must be put through a full range of movement several times a day. Local steroid injection into the shoulder joint may help in facilitating movement.

Bone Pain

Paget's Disease

Paget's disease is a disease of old age which is decreasing in frequency. The primary disorder is thought to be within bone osteoclasts, where virus particles have

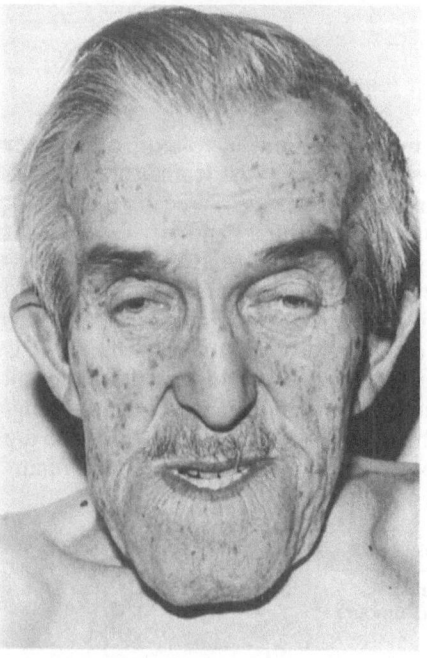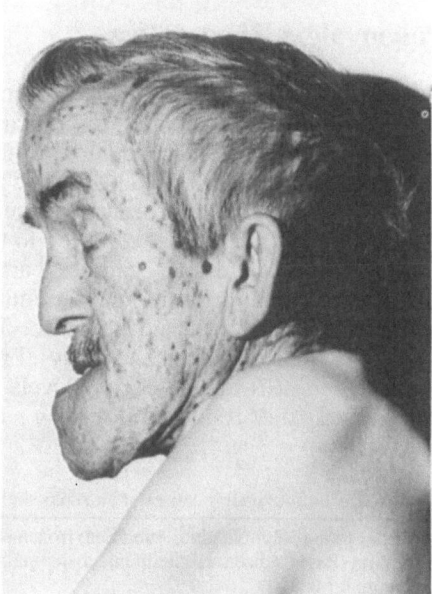

Fig. 6.5.   Paget's disease.

recently been demonstrated and may be causative. There is increased bone destruction followed by chaotic reformation resulting in softening, deformity and increased vascularity of bone. The skull, spine, pelvis and long bones are affected, leading to a large head, bent spine and bowed legs (Fig. 6.5). Sometimes only one bone is involved. Pain is the main symptom, though many severely affected bones are painless or only intermittently painful. Difficulty sometimes arises in distinguishing the pain of Paget's disease from that of osteoarthritis, which frequently accompanies the condition. The fact that pagetic pain is worse at rest, and is especially troublesome in bed at night, may help in differentiation. The course is variable and there may be long remissions. Deafness can result from stretching of the VIII nerve and other cranial nerves and the spinal cord and nerve roots may also be damaged. The bones easily fracture, but heal normally. About 2% of sufferers develop osteogenic sarcoma. The high blood flow may be an added embarrassment to a failing heart.

Diagnosis is confirmed by very high levels of blood alkaline phosphatase and hydroxyproline in the urine. Indeed, the diagnosis is often made incidentally by finding abnormal biochemical markers in an asymptomatic patient. Radiographic changes are pathognomonic. Treatment consists of pain relief and simple analgesics may suffice, though NSAIDs are helpful if the pain is primarily from joints. Specific measures include calcitonin, diphosphonates and methramycin and are used when pain is not relieved by simpler measures. They may be given prophylactically if the nervous system is endangered.

Osteopenia

Osteopenia (osteoporosis) refers to an age-related reduction in bone mass, the extent of which varies considerably between individuals. Its more rapid progression in women than in men reflects a disproportionate reduction in sex hormone production and there is a marked acceleration of bone loss after the menopause. Other risk factors include diseases such as multiple myeloma, hyperthyroidism and rheumatoid arthritis; drugs, especially corticosteroids and other influences such as immobility, low dietary calcium, alcohol abuse and cigarette smoking.

The patient loses height because of collapse and wedging of the vertebrae and spinal examination will reveal a kyphosis. In severe cases the lower edge of the thoracic cage can come to lie on the pelvic rim. Bones fracture often with trivial injury: first the wrists, followed by the hips and the vertebrae. The condition is not usually painful unless there is a fracture. Persistent backache as opposed to sudden localised severe pain associated with collapse of a vertebra is likely to be due to other causes. The presence of osteopenia should prompt a search for multiple myeloma by means of a protein electrophoresis and testing the urine for light chain immunoglobulin (Bence–Jones protein).

Treatment is difficult, and prevention may have more to offer than cure. Regular exercise is important and a low dose of combined oestrogen and progesterone at the time of the menopause and for some years thereafter may be of value in women at particular risk. When fractures do occur, analgesics should be given for the acute pain. No therapy has been shown to increase the amount of bone with the possible exception of sodium fluoride. The hope is to prevent further deterioration. Exercise is important in maintaining bone mass, anabolic steroids and calcium supplements being of unproven value.

Osteomalacia

Osteomalacia is due to calcium and vitamin D deficiency resulting from lack of exposure to sunlight, dietary insufficiency, malabsorption, renal failure and drug therapy (due to hepatic enzyme induction). There is a loss of bone mineralisation but in contrast to osteopenia, the amount of bone matrix is normal.

Classically, the patient presents with aching pain in the shoulder and pelvic girdles extending into the limbs. There is a proximal myopathy manifested by weakness and those affected may have a waddling gait, be unable to get upstairs or have difficulty combing their hair. The bones may have local areas of tenderness.

Diagnosis is established by finding reduced levels of calcium and phosphate and a raised alkaline phosphatase in the blood. Urinary calcium is low or absent. Pseudo-fractures (Looser's zones) may be demonstrated radiographically and bone biopsy may show typical features.

Treatment is with vitamin D and calcium, the dose required depending on the cause. In renal failure alfacalcidol must be given as a diseased kidney will not be able to metabolise cholecalciferol. When more than the normal daily requirement of vitamin D is given the dose should be carefully monitored as there is a risk of developing hypercalcaemia. The patient should be warned to stop treatment in the presence of nausea or vomiting and blood calcium levels should be checked.

Bone Tumours

Bone tumours can be either primary or secondary, but in practice, metastatic bone disease and multiple myeloma are the only neoplastic conditions regularly to involve the bones of old people. Metastases arise primarily from breast, prostate, lung, kidney or thyroid. Patients are generally unwell and may have pain at the site of the metastatic lesion. Backache is common. Radiographic changes are late, though a bone scan will show bone deposits earlier. Anaemia is often present due to replacement of haemopoietic tissue with tumour. The ESR may be raised and a monoclonal immunoglobulin is present in the serum with myeloma. Bence–Jones protein may be excreted in the urine.

Clinical Evaluation

The first step in evaluation of the patient is to take a detailed history. The site, onset and duration, character, severity, precipitating and relieving factors together with accompanying symptoms must all be elicited. A history of joint trauma is important as osteoarthritis commonly supervenes in later life. A family history of musculo-skeletal disorder is also important, haemophilia and rheumatoid disease being obvious examples of disorders with a strong genetic factor in their aetiology. A drug history must be elicited as thiazide diuretics, for example, can lead to hyperuricaemia and gout.

It is imperative to establish the source of the pain. Remember that non-rheumatological conditions such as myxoedema and Parkinson's disease may mis-

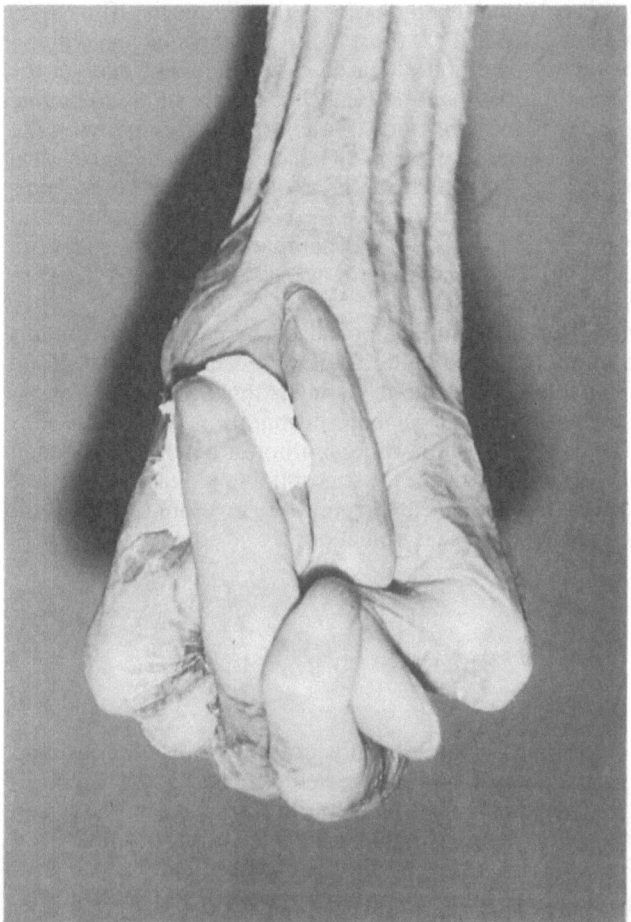

Fig. 6.6. Severe hand deformity in "burnt-out" rheumatoid disease. Despite bilateral involvement, the patient was totally self-caring.

leadingly present with muscle pain. Even if the pain is rheumatic in origin, there is often difficulty in deciding whether it arises from muscles, joints or bone.

Joint pain is felt on all movements (both active and passive) of the joint. It is often referred to the joint distal to the one involved (e.g. pain from the hip may be felt in the knee). When examining a painful joint, the corresponding joint on the other side and the joints above and below on the same side should be examined first. The joint should be inspected for signs of acute inflammation and deformity. On palpation, evidence of local heat, tenderness, crepitus and joint effusion should be sought. It should then be put through its full range of movement, both passive and active. It is of utmost importance to make a functional assessment by asking the patient to perform an everyday movement for which that joint is necessary. Not infrequently, useful function is preserved in joints which are very diseased, while those showing little disease activity can be almost useless (Fig. 6.6).

The distribution of joint involvement may indicate the diagnosis. Thus symmetrical peripheral involvement, especially of the metacarpo-phalangeal and proximal interphalangeal joints, favours rheumatoid disease, which rarely involves the carpo-metacarpal joint of the thumb. Asymmetrical changes are likely to be due to osteoarthritis or the seronegative arthritides, the latter usually involving the sacroiliac joints and spine. Associated features of the disorder may be so classical as to suggest the diagnosis. Thus osteoarthritis is associated with Heberden's nodes, tophi occur in chronic gout and nodules are present only in rheumatoid disease. It must be remembered that two or more rheumatological disorders can coincide in the same patient (Fig. 6.3). Rheumatoid disease and osteoarthritis are the conditions most commonly found together.

Pain from muscles and related structures is produced by certain movements only. The affected muscles are tender and entheses, if involved, acutely so. Bone pain is localised and worse on movement and on jarring from above or below.

It is important to assess the patient's general medical condition. Some musculo-skeletal disorders are confined to that system whereas others are part of a systemic illness. Thus muscle pain in an ill patient should suggest polymyalgia rheumatica; bone pain may be related to metastatic disease or multiple myeloma; while joint pain may be caused by rheumatoid disease or infection.

Management

The management of musculo-skeletal pain depends not only on the nature and severity of the underlying cause, but also on the patient affected with the condition. Management strategies that apply only to specific diseases have already been discussed. However, some general management principles apply to almost all patients with a musculo-skeletal disorder and are now described. The aims of treatment are to relieve pain and maintain function by the judicious use of rest, exercise and sometimes mechanical aids. The skills of many members of the multidisciplinary team will be required. Principles of rehabilitation are discussed in more detail in Chapter 25.

Pain Relief

In elderly people acute inflammatory episodes have often ceased, leaving the patient with chronic symptoms. Pain in these circumstances may be helped by simple analgesic agents such as paracetamol. Its effect may be further enhanced by combining it with dextro-propoxyphene or codeine. The efficacy of the former may be related to a change in mood rather than to additional analgesia. Codeine may cause constipation. Tolerance does not appear to be a problem with these preparations so that an increase in dose is not usually necessary.

The mainstay of drug treatment is NSAIDs; they are not curative as they do not modify the disease, but they do ease inflammatory symptoms. There are a large number of preparations from which to choose and it is wise to become familiar with a few from the different groups as no drug will suit all patients. The best drug is the one that produces the most relief and fewest side effects. Once commenced on therapy the patient should continue on that drug for at least 2 weeks, gradually increasing the dose until symptoms are controlled, side effects experienced or the maximum recommended dose reached. If symptoms are not controlled, an alternative agent should be tried. Total relief of symptoms is seldom achievable and the decision as to whether adequate symptom relief has been obtained can only be made by the patient. Combinations of NSAIDs will not be successful where single drug therapy has failed and will serve only to complicate the drug regimen.

The side effects of NSAIDs vary to some extent with the preparation. Salicylates are particularly likely to cause tinnitus and deafness while many others cause rashes, dizziness and headache. All upset the gastrointestinal tract, causing anything from mild nausea to peptic ulcer and haemorrhage, and should therefore be taken with meals. If drug therapy is necessary to keep the patient mobile it may need to be continued even in the presence of peptic ulceration. Healing will take place if an H_2 blocker is given, possibly combined with a mucosal protective agent. The H_2 blocker will need to be continued as long as the NSAID. Fluid retention, causing heart failure, is another side effect of NSAIDs and is dose dependent. Some alter anticoagulant requirement while the fenamates may cause an haemolytic anaemia.

Steroids are now rarely used systemically. The only indication for their use is the occasional patient who develops severe progressive disease for the first time in old age. The dose should not exceed 5–7.5 mg of prednisolone daily so as to minimise Cushing's syndrome and other side effects. They should be discontinued if there is no improvement within 2 weeks. Otherwise the dose should gradually be reduced by 1 mg a month and stopped as soon as possible. The object is to prevent the patient becoming immobile or even bedfast.

Local steroid injections on one or two occasions in conditions such as frozen shoulder can produce dramatic results. However, this is of no long-term value if not followed by passive and active exercises. With joint effusions, aspiration followed by a single injection of intra-articular steroid is helpful. Multiple intra-articular steroid injections for more chronic disease, especially of the knees, have been shown not to be of long-term benefit, though they may help an individual patient to remain mobile. Too frequent injections may be associated with further joint damage.

Local heat, wax baths, application of various forms of electrical and thermal energy and counter-irritants to the skin are helpful in easing pain so that exercises can be more readily undertaken. Special diets, copper bangles, herbal remedies and acupuncture have as yet no scientific evidence in their favour, except that acupuncture does ease some pain.

Surgery

Surgery may be necessary to relieve pressure in the carpal tunnel and on tendon sheaths in rheumatoid disease. Ruptured tendons can be repaired, but prevention has better results. Hallux valgus and hallux rigidus can be corrected and excision arthroplasty of the metatarsal heads is indicated in the rare event of insoles and proper shoes failing to keep the patient mobile. Joint replacement has revolutionised the treatment of disease of the hip. Results can be excellent with good movement and pain relief in 95% of patients. As better prostheses become available results are improving with other joints. Sudden spinal cord compression for a prolapsed disc is a surgical emergency. Apart from this, disc lesions are rarely treated surgically in the older patient. Very occasionally an atlanto-axial subluxation may have to be stabilised. Timing of surgery is important and when many joints are involved careful thought has to be given as to which to do first. The cervical spine should always be X-rayed in flexion before undertaking any surgical operation in a patient with rheumatoid disease. If there is any atlanto-axial instability a collar should be worn during the operation.

Rest and Exercise

Bed rest, while helpful during periods of inflammation and constitutional disturbance, should be prescribed very sparingly in the elderly. Even a few days in bed can lead to stiffening up which may take many months to correct. Patients with active rheumatoid disease may benefit from a few hours rest at midday and it is better that this is taken on the bed rather than in a chair so that knees and wrists can be kept in extension. Acutely swollen joints are immobilised in the position of maximum function; knees, for instance, should be rested by splinting in extension and never by putting a pillow behind them. Wrists should be splinted in slight dorsiflexion. Splints should be light and well-fitting and avoid pressure on surrounding tissues. Joints should not be immobilised for long as relevant muscles waste very rapidly with disuse.

Splints can be worn for short periods to protect specific joints (e.g. on the wrists while performing household tasks). A cervical collar at night may enable a patient with osteoarthritis of the cervical spine to get a good night's sleep. At the same time advice should be given on posture and avoiding carrying heavy weights. The neck should be put through a full range of movement three or four times a day and only one pillow used at night. Patients should not become too dependent on a collar as better long-term results follow strengthening of the muscles. In rheumatoid disease, if there is atlanto-axial instability, a collar may have to be worn permanently. Back supports during the day can be used in the same way as collars are used at night. Good posture, avoidance of lifting objects from the stooping position and exercises to strengthen the abdominal muscles are important. Many older patients are unable to tolerate a back support or a cervical collar.

Isometric exercises should be encouraged from the start and active exercises undertaken as soon as possible. Swimming is a very good general exercise as it involves moving most joints. Movements are easier in water, especially if it is warm. Some swimming pools have special sessions for pensioners.

Aids

Simple aids will enable some tasks to be accomplished, but proper assessment is necessary and the advice of an occupational therapist is often invaluable. Aids such as a walking-stick held in the opposite hand can relieve pressure on the hip, but may place additional strains on the joints in the upper limb. Raising the shoe will correct shortening and enable the other knee to be held straight. A metatarsal bar placed behind the metatarsal heads will enable a patient with severe rheumatoid disease to walk more comfortably. Special shoes can be ordered, but are often unsatisfactory although, fortunately, wide fitting, low heeled shoes are more readily available nowadays. Regular chiropody is important as it is difficult for patients with hip and knee disease to attend to their own feet.

Further attempts to keep the patient independent can be achieved by adapting the environment. Stairs produce a lot of strain on the weight-bearing joints so single-floor accommodation or a stair lift should be considered. High and low shelves should be avoided and light and power switches should be at an easily accessible height. Patients with hip disease need higher chairs and a raised toilet seat; toilet and bath rails may also be necessary. Mobility and some degree of independence can be achieved in severe disease by using an electric wheelchair. Finally, it should be remembered that arthritis inevitably restricts activities and that this can lead to isolation and depression.

Counselling

The confidence and cooperation of the patient and relatives must be gained. They need to know the probable course of the disease and realistic management goals should be established. Too much gloom should be avoided as much can be achieved by treatment even when it is only palliative. Not everybody gets worse and exacerbations are usually followed by remissions. Maintenance of good general health and the avoidance of undue stress, exposure to extremes of temperature or sudden excessive exercise is sensible advice. Patients should be encouraged to be as mobile as possible and to maintain their hobbies and interests. If this is not feasible, new interests should be encouraged. Organisations such as Arthritis Care can provide diversion for the sufferer and support for the carer. The Arthritis and Rheumatism Council (ARC) produces many instructive leaflets.

Further Reading

Capell HA, Daymond TJ, Dick WC (1983) Rheumatic disease. Springer-Verlag, Berlin Heidelberg New York

Griffiths ID (1984) Drug and non-drug management of chronic inflammatory joint disease. In: Evans JG, Caird FI (eds) Advances in geriatric medicine 4. Pitman, London

Medicine International (1985) Rheumatology, vols 22 and 23. Medical Education (International), Oxford

Pal B, Dick WC (1984) Some thoughts on the aetiopathogenesis of chronic inflammatory joint disease. In: Evans JG, Caird FI (eds) Advances in geriatric medicine 4. Pitman, London

Platt P (1984) Diagnosis and treatment of crystal-induced diseases. In: Evans JG, Caird FI (eds) Advances in geriatric medicine 4. Pitman, London

Weatherall DJ, Ledingham JGG, Warrell DA (1987) The Oxford textbook of medicine, 2nd edn. Oxford University Press, Oxford, pp 16.1–17.38

Chapter 7

Dyspnoea

P. Finucane

Dyspnoea is the subjective sensation of difficulty in breathing. Chronic dyspnoea is one of the commonest disabilities reported by old people and in one survey, 29% of those aged between 65 and 75 years complained of being breathless after any effort. The prevalence rose to 35% for those aged over 75 years. Acute dyspnoea is a highly distressing complaint and those affected often fear death through suffocation. The importance of dyspnoea as a symptom in terminal illness is discussed in Chapter 26.

Dyspnoea is due to an increased ventilatory rate following stimulation of the respiratory centre. Normal people become aware of shortness of breath when the ventilatory rate is doubled; when the rate is tripled or quadrupled breathing becomes uncomfortable. In disease states, a given ventilatory rate will become increasingly uncomfortable with a lowering of respiratory reserve and with an increase in the work of breathing. The ventilatory rate increases with exercise so that dyspnoea of gradual onset will initially be present only on exertion. Should the underlying disease progress and further diminish respiratory reserve or increase the work of breathing, dyspnoea will be experienced with progressively less exertion and eventually be present at rest.

Age-related structural and physiological changes in the respiratory system (see Chap. 1) predispose to dyspnoea. The respiratory reserve is decreased and stiffness of the chest wall together with reduced lung compliance increases the work of breathing. The ventilatory response to exercise is also exaggerated. Despite these changes, shortness of breath is an important symptom of underlying disease and must not be ascribed to old age.

Stimulation of the respiratory centre can be due to disease of the lung, airways, pleura or chest wall as outlined in Fig. 7.1. These in turn may be due to a variety of disorders, the commonest of which are listed in Table 7.1. As with so many problems in the medicine of old age, two or more conditions may combine to cause symptoms in a given patient. Psychogenic factors are important both as a cause of dyspnoea and in regulating the body's response to it.

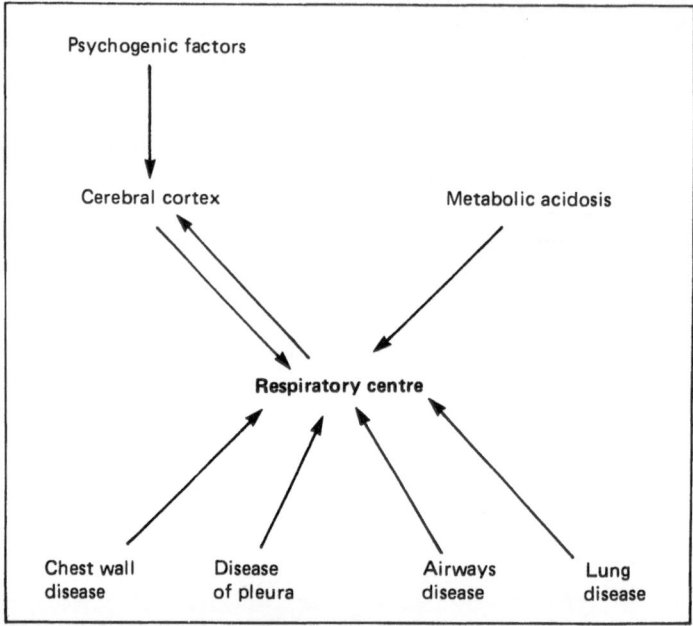

Psychogenic factors

Cerebral cortex   Metabolic acidosis

Respiratory centre

Chest wall   Disease   Airways   Lung
disease   of pleura   disease   disease

Fig. 7.1.   Factors which stimulate the respiratory centre and thereby cause dyspnoea.

Table 7.1.   Common causes of dyspnoea

Lung disease (pneumonia, lung collapse, pulmonary fibrosis,
   pulmonary oedema, pulmonary embolism)
Airways disease (chronic bronchitis, asthma)
Disease of the pleura (pleural effusion, pneumothorax)
Chest wall disease (bone and joint disorders, neuromuscular disorders)
Psychogenic factors (anxiety, hysteria,)
Metabolic acidosis (diabetic ketoacidosis, renal failure)

Lung Disease

Pneumonia

Pneumonia is the commonest cause of death in very old people; 80% of all who die of pneumonia are aged over 60 years. Pulmonary sepsis is often the terminal event in people with end-stage non-respiratory disease. Its increased prevalence in old age is due to a combination of hypostasis and impaired immunity. The virulence of the infective organism is of lesser importance except in hospital populations where nosocomial chest infections are a particular problem among elderly patients.

Dyspnoea is the single most important symptom and tachypnoea the cardinal sign. Expected associated features such as pyrexia may be entirely absent, particularly in the early stages. When they exist, associated findings are often non-specific and include acute confusion, drowsiness and impaired mobility. Localising signs are usually apparent on chest examination, though they may be masked by concomitant chronic chest abnormalities.

The choice of antibiotic and mode of administration will depend on the severity of the infection and on the general condition of the patient. Particularly with nosocomial infections, sputum samples should be taken for culture and sensitivity prior to antibiotic therapy.

Associated chest pain and hypoxia should be treated with analgesia and oxygen respectively. In elderly patients the possibility that infection may be due to un-usual organisms (e.g. tubercle bacillus) should be kept in mind and appropriate investigation instigated should the response to treatment not be prompt.

Lung Collapse

Lung collapse follows obstruction of a major airway due to an intrinsic lesion or to extrinsic compression. Intrinsic lesions can be stenosing as occurs with a bron-chogenic carcinoma. Alternatively, airways obstruction can result from foreign body inhalation or from a mucous plug.

Lung cancer is the commonest malignancy in males and is replacing breast cancer as the commonest malignancy in females. The peak age at presentation is about 70 years and in most patients reflects many years of cigarette smoking. Res-piratory symptoms include cough, haemoptysis and chest pain in addition to dyspnoea. Weight loss is a prominent association (see Chap. 10). The clinical signs and radiological features depend on the extent of the disease and on whether com-pression of local structures or metastatic spread has occurred. The diagnosis can be confirmed by sputum cytology. Central lesions can be visualised and biopsied at bronchoscopy and lesions in the lung periphery can be biopsied percutaneously.

Irrespective of the age of the patient, the prognosis is poor and palliation is all that can be offered to the majority of patients. Lung resection is often precluded by the extent of the lesion or the presence of other chest disease, particularly chronic airways disease. Some 15% of patients may benefit from surgical excision. Palliative radiotherapy will usually stop haemoptysis, shrink obstructing tumours and relieve metastatic bone pain. Squamous cell carcinoma responds best. Small (oat) cell carcinomas respond to chemotherapy, though the potential benefits of treatment may be outweighed by its side effects.

Pulmonary Fibrosis

Pneumoconioses, chronic allergic alveolitis, fibrosing alveolitis and chronic sarcoidosis are among a group of relatively uncommon lung diseases which cause pulmonary fibrosis in old people. If symptomatic, dyspnoea is the principle complaint, though a chronic non-productive cough is often found in advanced disease. With conditions such as asbestosis and fibrosing alveolitis, finger clubbing may be seen. Late inspiratory crackles are a common finding on chest auscultation. Diffuse radiological opacities are found (Fig. 7.2). Respiratory function tests show a restrictive defect, the decline in FEV_1 paralleling that in the FVC.

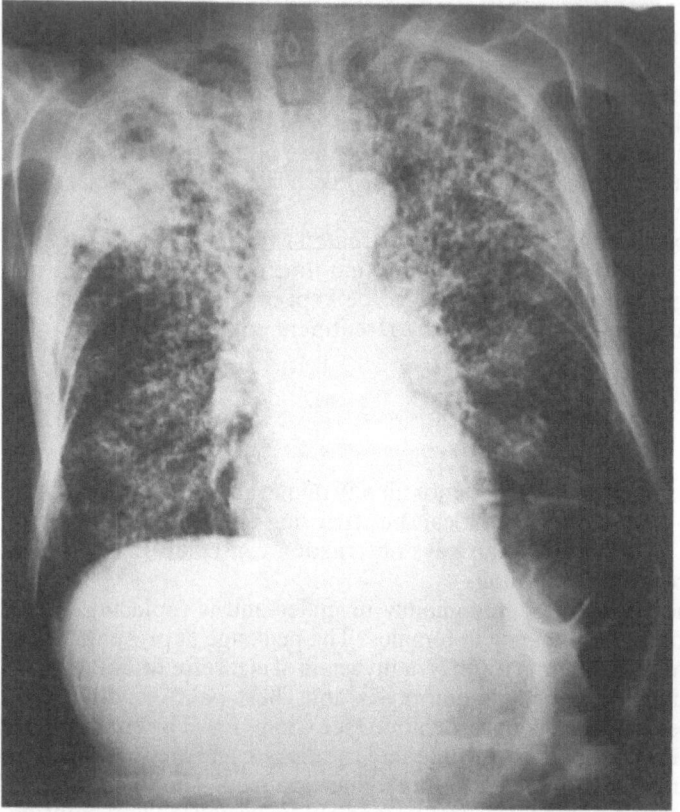

Fig. 7.2.   Pulmonary fibrosis with co-existing old tuberculous scarring of the right lung apex. (By permission of Dr. D. Cochlin.)

Pulmonary Oedema

Pulmonary oedema is usually due to cardiac failure though non-cardiogenic oedema occurs in adult respiratory distress syndrome. The left ventricle may fail when it is diseased or when its work load is increased. The cardiac components which become diseased are its pericardium, myocardium or valves. Alternatively its function can be affected by dysrhythmia. An increased venous return to the heart increases the *pre-load*, while its having to work against a pressure gradient (as in hypertension and aortic stenosis) increases the *after-load*. In a given patient, the cause of failure is often multifactorial. For example, when cardiac output is diminished due to heart muscle disease, fluid retention occurs and pre-load is increased, further exacerbating the heart failure.

Dyspnoea and fatigue are the commonest symptoms of cardiac failure, the latter being secondary to a reduced cardiac output. Signs of pulmonary congestion or effusion will be present, a tachycardia is usual and auscultation of the heart may reveal a gallop rhythm. Signs of right ventricular failure are often found in association. Chest radiography will confirm the presence of congestion of the upper lobe veins, oedema of the inter-lobular septae, fluid in the horizontal fissure, bilateral pleural effusion and perhaps frank pulmonary oedema (Fig. 7.3).

The treatment of cardiac failure involves optimising cardiac function while decreasing pre-load and/or after-load. The therapeutic strategy will depend on the underlying cause. Treating cardiac factors may involve controlling an arrhythmia, replacing a diseased valve or draining a pericardial effusion. Pre-load is reduced by diuretic therapy and with venodilators (e.g. nitrates) and is effective when fluid overload is a significant factor. After-load is reduced by vasodilator drugs and angiotensin converting enzyme inhibitors are now the drugs of choice.

Pulmonary Embolism

Pulmonary embolism is discussed in Chapter 4. Dyspnoea is a prominent feature, irrespective of the size of the embolus. Occasionally, small recurring emboli may be silent until pulmonary hypertension results and presents with dyspnoea. Associated clinical features include a parasternal heave and a loud second heart sound.

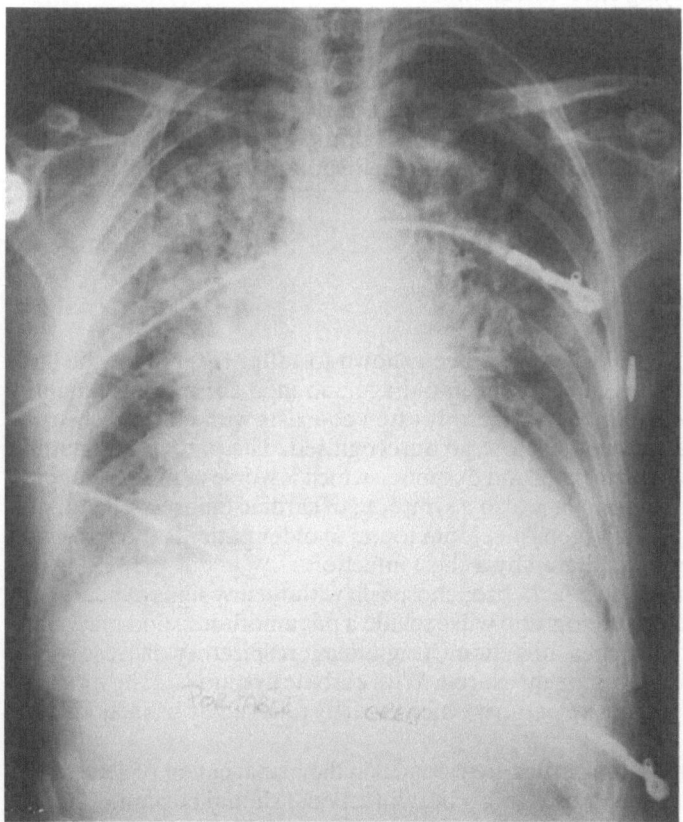

Fig. 7.3. Severe acute left ventricular failure. (By permission of Dr. D. Cochlin.)

Airways Disease

Chronic Obstructive Airways Disease

Chronic obstructive airways disease is usually related to cigarette smoking, though exposure to other pollutants is responsible in some patients. Its prevalence peaks between the ages of 50 and 80 years; in Britain about one quarter of all elderly males and one eighth of females are affected. Acute exacerbations of chronic diseases are usually triggered by a chest infection.

The clinical spectrum ranges from chronic bronchitis where sputum production and recurring chest infections predominate, to emphysema where progressive dyspnoea is the main symptom. The majority of patients will have elements of both conditions. In mild disease clinical signs will not be obvious, whereas in moderate or severe disease, a hyperinflated chest, diminished chest expansion, diminished air entry to the lung fields together with an expiratory wheeze and inspiratory crackles may be found. Signs of right ventricular failure reflect chronic hypoxaemia and resulting pulmonary hypertension. Chest radiography will confirm that the chest is hyperinflated and, in acute exacerbations, may reveal evidence of an underlying chest infection.

In most patients with chronic airways disease, airflow obstruction is at least partly reversible with bronchodilating drugs. Antibiotic therapy and oxygen will be required to treat infection and hypoxia. Short courses of corticosteroids are useful in severe exacerbations of disease and a minority of patients will need maintenance steroid therapy. Patients who are prone to frequent acute attacks should be educated to take antibiotics should their sputum become infected.

Bronchial Asthma

Over 5% of people over 70 years have been shown to suffer from reversible airways obstruction. Asthma can present in old age and men are more frequently and more severely affected than women. It often co-exists with chronic obstructive airways disease and may therefore go unrecognised. The paroxysmal nature of attacks, together with wheezing and dyspnoea which is worse at night is suggestive, though nocturnal dyspnoea is also a symptom of cardiac failure. A history of susceptibility to extrinsic allergens is seldom found in older patients though acute attacks are sometimes precipitated by a chest infection.

During an acute asthmatic attack, bronchospasm without any signs of heart failure will be found. A chest radiograph will exclude a pneumothorax and may show evidence of an underlying chest infection. If significant respiratory distress is evident arterial blood gases must be measured. With chronic dyspnoea, lung function studies will show an obstructive pattern which is partly relieved by bronchodilator therapy.

Oxygen and bronchodilating drugs are essential in the management of acute asthmatic attacks. Predisposing causes (e.g. chest infections) should be identified and treated. As in younger patients, maintenance treatment is with bronchodilating drugs. Inhaled agents are preferable as they have fewer side effects than oral drugs, though old people often have difficulty in using traditional puffers. New delivery systems which facilitate inhalation are now increasingly being made available. A therapeutic trial of corticosteroids should be considered for those patients who continue to have significant dyspnoea following optimal bronchodilator therapy. Many physicians are unduly reluctant to maintain their asthmatic elderly patients on adequate doses of corticosteroids.

Disease of the Pleura

Pleural Effusions

Pleural effusions can be attributable to exudates which have a high protein content (>30 g/l) and are most often caused by chest infection, pulmonary embolism, lung and pleural neoplasms and chest trauma. Alternatively, they can be due to transudates, which have a relatively low protein content and occur in cardiac failure and in hypoproteinaemic states.

Dyspnoea is the chief symptom though effusions must be quite large before they alone cause symptoms. However, dyspnoea is seen with relatively small effusions when they are associated with underlying lung disease. Chest pain is an associated feature if the parietal pleura is inflamed (see Chap. 4). Examination reveals diminished chest expansion, impaired tactile vocal fremitus and decreased breath sounds over the affected area. Unless there is collapse of the underlying lung, a large pleural effusion will cause mediastinal shift, detected clinically as a deviated trachea and a displaced cardiac apex beat. The underlying cause of the effusion may be clinically apparent.

If the underlying cause is not apparent following clinical and radiological evaluation, a sample of pleural fluid should be aspirated and sent for biochemical and bacteriological examination. Haemorrhagic fluid suggests a malignant process or pulmonary infarction or trauma. Pleural fluid may obscure radiological evidence of disease (e.g. an underlying neoplasm), so chest radiography should be repeated after pleural aspiration. At the time of aspiration, the pleura can be biopsied, though the diagnostic yield from this procedure is low.

The management of pleural effusion depends on its size and on the underlying cause. Large effusions can cause respiratory distress even at rest and need urgent drainage. It is best to remove fluid in volumes of about one litre as the removal of larger amounts can cause pulmonary oedema. Large effusions should be drained gradually using an intercostal drain and an underwater seal. With malignant disease, fluid tends to reaccumulate. Repeated drainage of protein-rich fluid depletes body stores and resulting hypoproteinaemia will exacerbate the problem. Reaccumulation can be prevented by injecting an irritant substance into the pleural space, so causing a chemical inflammation of the visceral and parietal layers which subsequently become adherent. Corynebacterium parvum, talc, bleomycin and tetracyclin are frequently employed.

Spontaneous Pneumothorax

Spontaneous pneumothorax in old people is usually due to rupture of an emphysematous bulla and is often associated with obstructive airways disease. Other underlying conditions include a lung abscess or a cavitating tumour. Often it presents with an exacerbation of chronic dyspnoea only, though chest pain is also common (see Chap. 4).

Chest Wall Disease

Bone and Joint Disorders

Diseases which cause a thoracic spinal kyphosis and/or scoliosis can limit respiratory movements. These alone are rarely a cause of dyspnoea but they may further compromise respiratory function in the presence of other chest disorders. Ankylosing spondylitis is a disease of relative youth though it can present in old age. When it does so, clinical features are comparatively mild and costo-vertebral joint involvement seldom compromises respiratory function.

Neuromuscular Disorders

Post-infective polyneuropathy (Guillain–Barré syndrome) and myasthenia gravis are very unusual causes of dyspnoea and poliomyelitis is now largely of historical interest. Occasionally, dyspnoea is an early symptom of motor neurone disease.

Psychogenic Factors

Some 20% of old people suffer from neuroses and in half of these such problems first become apparent after the age of 65. Psychogenic factors can be the sole cause of dyspnoea; in one large study of elderly patients dyspnoea was not attributable to specific organic disease in about one third of sufferers. Psychogenic factors can also influence the patient's response to dyspnoea due to organic disease.

Anxiety

Anxiety states are characterised by dyspnoea and tachypnoea and are usually associated with a depressive illness (see Chap. 19). With acute attacks, signs of autonomic dysfunction include palpitation and tachycardia, sweating, tremulousness and a dry mouth. Hyperventilation causes a respiratory alkalosis, which in turn results in hypocalcaemia and paraesthesia in the hands and feet.

People who are acutely breathless due to organic disease are usually anxious. It is often difficult to decide on the extent to which respiratory distress is due to hyperventilation from anxiety. By talking to and reassuring the patient, dyspnoea will often significantly improve. However, it is important not to underestimate the severity of symptoms and thereby delay the institution of potentially life-saving treatment.

Management strategies should attempt to identify and remove any underlying cause. The nature of the attacks should be explained to the patient and reassurance given. Relaxation exercises and behavioural psychotherapy benefit many patients. Anxiolytic drugs have an important role in the management of acute and severe episodes of anxiety. Ideally, once the acute stage has passed, they should be gradually withdrawn. Benzodiazepines (e.g. diazepam) are the agents of choice.

Metabolic Acidosis

In this condition the decrease in pH stimulates the respiratory centre, in an attempt to cause a compensatory respiratory alkalosis. Profound dyspnoea of a deep sighing nature (Kussmaul breathing) can result. It is most often seen with acute renal failure and diabetic ketoacidosis. Treatment is that of the underlying disease, though with profound acidosis, bicarbonate infusion will sometimes be necessary.

Clinical Evaluation

A detailed description of the patient's respiratory problem is the chief requirement for accurate diagnosis. The history should elicit whether dyspnoea is of sudden or gradual onset and whether it is persistent or paroxysmal. Does it vary in intensity throughout the day? Note any associated symptoms. The presence of a wheeze, for example, suggests airways disease while paraesthesia and palpitation point to an anxiety attack.

It is useful to quantify the severity of dyspnoea. A subjective assessment of severity is often unreliable. Smokers for example, may disregard significant shortness of breath if the symptom has been of gradual onset. A more reliable assessment is obtained if dyspnoea is related to activities of daily living. Does shortness of breath impair the patient's ability to dress, do housework or go outdoors? To what extent does dyspnoea interfere with speech? When dyspnoea follows exertion, the interval between stopping the exertion and recovery is a useful indicator of its severity.

On examination the rate and pattern of respiration can be of diagnostic and prognostic importance. Kussmaul's respiration due to metabolic acidosis is distinctive. Cheyne–Stokes respiration is seen in a variety of severe neurological and cardio-respiratory disorders and carries a poor prognosis. Note the presence of finger clubbing, cyanosis and evidence of carbon dioxide retention on general medical examination. Systematic examination of the respiratory and cardiovascular systems should follow.

Further Investigation

Chest Radiology

Chest radiology can be regarded as an extension of the clinical examination and a plain radiograph is mandatory in all patients with an acute chest problem. Active chest disease is not always clinically apparent and its presence may be masked by other coincidental chest disease. For example, a clinically important pneumothorax could go unnoticed in an asthmatic patient without radiological examination. X-ray tomography and CT scanning are often employed to clarify the nature of shadows identified by plain radiography.

Arterial Blood Gases

The most important test of lung function in acutely ill patients involves measurement of the arterial blood gases. The arterial PO_2 allows an assessment of oxygen saturation. Respiratory failure refers to a drop in PO_2 below 60 mmHg (8 kPa), at which stage the oxygen saturation drops precipitously. PCO_2 is inversely related to the patient's ventilatory status. Type 1 respiratory failure refers to hypoxaemia in the presence of normal or hyperventilation (normal or low PCO_2) whereas in type 2 failure, hypoxaemia is associated with impaired ventilation (elevated PCO_2).

Respiratory Function Tests

Respiratory function tests are used to distinguish those diseases which cause chronic airways obstruction from those which cause chronic airways restriction. Measurement of peak expiratory flow rate (PEFR) using a flow meter is useful in monitoring a response to bronchodilator therapy in chronic obstructive airways disease and asthma.

Management

Whatever their age, those who smoke or who are obese should be given appropriate advice on modifying their life style. Irrespective of the underlying cause, people with dyspnoea should be encouraged to take exercise. Those with chronic symptoms often avoid exertion, become unfit and so compound the problem. A programme of exercise with a gradual increase in the degree of exertion should be drawn up. This will usually involve walking on the flat initially, but more robust exercise may later be possible. The psychological benefits of an exercise programme are often substantial and may be largely responsible for any perceived improvement in respiratory function.

Oxygen Therapy

Oxygen therapy is essential for acutely dyspnoeic patients and especially for those in respiratory failure (see above). Those with type 1 respiratory failure can safely be given oxygen in sufficient concentration to raise the PO_2 above 60 mmHg (8 kPa). Patients with type 2 respiratory failure have a blunted hypercapnic stimulus to ventilation. They are therefore dependent on their hypoxic stimulus to ventilation and rapid correction of hypoxaemia can depress ventilation further. Judicious use of oxygen in low initial concentrations is essential.

In those with chronic hypoxaemia, both the prospect of survival and the quality of life can be improved by continuous oxygen therapy. Relief of hypoxaemia also reduces pulmonary hypertension and consequent cor pulmonale. Oxygen needs to be given for prolonged periods (at least 15 hours a day). Oxygen concentrators are the best source in a domestic environment and machines are becoming increasingly more compact and silent. Oxygen from the machine (or from oxygen cylinders) is best delivered through nasal prongs.

Further Reading

Davies B (1985) The respiratory system. In: Pathy MSJ (ed) Principles and practice of geriatric medicine. John Wiley & Sons, Chichester
Freeman E (1985) The respiratory system. In: Brocklehurst JC (ed) Textbook of geriatric medicine and gerontology (3rd edn). Churchill Livingstone, Edinburgh
Landahl S, Steen B, Svanborg A (1980) Dyspnoea in 70-year-old people. Acta Med Scand 207:225–230

Chapter 8

Hypertension

A. B. Davies

"Primum non nocere"

Hypertension, defined as a systolic pressure of 160 mmHg or more, a diastolic pressure of 95 mmHg or more, or both, is encountered in approximately 50% of all people over the age of 65 years. In most population groups, apart from some primitive cultures, systolic pressure increases with age in a linear fashion until the eighth decade. This is primarily related to the loss of elasticity of the major arteries. Diastolic pressure also increases with age until the seventh decade, at which stage it tends to level off.

It used to be argued that elevated blood pressure in the elderly was physiological rather than pathological and was best left untreated. Case reports attributed profound hypotension, amblyopia and transient cerebral disturbances to antihypertensive agents and suggested that such therapy was meddlesome. Small scale studies from Britain found no increased risk from hypertension in old age and even suggested that it might have a "protective effect" in the very old. As recently as the 1960s the only stated indication for antihypertensive agents in old people was the presence of heart failure.

More recently evidence that antihypertensive therapy benefits the old has been accumulating. Early data were gleaned from sub-groups of elderly patients involved in therapeutic trials. The small numbers, the design of the trials and the statistical methods used failed to impress many clinicians. Nevertheless, taken as a whole they gave a favourable impression of antihypertensive therapy. There is now a wealth of evidence from insurance company actuarial tables and from clinical studies indicating that systolic hypertension is an independent major risk factor for myocardial infarction, stroke and heart failure. The higher the pressure the greater is the risk and this risk does not diminish with advancing age. Cardiovascular mortality is tripled in the hypertensive elderly patient when compared with normotensive subjects of the same age. An elevated diastolic pressure is an independent risk factor for stroke and premature cardiovascular death. Therapy

which lowers blood pressure decreases such risks, although a major disappointment has been the failure to make an impact on the incidence of acute myocardial
infarction in the hypertensive patient.

The results of the only controlled therapeutic trial dedicated specifically to the
study of an elderly population, by the European Working Party on Hypertension
in the Elderly (EWPHE), have become available in recent years and deserve
special consideration. A significant overall reduction of 27% in cardiovascular
mortality was found in the actively treated group, though the overall mortality
was not significantly lowered. Deaths from acute myocardial infarction were significantly reduced but deaths from cerebrovascular disease were not. However,
non-fatal strokes were significantly reduced as was the incidence of severe congestive cardiac failure. In patients aged over 80 years (mainly female) no benefit
from active therapy was seen. In the light of the effect of therapy on cardiovascular
mortality, the trial was terminated on ethical grounds.

Considerable interest has been aroused by the possibility of stroke prevention
in the elderly population among whom stroke is relatively common and where a
non-fatal stroke may be feared more than a fatal one. It has been estimated that
treatment of 60 elderly patients for one year may prevent one stroke, whereas a
recent Medical Research Council trial suggested that it would require treatment
of 280 younger patients for one year to achieve the same result.

Various trials have been criticised on the basis of patient selection and data interpretation, but it seems unlikely that any other trial of the same scale as that of
the EWPHE will be repeated and so the individual clinician will have to determine
his or her policy upon the available evidence. Controversy continues, but it is now

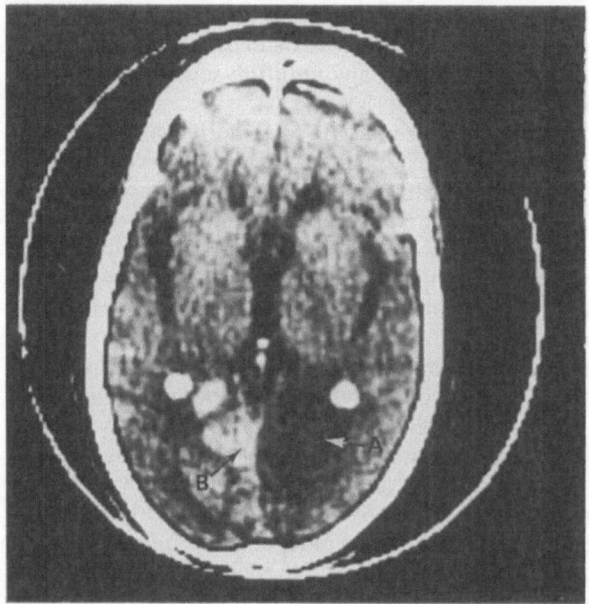

Fig. 8.1. CT scan of an 81-year-old hypertensive male presenting with cortical blindness. There is
infarction (low density) in the right visual cortex (A) and haemorrhage (high density) in the left visual
cortex (B).

apparent that a commonsense approach steering a course between therapeutic nihilism and iatrogenic catastrophe can be pursued with the probability of benefit. A useful concept in the evaluation of blood pressure is not to think of what is or is not normal for a patient's age, but whether a particular level of blood pressure is associated with an unacceptably high risk of future morbid events or of premature death.

Most physicians would agree that elderly patients whose diastolic pressure exceeds 110 mmHg warrant treatment. Those whose diastolic pressure is less than 90 mmHg are best left untreated. The difficulty arises in deciding when to initiate treatment when the diastolic pressure is between these values. Such patients need to be assessed individually. A patient who is robust or who has evidence of end-organ hypertensive damage is likely to benefit from treatment. Factors such as frailty, existing polypharmacy, erratic drug compliance and orthostatic hypotension will bias the physician against treatment.

Though systolic pressure is more reliable as a predictor of risk, guidelines regarding the levels at which treatment is likely to be beneficial are lacking as clinical trials in the past have focussed on diastolic pressure. Particular problems arise in relation to isolated systolic hypertension (i.e. where diastolic pressure is normal). Often isolated systolic hypertension is due to "pseudohypertension" (see below). Attempts to lower such pressure are often unrewarding, the patient developing drug toxicity before the pressure comes under control.

Complications of Hypertension

Stroke

Stroke is defined as an impairment of brain function of vascular origin lasting for 24 hours or more. The World Health Organization definition includes intracerebral haemorrhage, cerebral infarction and also subarachnoid haemorrhage and transient ischaemic attack. Cerebral infarction accounts for the major proportion of "hypertensive stroke" and haemorrhage for only approximately 20%. They may occur together (Fig. 8.1).

There is a wealth of evidence suggesting that the major reversible risk factor associated with stroke is hypertension. This accelerates the formation of atheroma with medial hypertrophy in the larger vessels predisposing to thrombus formation, embolism and occlusion. The smaller vessels are subject to a degenerative lipohyalinosis and also occlusion resulting in "lacunar" infarcts. Rupture of Charcot–Bouchard aneurysms produces cerebral haemorrhage. The relationship between hypertension, rupture of berry aneurysms and subarachnoid haemorrhage is not so well-defined.

The autoregulatory mechanism governing cerebral circulation is thought to be "reset" in hypertension, theoretically making cerebral perfusion more pressure dependent at lower pressures. Aggressive drug therapy can result in decreased cerebral perfusion and cause stroke. The autoregulatory response is damaged in the acute phase of a stroke and results in an initially elevated blood pressure, which falls spontaneously over 48 hours. Treatment of hypertension in the acute stage of a stroke is generally harmful and can occasionally have catastrophic results.

The benefit of antihypertensive therapy in primary stroke prevention has been demonstrated by various trials including the EWPHE trial previously mentioned. Antihypertensive therapy is also probably effective in secondary stroke prevention (i.e. following a completed stroke), though this has been studied less extensively. Aspirin should probably be included in the drug regimen when attempting secondary stroke prevention provided there is no contraindication to its use.

Myocardial Infarction

Myocardial infarction occurs predominantly as a result of thrombotic occlusion of an atheromatous coronary artery. Hypertension, in association with other factors (e.g. diet, smoking), accelerates the development of atheroma. It also alters the relationship between the metabolic demands of cardiac muscle and its blood flow because of the chronically increased systolic load and resultant hypertrophy.

Infarction is often thought of as an affliction of middle age, but in England and Wales the majority of deaths from acute myocardial infarction occur in the sixth and seventh decade in men and the seventh and eighth in women. Antihypertensive therapy is best avoided in the acute stage of myocardial infarction because of the tendency to spontaneous hypotension from pump failure. Existing antihypertensive therapy should be stopped. Occasionally the presence of left ventricular failure causes previous high blood pressure to be "decapitated" in the post-infarction period.

Although previous hypertension is a major risk factor for myocardial infarction, the results of therapeutic trials of antihypertensive agents have on the whole been disappointing in terms of reducing risk. Two studies, however, have shown that controlling blood pressure does reduce the risk among a sub-group of young, non-smoking men. With regard to elderly subjects, the EWPHE study revealed no reduction in non-fatal infarction but a reduction in fatal infarction. While beta-blockers have been shown to be of use in secondary prevention following a myocardial infarction, the effect is not related to their antihypertensive properties.

Heart Failure

The left ventricle responds to a chronically increased pressure load by hypertrophy and then dilatation. With the onset of dilatation the physical signs of heart failure appear with atrial or ventricular gallop rhythms and signs of fluid retention (elevation of venous pressure and dependent oedema). Pleural effusions are not uncommon. Coronary artery disease, with associated "segmental" ischaemia and/ or infarction, is responsible for a large proportion of hypertensive heart failure. In the elderly patient diminished activity and reduced expectations of exercise tolerance may result in physical signs predominating over symptoms (Fig. 8.2). Clinical, ECG or echocardiographic evidence of left ventricular hypertrophy is associated with an increased risk of a morbid event or death and the presence of heart failure further worsens the prognosis.

Although it makes little difference to the planned therapy, one should consider the coexistence of a cardiomyopathy and mild hypertension in the differential

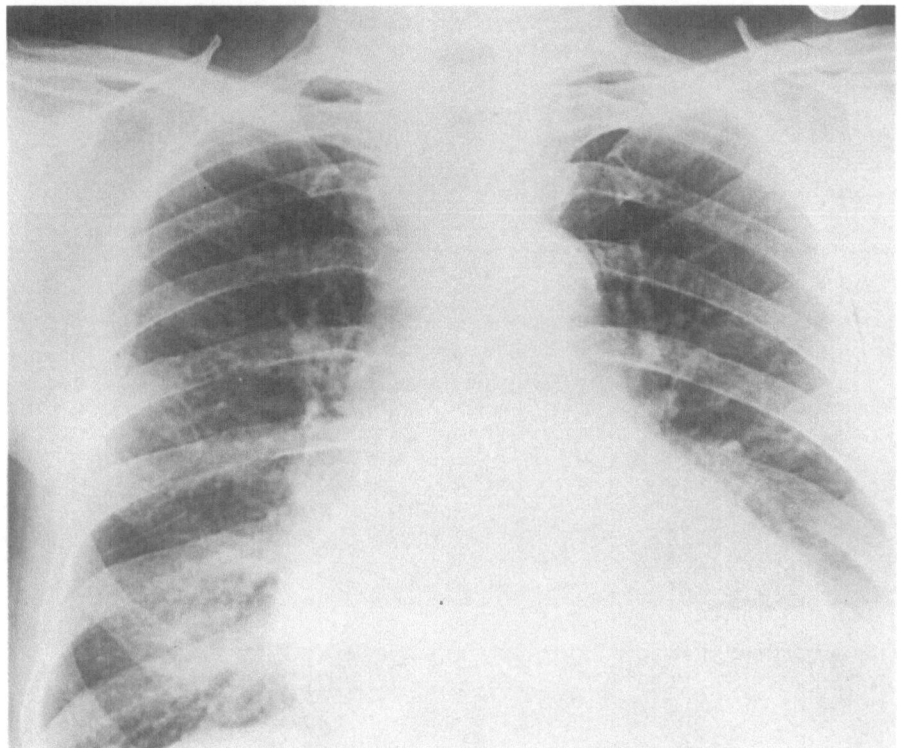

Fig. 8.2. Postero-anterior chest radiograph of an 80-year-old hypertensive male who denied shortness of breath. There is an enlarged cardiac silhouette and a left-sided pleural effusion.

diagnosis of hypertensive heart failure. Therapy is aimed at reduction of the systolic load with vasodilators as well as the production of a diuresis. Chronic antihypertensive therapy may reverse or halt hypertrophy.

Aortic Aneurysm

Aortic aneurysm (Fig. 8.3a, b) results primarily from abnormality of the medial layer of the vessel wall. Thoracic aortic aneurysms may be related to either inflammatory aortitis (e.g. in syphilis or ankylosing spondylosis) or there may be a genetic predisposition in Marfan's syndrome. The majority are caused by a non-specific medial degeneration which is not associated with atheroma. There is a clear relationship with age, previous hypertension and possibly a bicuspid aortic valve. When aortic dissection occurs there is often no obvious histological abnormality. Aneurysms of the distal aorta, on the other hand, are nearly always related to intimal atheroma and associated medial destruction. There is a relationship to age, but not so clearly to hypertension.

The site of the aneurysm or dissection will govern the mode of presentation (e.g. dysphagia, abdominal pain, shortness of breath). It will also determine the related physical signs (e.g. aortic regurgitation, absent peripheral pulses, pulsatile

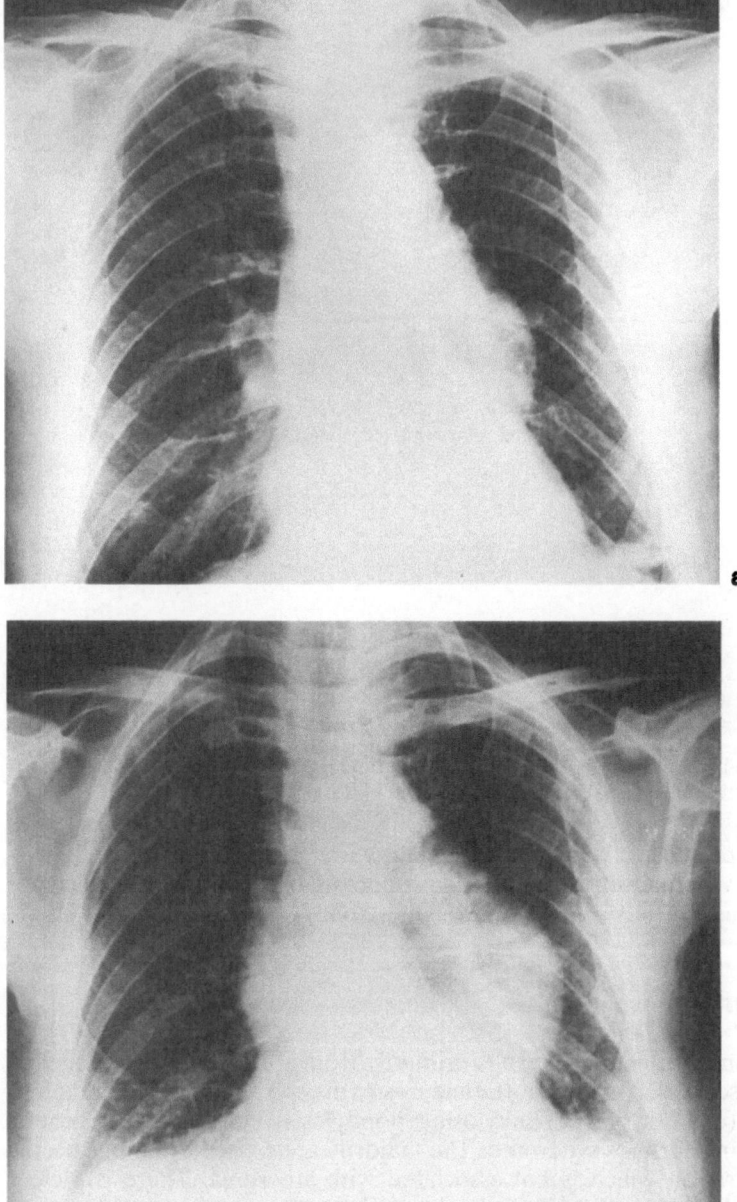

Fig. 8.3a, b.   The progression of an asymptomatic aortic aneurysm over a period of 3 years in a hypertensive septuagenerian.

abdominal mass). The medical management of an aneurysm of any aetiology is aimed at prevention of expansion or dissection by reduction of intramural wall stress. This is related to intra-arterial pressure and possibly its rate of change (i.e. blood pressure reduction). Where there is evidence of rapid enlargement or recent dissection, with or without associated occlusion of major arterial branches or aortic valvar regurgitation, surgery is indicated if the general condition of the patient is otherwise satisfactory.

Malignant Phase Hypertension

This aptly named variant of hypertension is pathologically characterised by fibrinoid necrosis in the arterial and arteriolar walls with muscular hypertrophy. This leads to rapid occlusion of small vessels causing micro-infarcts and haemorrhages in various organs, particularly the kidney, brain and intestine. Clinically it can be recognised by the presence of papilloedema, usually accompanied by fluffy retinal exudates and haemorrhages.

Malignant or accelerated phase hypertension is usually quoted as occurring in approximately 1% of all hypertensives. In the EWPHE trial, 5 of 424 elderly patients developed this complication, having been on placebo for an average of 3 years. Untreated malignant hypertension has a very poor prognosis and death occurs within months, almost always as a result of renal failure.

Evidence that aggressive control of blood pressure leads to clinical improvement and reversal of damage (including retinopathy) is so conclusive that no controlled therapeutic trial has ever been contemplated. As with benign hypertension, hasty reduction of pressure levels may result in neurological impairment and very rapid pressure reduction is now only advocated in the presence of an acute aortic dissection. Blood pressure should be reduced over hours rather than minutes. Although agents such as hydralazine, diazoxide or sodium nitroprusside can be given by slow infusion or repeated intravenous boluses, rapidly effective oral agents (e.g. labetalol or captopril) can also be used.

Renal Disease

Unlike malignant phase hypertension, uncomplicated essential hypertension is unlikely to be the cause of severe deterioration in renal function. Impaired renal function does occur, however, and is more likely in the presence of coexisting disease such as prostatic outflow obstruction. Renal function can be preserved by the removal of any reversible elements, and there is growing evidence that aggressive antihypertensive therapy itself will preserve renal function.

Probably well over 90% of hypertension is "essential" in all age groups. In old age, renovascular and renal parenchymal disease are the major causes of secondary hypertension, with endocrine abnormalities such as Cushing's syndrome, phaeochromocytoma and aldosterone and renin-secreting tumours being rarities. Underlying renal parenchymal diseases include chronic pyelonephritis, obstructive uropathy, chronic analgesic abuse and polycystic disease. The degree of renal impairment seems to be a factor in blood pressure elevation and this may be related to salt and water retention.

Clinical Evaluation

Hypertension is generally an incidental finding as it tends to be asymptomatic. In taking the history, particular reference should be made to those diseases (e.g. renal disorders) which are known to lead to secondary hypertension. A drug history is important as some agents (e.g. NSAIDs, corticosteroids) can elevate blood pressure. Social and dietary habits should be enquired about as excessive alcohol or salt intake also elevate blood pressure. Liquorice addiction is much quoted as a cause, but is seldom found in practice. Symptoms of hypertensive complications (e.g. transient ischaemic attacks) should also be sought.

Measurement of the blood pressure is usually undertaken by the doctor although general population screening by a trained nurse has been shown to be perfectly feasible. Many factors can spuriously elevate or lower the blood pressure as measured by sphygmomanometry: the position of the patient's arm, obesity, the size of the arm cuff and the quality of the equipment used can all influence the recording. It is now common practice to record the first and fifth phases of the Korotkoff sounds (i.e. the appearance and complete disappearance of the sounds). Pressures should always be taken in both arms on the initial visit as artefactual low recordings in one arm can be produced by arterial stenosis. Systolic pressure differences as great as 40–50 mmHg can be found. It is important to measure blood pressure with the patient both supine and standing. Impaired neurohumoral control can result in the postural drop of blood pressure with an absence of the normal compensatory tachycardia. Such postural hypotension is a major cause of falls and syncope in elderly patients.

The physician should interpret a single elevated blood pressure reading with caution. Blood pressure changes continuously throughout the day. There is diurnal variation with maximal readings found in the morning, falling to a nadir during sleep. It is now well recognised that the very act of measuring blood pressure will produce a "defensive" elevation of pressure which is transient. This is most likely to occur in anxious people. Furthermore, it has been shown that if people whose "hypertension" is newly diagnosed are left untreated, blood pressure will return to normal in as many as a third. In order to reduce the likelihood of inappropriate drug therapy and follow-up for such patients, assessment should be based on readings obtained on at least three occasions during a 2–3 month period.

Sometimes, atherosclerosis results in a spuriously elevated blood pressure being recorded with sphygmomanometry. This "pseudohypertension" should be suspected if the elevated pressure is predominantly or exclusively systolic. Another pointer is the absence of end-organ hypertensive damage. Direct measurement of intra-arterial pressure will confirm the problem, though it can be suspected clinically by performing Osler's manoeuvre. The radial artery is compressed proximally so as to obliterate pulsation; if the vessel can be palpated by rolling a finger over it, this indicates atherosclerosis.

Physical examination should be performed in order to elucidate underlying disease causing secondary hypertension. For example, an abdominal bruit may suggest underlying renal artery stenosis. In addition, evidence of end-organ hypertensive damage should be sought. Particular attention should be paid to the heart (looking for cardiomegaly and heart failure) and the eyes (looking for retinopathy). If such end-organ damage is found, it places the patient in a category with a poorer prognosis and will affect the decision whether or not to treat.

Finally, the patient's assessment should include a search for other atherogenic risk factors. While it is suggested that serum cholesterol declines in importance with age, obesity, as well as having an effect on blood pressure, remains an independent atherosclerotic risk factor.

Further Investigation

Complex screening procedures to elicit any underlying cause of hypertension invoke the law of diminishing returns. Also, the reluctance of many elderly patients to undergo major operative procedures should temper one's investigative enthusiasm in some cases. For most patients, a full blood count, measurement of serum electrolytes, urea, creatinine and glucose, urinalysis and urine culture, chest X-ray and ECG are all that is required.

Should the history, physical examination or screening tests suggest that underlying pathology is likely, further tests may be indicated. For example, the presence of a rapid deterioration in blood pressure control, the development of urinary abnormalities, the presence of a bruit or unexplained hypokalaemia should prompt a search for renal artery stenosis. A further indication for more detailed investigation is blood pressure which is apparently unresponsive to standard therapy. Almost always, however, such "resistant" hypertension reflects poor drug compliance. Abnormalities found on screening will often have a simple explanation. Thus hypokalaemia is more likely to reflect diuretic therapy rather than Cushing's syndrome. Recent therapeutic advances have prompted a more aggressive approach towards the diagnosis of hypertension in old age. For example, renal artery stenosis can now be reversed by percutaneous transluminal angioplasty. However, routine screening for renovascular disease is not recommended because of the low detection rate.

Visualisation of the renal tract has been facilitated by ultrasound techniques which give information on renal size, the presence of cysts and obstructive problems. Rapid phase urography and isotope renography can be used to diagnose renal artery stenosis, though the investigation of choice is still arteriography, especially if angioplasty is to be considered.

Management

Any source of secondary hypertension should be identified and where possible removed. Percutaneous transluminal angioplasty is being increasingly used in elderly patients with renovascular hypertension (Fig. 8.4). It carries a small but definite morbidity of 5% and there is occasional associated mortality. The success rate regarding its ability to lower blood pressure varies from 40% to 80%. Restenosis commonly occurs and requires further dilatation which tends to be less successful than the initial one.

In the case of essential hypertension, the management aims are to eliminate associated atherogenic risk factors and to lower the blood pressure. With regard

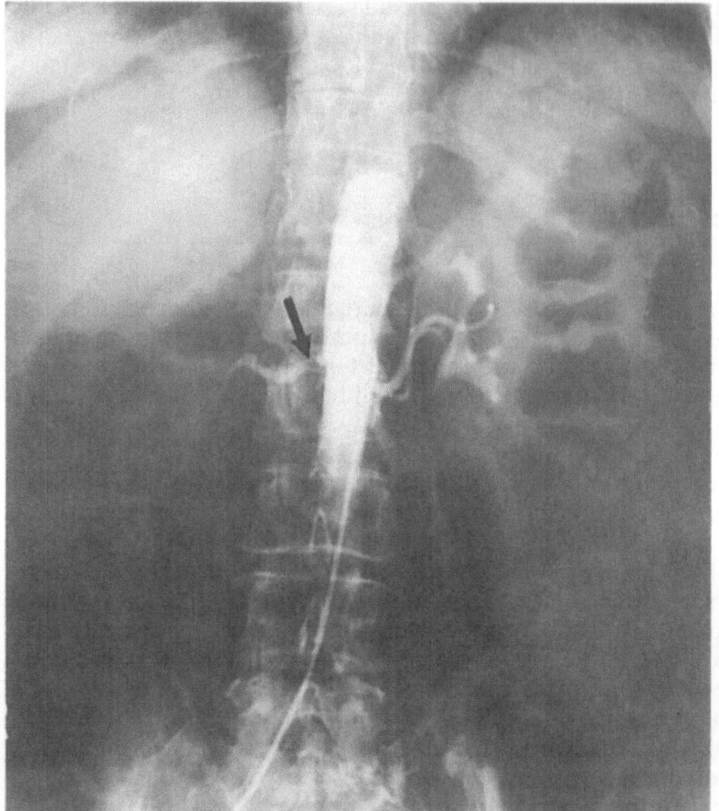

a

Fig. 8.4. **a** Tight atheromatous stenosis of the right renal artery demonstrated at angiography. **b** After successful dilatation, there is also a small iatrogenic dissection.

to the former, advice to stop smoking and to moderate alcohol intake should be given when appropriate. Reduction of obesity is a worthwhile goal and every assistance should be given in terms of dietary advice.

Non-drug Treatment

Despite some experimental and clinical data suggesting that strict dietary sodium restriction, calcium and potassium supplementation, yoga and regular physical exercise can reduce blood pressure levels, there is little or no evidence that these measures may produce any prolonged benefit.

Drug Treatment

The age-related changes in drug handling are outlined in Chapter 24. Antihypertensive agents are a major cause of iatrogenic morbidity in the elderly. This can be

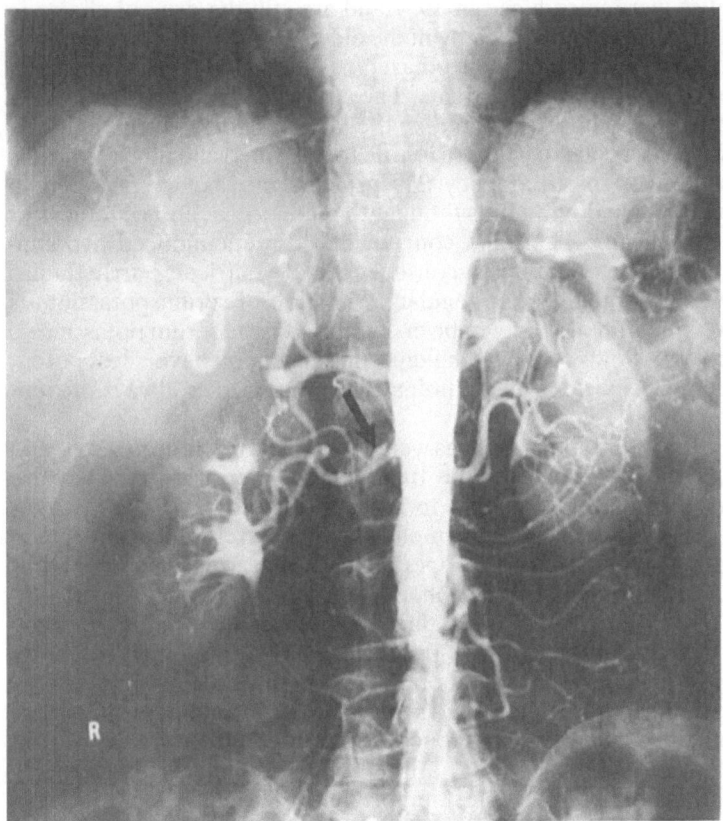

Fig. 8.4b

minimised if adequate consideration is given to the need for antihypertensive medication in the first place and if the drug dosages are titrated against blood pressure response. There is as yet little evidence that antihypertensive agents are tolerated less well because of age alone, but therapy may interact with conditions more prevalent in the elderly. The choice of antihypertensive agent will be governed by the necessity of avoiding adverse effects, for example: beta-blockers are contraindicated in heart failure or obstructive airways disease; diuretics are contraindicated in a patient prone to gout.

The "stepped care" approach consisting of diuretic, diuretic + beta-blocker, diuretic + beta-blocker + vasodilator has been advocated in the last 10 years. It arose from a consensus opinion and, although it attempts to reduce single drug toxicity, has no other rational basis. More recently it has become widely appreciated that essential hypertension is a heterogeneous entity and that it may be possible to predict the hypotensive effect of drugs in certain sub-groups; for example, elevated basal serum renin concentrations may provide a more rational basis for beta-blockade. Certainly increased understanding of the renin–angiotensin system makes it possible to predict synergy between drug groups such as thiazide diuretics and angiotensin-converting enzyme (ACE) inhibitors. Newer and more potent drugs with a lower incidence of unwanted effects make mono-therapy available to a larger proportion of patients.

Thiazide diuretics were introduced in 1957 and are still the drug of choice in mild to moderate hypertension, especially in the elderly. Virtually all therapeutic trials have included them and after benzodiazepines they are probably the most used, and misused, drugs in elderly patients. The antihypertensive effect outlasts the diuretic effect by many hours, and unlike the latter, is not dose-related. The unwanted effects are dose-related so there is little to be gained and much to be lost by increasing total dose or dose frequency. The principal mode of action in reducing blood pressure is still in doubt but is thought to relate to salt and water loss or their vasodilator properties. The main concern that diuretic-induced hypokalaemia may result in sudden death as a consequence of ventricular arrhythmias has not been well substantiated, but regular estimation of serum potassium is mandatory. Arrhythmias are unlikely to be encountered if the serum potassium is greater than 3.0 mEq/l. Potassium-sparing diuretics in general have a less potent antihypertensive effect, nor does the combination with thiazides always prevent hypokalaemia.

Beta-adrenergic receptor blocking drugs were introduced in the early 1960s and heralded a radically new approach to the treatment of hypertension. They are frequently preferred to diuretics in mild to moderate hypertension in younger patients. All beta-blockers have similar molecular structures which have been manipulated to produce a variety of properties such as cardioselectivity (thus minimising bronchoconstriction and peripheral vasoconstriction), intrinsic sympathomimetic activity (thus minimising the risk of bradycardia), membrane stabilising activity (giving antiarrhythmic properties) and altered lipid solubility (minimising CNS side effects). The only one of these properties of real importance in the context of hypertension is lipid solubility. For example, propranolol, with high lipid solubility, has a high incidence of unwanted effects on the central nervous system; atenolol, with low lipid affinity, may accumulate dangerously when there is renal impairment. The most important cardiac effect is bradycardia and is independent of the antihypertensive effect which is predominantly a central one, although resetting of baroreceptors and reduction of renin levels may also occur. In old age there is some evidence of decreased responsiveness to adrenergic stimulation and thus reduced efficacy of beta-blocking drugs.

The first calcium channel blocking agent, verapamil, was synthesised in 1962 and was originally thought to be a beta-blocker. It was subsequently found to be a coronary and peripheral vasodilator and underwent trials as an antianginal agent. After initial dosage problems, successful clinical trials have resulted in the availability of an increasing number of "calcium antagonists" which are not necessarily chemically related. Calcium is essential for muscular contraction and unlike skeletal muscle, myocardial and smooth muscle do not have large stores of intracellular calcium ions. These agents prevent the inward flux of ionic calcium associated with depolarisation of the cells and so alter their contractile properties. Their profiles of action are also varied, with effects on cardiac conduction tissue and cardiac muscle being found particularly with verapamil and diltiazem, while nicardipine and nifedipine have predominantly vasodilator properties.

Various other vasodilator drugs are available, hydrallazine and prazosin being examples, but they have a tendency to cause a reflex tachycardia which offsets their antihypertensive effect. They are therefore best used in conjunction with a beta-blocker, rather than as single antihypertensive agents.

ACE inhibitors came into use with the development of orally active captopril in the late 1970s. Enalapril, which is longer acting, has since been introduced and many new agents are in the process of being developed. These agents have rapidly gained a place in the treatment of moderate to severe hypertension and although originally thought to be of special use in the renovascular variety they are effective in all grades and types of hypertension. Initial dose-related problems of profound hypotension have largely been eliminated. These agents prevent the formation of vasoconstrictor octapeptide angiotensin II from its inactive decapeptide precursor angiotensin I. They have a powerful vasodilator effect and have also been shown to increase cardiac output slightly and so have a particularly useful role in hypertensive heart failure. In combination with thiazides and loop diuretics they have a synergistic antihypertensive effect as well as having a balanced effect on potassium excretion. Caution must be advocated at the initiation of therapy as it has come to be appreciated that rapidly deteriorating renal function and profound prolonged hypotension can occur in subjects with previously undiagnosed bilateral stenosed renal arteries.

The more recently available antihypertensive agents are potent yet less toxic than their predecessors. At present choice of therapy is empirical, but a rational basis may emerge. Ideally medication should involve the minimum number of tablets to maximise compliance and reduce the likelihood of accidental toxicity in a population with a high incidence of memory disturbance and a propensity to confusional states.

Further Reading

Amery A, Birkenhager W, Bulpitt C et al. (1985) Mortality and morbidity results from the European Working Party on High Blood Pressure in the Elderly trial. Lancet I:1349–1354

Editorial (1986) The risks of antihypertensive therapy. Lancet II:1075–1076

Kannel WB (1986) Prevalence, incidence and hazards of hypertension in the elderly. Am Heart J 112:1362–1363

Kannel WB, Dawbe TR, McGee DL (1980) Perspectives on systolic hypertension: the Framingham study. Circulation 61:1179–1182

Petrie JC, O'Brien ET, Little WA, DeSwiet M (1986) Recommendations on blood pressure measurement. Br Med J 293:611–615

Pickering G (1968) High blood pressure, 2nd edn. Churchill Livingstone, Edinburgh

Chapter 9

Lower Limb Oedema

T. Rudra

Elderly patients with lower limb oedema may present themselves to their General Practitioners or to a variety of hospital departments. This reflects the diverse nature of conditions which can underlie the problem. Its diagnosis and management is usually straightforward and yet at times it may tax the ingenuity of the most experienced clinician. While all clinicians involved in the care of old people realise that the problem is common, there are surprisingly few published studies on its actual prevalence.

Anatomy and Physiology

An understanding of the basic anatomy of the venous system in the lower limb and the physiological principles of oedema formation are essential if one is to appreciate the different causes, make an accurate diagnosis and offer rational therapy.

Venous drainage of the lower limbs occurs via a network of superficial and deep veins, connected by communicating veins. Blood normally flows from superficial to deep veins and thence to the heart. Venous return is greatly dependent on the contraction and relaxation of limb muscles which exerts a pumping effect on the deep veins. The generation of a negative intra-thoracic pressure during inspiration and transmitted pressure from adjacent arteries are of much lesser importance in promoting venous return to the heart.

Uni-directional flow of blood towards the heart is dependent on the presence of valves in both the deep and communicating veins. Such valves are particularly important in the lower limbs of man where an erect posture generates considerable hydrostatic pressure opposing venous return.

Loss of the pumping action of leg muscles, as occurs with hypostasis, will impair venous return to the heart and promote limb oedema. Valvular incompetence of the deep and/or communicating veins also results in oedema. When valves in the deep veins are incompetent, the hydrostatic pressure increases, while with incompetence of valves in the communicating veins, the flow of blood from superficial to deep veins is reversed. The contraction of leg muscles exacerbates the abnormal pattern of blood flow so that oedema is more evident following a period of exercise and especially towards the end of a day's activities.

Excessive accumulation of interstitial fluid also results in oedema formation. Interstitial fluid forms as a result of the physiological processes of filtration and re-absorption that occur respectively at the arterial and venous ends of the capillary system. Normally these two processes of filtration and re-absorption are in equilibrium, thus keeping the amount of interstitial fluid constant. The following factors affect this equilibrium:

1. *Capillary blood pressure*. The arterial blood pressure is the main driving force for the process of filtration at the arterial end of the capillary. As the blood passes through the network of capillaries most of this pressure is dissipated and at the venous end is therefore much lower.

2. *Plasma colloid oncotic pressure*. The relatively large protein molecules of the plasma do not pass through the capillaries and therefore exert the main osmotic influence within the capillary. The electrolytes, glucose and urea are also osmotically active but, as they are normally present in equal concentrations on both sides of the capillary, they do not contribute to plasma oncotic pressure.

3. *Interstitial colloid oncotic pressure*. In the normal state there is only a small concentration of protein molecules in the interstitial fluid. However, alterations in capillary membrane permeability or lymphatic obstruction could increase the protein content of the interstitial space.

4. *Interstitial fluid pressure*. The space available for the interstitial fluid volume is small. If the volume increases above normal the pressure within the space increases.

5. *Capillary membrane permeability*. The capillary membrane is semi-permeable. It is permeable to all normal constituents of plasma except protein, the major factor favouring re-absorption of interstitial fluid. Any alteration in permeability which allows protein to escape into the interstitial space will favour oedema formation.

Table 9.1. The causes of lower limb oedema

Local disorders
Dependent oedema
Vascular disorders (chronic venous insufficiency, occlusion of large viens, deep vein thrombosis, arterial reconstruction)
Popliteal (Baker's) cyst
Gastrocnemius rupture
Lymphoedema
Lipoedema
Infection

Systemic disorders
Cardiac disease (congestive cardiac failure, constrictive pericarditis)
Hypoproteinaemic states (hepatic cirrhosis, nephrotic syndrome, acute glomerulonephritis, starvation)
Thyroid dysfunction (hyper- and hypothyroidism)
Drugs (corticosteroids, NSAIDs, vasodilators)
Exposure to extremes of temperature

---

6. *Lymphatic flow*. The lymphatic system drains some of the interstitial fluid. Lymphatic fluid contains large quantities of protein and any obstruction of lymphatic outflow will result in leakage of this protein content, thus favouring oedema formation.

The causes of lower limb oedema are outlined in Table 9.1 and can usefully be classified as local or systemic in nature.

Local Disorders

Dependent Oedema

Old people have lax skin and low interstitial pressure, allowing the accumulation of large quantities of interstitial fluid. Sitting or standing for prolonged periods without any accompanying muscular activity can cause leg oedema even in the absence of any other predisposing factor. Some elderly patients with conditions which restrict mobility (see Chap. 15) are thus particularly susceptible to dependent (hypostatic) oedema. Dependent oedema is usually bilateral. It is often mistakenly attributed to cardiac failure and is therefore inappropriately treated with diuretics. It is also seen in patients with severe peripheral vascular disease. Some patients who experience rest pain may hang a foot over the edge of the bed at night to enable them to sleep, so oedema may be more noticeable in that leg.

The most important step in the correct management of dependent oedema lies in correct diagnosis, thus avoiding irrational therapy. Gravity will assist venous drainage if the legs are raised above the level of the trunk. Where possible, therefore, the legs should be elevated regularly during the day, the exact frequency and duration of elevation depending on the severity of the problem and its underlying cause. Patients with impaired hip and knee movement may need to lie supine to facilitate drainage. Explanation, reassurance and the encouragement of mobility are important.

Vascular Disorders

A common cause of leg oedema that is also misdiagnosed in many elderly patients is *chronic venous insufficiency*. Following a single or multiple episodes of thrombosis, damage to the valves of the deep and communicating veins renders them incompetent. Venous hypertension occurs when in an upright posture and oedema gradually develops. The increased venous pressure also distends the endothelial pores in the capillaries, thus altering their permeability and allowing the leakage of red cells, fibrinogen and other macromolecules. These are broken down in the tissue spaces, leading to inflammatory changes which manifest clinically as pigmentation, induration and inflammation within the skin and subcutaneous tissues. These changes are referred to as lipodermatosclerosis and precede the development of venous ulceration in the affected leg (Fig. 9.1).

Treatment is aimed at reducing venous hypertension and preventing complications. Properly fitted elastic stockings should be worn during the day and mobility

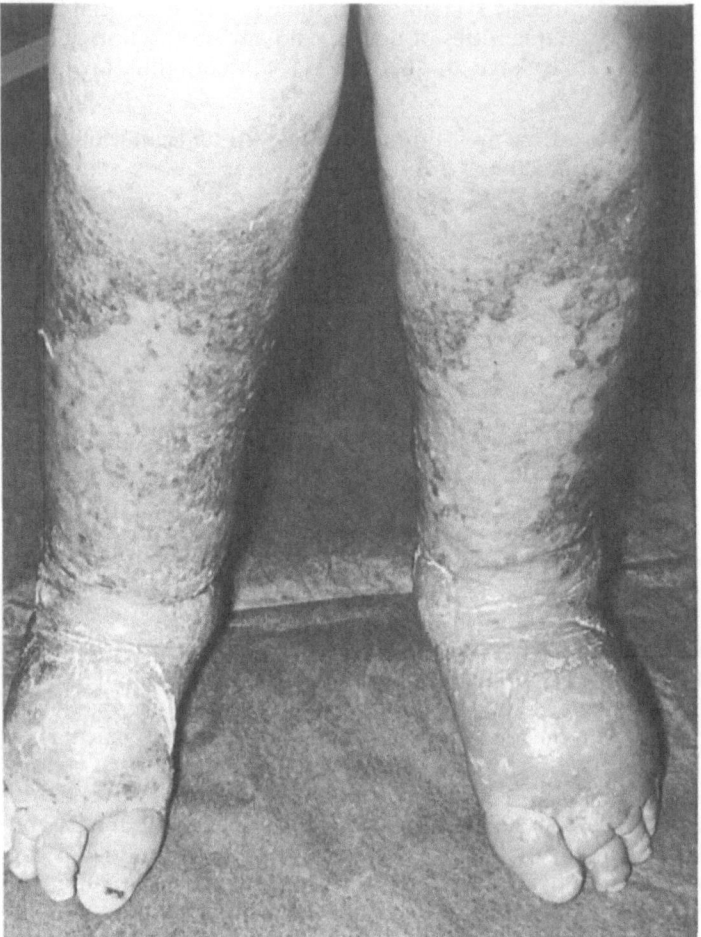

Fig. 9.1.   Lipodermatosclerosis.

encouraged. Any signs of eczematisation or ulceration should be looked for and promptly treated. Drugs, ligation of varicose veins and sclerotherapy have little to offer in management.

Occlusion of large veins such as an iliac vein or the inferior vena cava can cause swelling of one or both legs. The venous occlusion may be due to external compression from a pelvic or abdominal tumour, a distended bladder or lymph nodes and can also result from thrombus formation. Due to the level of occlusion, the swelling involves the whole of the leg.

If large vein occlusion is suspected, it is mandatory to palpate the abdomen, perform a rectal examination and a vaginal examination in the female patient. Ultrasound examination of the abdomen and pelvis will often identify an obstructing lesion which is not obvious on palpation. It can help clarify the nature of a palpable lesion and can aid confirmation of the presence of ascites. A CT scan is indicated when an obstructive lesion in the abdomen or pelvis is very likely and the ultrasound examination is unhelpful or inconclusive.

Treatment consists of removing any underlying cause together with anticoagulation (see below).

Deep vein thrombosis is one of the commonest causes of an acutely swollen leg in the elderly. Occlusion of the deep veins by thrombus results in an increase in the venous pressure at capillary level. When the venous pressure is high enough to overcome the factors favouring re-absorption of the interstitial fluid, oedema is produced. Oedema usually develops within 24–48 hours of the occlusion. The commonest symptoms are pain and swelling in the leg, together with general malaise and fever. It is accompanied by localised warmth and tenderness to deep palpation. The swollen leg may also have a slight cyanotic hue and some superficial veins may be prominent.

Venography is the most definitive test for diagnosing a deep vein thrombosis. Its disadvantages lie in the fact that it is invasive, may be painful, may induce phlebitis and is relatively expensive. Other non-invasive diagnostic tests include impedance plethysmography, Doppler ultrasonography and labelled fibrinogen scans. Many clinicians feel that before a patient is committed to anticoagulation following deep vein thrombosis, it is mandatory to confirm the diagnosis by one of these tests.

Treatment is by anticoagulation, provided that there is no contraindication. Immediate anticoagulation is achieved with either intravenous or subcutaneous heparin and is continued with warfarin. Close monitoring of coagulation and titration of dosage is essential. The usual course of treatment lasts for about 6 weeks, though this must be prolonged should the thrombus have embolised to the lungs. Several studies have shown that age alone is no barrier to successful anticoagulation, although old people require smaller dosages of warfarin than do young adults. Many elderly patients are on multiple drugs and the possibility of drug interactions which could affect anticoagulation should be borne in mind. The dangers of this should be explained to patients and their relatives.

When blood flow is re-established to an ischaemic limb by *arterial reconstruction*, oedema can develop in that limb. This is due to alteration in capillary membrane permeability. Occasionally, the oedema can be severe enough to cause generalised swelling of the limb with bulla formation.

Popliteal (Baker's) Cyst

A popliteal synovial cyst can cause the leg to swell due to a variety of reasons. The cyst may cause compression of the popliteal vein and lead to oedema of the leg. It may dissect into the calf muscles and cause pain and swelling. Rupture of the cyst can cause an acutely swollen, painful leg and the symptoms and signs may be difficult to distinguish from a deep vein thrombosis. Indeed, a persistent popliteal cyst, by compressing the popliteal vein, can lead to a deep vein thrombosis.

Arthrography is the most definitive way to identify a popliteal cyst. Ultrasound scanning is also used and has the advantage of being non-invasive.

Localised popliteal cysts are often painless and do not require specific treatment. If they are symptomatic the cyst should be aspirated via the knee joint and injected with corticosteroids.

Gastrocnemius Rupture

A tear of the medial head of the gastrocnemius muscle is associated with a distinct clinical picture. Typically there is sudden onset of pain in the calf while engaged in some activity and the patient often hears a "snap" or "pop" in the affected leg. There is rapid development of swelling and within a few days ecchymosis appears around the ankle and foot.

Treatment during the first 2 days consists of application of ice packs and elevation of the leg. This is followed by progressive ambulation, initially avoiding weight-bearing on the affected leg. When weight-bearing begins, a lift in the heel of the shoe avoids excessive stretching and re-injury of the gastrocnemius. This is followed by progressive proper stretching exercises until maximum recovery is obtained.

Lymphoedema

Lymphoedema is due to obstruction, or a deficiency in the numbers, of lymphatic vessels. An accumulation of the protein-rich lymphatic fluid results, which leads to a rise in the fluid pressure and colloid oncotic pressure within the interstitial space. Oedema is formed, lymphoedema characteristically beginning in the most distal portion of the foot and producing a dorsal lump. It is initially soft and pitting but when it persists, fibrosis occurs and results in thickening and induration of the skin. The oedema is then non-pitting. Longstanding lymphoedema of any cause can become secondarily infected (lymphangitis) and this eventually leads to further scarring and thickening of the skin. These skin changes give a characteristic appearance, often referred to as "pigskin".

Lymphoedema may be classified as primary (idiopathic) or secondary (obstructive). Primary lymphoedema may be congenital or acquired and usually, though not always, begins early in life. Women are affected almost ten times more frequently than men. Secondary lymphoedema is due to obstruction and may be further classified as inflammatory or non-inflammatory. Secondary non-inflammatory lymphoedema may result from metastatic carcinoma involving the regional lymph nodes, irradiation or surgical removal of lymph nodes. Secondary inflammatory lymphoedema is the result of recurrent lymphangitis or cellulitis, the inflammatory process causing lymphatic occlusion.

Although lymphangiography may be of diagnostic use in some cases of lymphoedema it is rarely performed because of its invasive nature, risk of infection, scarring and the potential risk of embolisation.

While lymphoedema is reputedly difficult to treat, adherence to basic principles can help the patient immensely. Even though the limb may not return to normal, the improvement which follows good management encourages both patient and doctor. The idea is to rid the limb of as much oedema as possible and to then teach the patient to maintain this situation. Elevation of the limb, external compression with elastic stockings, intermittent diuretic therapy, infection control with prompt treatment of lymphangitis and fungal infections of the feet and toes are all aimed at achieving this goal. Surgical measures for treating lymphoedema are disappointing and hardly ever employed in the elderly.

Lipoedema

Lipoedema is characterised by the bilateral and symmetrical deposition of fat in the lower extremities and its occurrence in women only. It is associated with obesity from the waist down and the legs are non-pitting. A distinguishing feature of lipoedema is that the foot is not involved. Although the patient complains of swollen legs there is no real "oedema" in the physiological sense.

Infection

Infections can cause a swollen leg by a variety of mechanisms. An acute onset of warm, erythematous, painful swelling, often accompanied by fever and chills, is typical of cellulitis. Tender regional lymph nodes are an important clue. Fungal intertrigo of the feet can be a portal of entry leading to secondary bacterial infections, causing cellulitis or lymphangitis. Recurrent attacks of lymphangitis can lead to lymphoedema (secondary inflammatory lymphoedema).

Filariasis is a parasitic infection involving the lymphatics in tropical countries. The oedema produced is frequently considerable and the pachydermatous skin may resemble that of an elephant (elephantiasis).

Cellulitis is most often due to streptococcal organisms and penicillin is the antibiotic of choice. Uncommonly *Staphylococcus aureus* is responsible, when flucloxacillin should be used. In those who are sensitive to penicillin, erythromycin is the drug of choice.

Systemic Disorders

Congestive Cardiac Failure

Congestive cardiac failure becomes more prevalent with increasing age. It is generally found in a patient with cardiac ischaemia or hypertension, though respiratory problems such as chronic bronchitis and recurring pulmonary emboli are other important underlying factors. Right- and left-sided heart failure (see Chap. 7) often coincide. With right-sided heart failure, patients may complain of ankle swelling, and have difficulty wearing shoes and mobilising. Nausea and abdominal pain may be secondary to congestion of the gut and liver. Symptoms of vague tiredness and weakness are particularly common. On examination, an elevated jugular venous pulse, sacral oedema, hepatomegaly and ascites may be found in addition to ankle oedema.

The treatment of cardiac failure is discussed in more detail in Chap. 7. When right-sided heart failure predominates, decreasing pre-load on the heart with diuretic therapy is the main-stay of treatment. However elevation of the limbs will hasten resolution of ankle oedema and should not be neglected.

Hypoproteinaemic States

The causes of hypoproteinaemia are protean and include kwashiorkor (chronic protein malnutrition), hepatic dysfunction and protein-losing syndromes. The latter include the nephrotic syndrome and protein-losing enteropathy. Serum albumin, which measures visceral protein mass, will be low.

Treatment consists of reversing the underlying cause. Intravenous administration of salt-poor albumin will transiently elevate the serum albumin and help to initiate a diuresis. Such treatment is expensive and is not a long-term solution in hypoproteinaemic states.

Thyroid Dysfunction

Some 50% of thyrotoxic old people will have leg oedema at presentation. In only half of these is the oedema attributable to congestive cardiac failure. The management of hyperthyroidism is discussed in Chapter 10.

Leg oedema is also found in hypothyroidism as it precipitates cardiac failure. When initiating treatment of long-standing hypothyroidism with L-thyroxine, cardiac failure can be precipitated. To avoid this risk small doses of L-thyroxine must be given initially and the dose gradually increased.

Drugs

With many problems in geriatric medicine, the underlying cause is iatrogenic. Ankle oedema is no exception. The drugs which are implicated cause fluid retention, peripheral vasodilatation or exacerbate heart failure. Among the drugs causing fluid retention are corticosteroids and NSAIDs, sex hormones, carbenoxolone and the centrally acting antihypertensive agents methyldopa and clonidine. The peripheral vasodilators include nifedipine, hydralazine and diazoxide. Drugs which have a negatively inotropic effect include all anti-arrhythmic agents and beta-blockers. Ankle oedema will be produced as a manifestation of heart failure. With some of these drugs (e.g. nifedipine), the advent of ankle oedema is unimportant and the patient can be reassured. With others however (e.g. beta-blockers), oedema signals the onset of serious problems which will necessitate stopping treatment.

Exposure to Extremes of Temperature

When the lower limbs are exposed to extremes of temperature it can alter capillary membrane permeability thus leading to oedema formation. The history provides the vital clue in these cases.

Clinical Evaluation

In patients presenting with lower limb oedema, the basic tools of clinical medicine, the history and the physical examination, remain the cornerstones of diagnosis. The history alone can provide many valuable clues. The speed of onset of oedema can suggest the underlying cause (e.g. an onset over a period of hours makes lymphoedema unlikely, whereas a gradual onset over several days, weeks or months suggests the opposite). The duration and pattern of the oedema can also be helpful. Recurring oedema which suddenly appears and disappears suggests an underlying infection or recurrent injury. A variable degree of swelling throughout the day is a feature of oedema of recent onset. Maintenance of a standing or a seated posture causes oedema to increase. Thus it is least apparent in the morning and worst in the evening. Even lymphoedema shows this variation in its early stages, but as the condition becomes more chronic the variation diminishes.

When lower limb oedema is associated with pain it is likely to be due to local disease. Cellulitis, a ruptured Baker's cyst or a ruptured gastrocnemius muscle can cause various degrees of pain. With the latter, an audible snap sometimes precedes the pain and swelling. Deep vein thrombosis is usually accompanied by pain but its absence does not exclude it. In the history it is important to enquire about any associated symptoms relating to cardiovascular disease, renal disease, hepatitis and malabsorption. A history of trauma, previous surgery and of drug therapy should also be sought. Drugs are a common and often forgotten cause of oedema.

On inspection the distribution of the swelling should first be noted. Unilateral oedema suggests a local cause. When secondary to an underlying general disorder, the swelling is bilateral and is usually symmetrically distributed. The latter is generally soft and pitting in nature and is accompanied by oedema in other dependent parts. In patients who are confined to bed, sacral oedema may be more prominent than leg oedema. These features should alert the physician to look beyond the lower extremities for its cause.

Certain skin changes are of diagnostic significance. A thickened, taut and fibrotic skin indicates that the problem is chronic, whereas a soft skin which easily pits on pressure suggests a recent onset. When the swelling is accompanied by warmth, redness and a lymphangitic streak, the diagnosis is cellulitis. An ecchymotic area on the calf is found with a tear of the medial head of the gastrocnemius muscle. Skin ulceration in an oedematous leg is usually due to chronic venous hypertension. Such ulcers are found most commonly in the region of the medial malleolus. The legs should be examined for associated varicose veins, usually involving the long or short saphenous veins or their tributaries. These are best seen when the patient is standing.

When oedema is not apparent the patient should be asked to identify the affected area because the "swelling" referred to may be fat (lipoedema).

Physical examination should include, in addition to the lower limbs, a search for different signs relating to the different causes of secondary oedema. Remember to look for disorders which restrict mobility (see Chap. 15) as oedema is commonly attributable to the resulting dependent position of the lower limbs.

Management

Lower limb oedema signifies an underlying disease process with many possible causes. With a proper understanding of the anatomical and physiological basis for the problem and with information obtained from the history and physical examination, it is possible in the majority of cases to identify the underlying cause.

Treatment should be aimed primarily at reversing the cause, though irrespective of this, local measures will help reduce the oedema. The importance of elevation of the oedematous limb so that gravity can assist drainage has been previously mentioned. Should elastic stockings be issued, more than one pair will be required allowing one pair to be in use while the other is being washed. If the stockings succeed in reducing limb swelling, this in itself will render them too large and ineffective and, in any case, stockings will lose their elasticity in time. Patients with elastic stockings need to be followed up, therefore, and have their stockings changed as required.

Especially in conditions in which lower limb oedema is likely to be persistent or recurrent it is important to inform and educate the patient as to the nature of the problem and how it is best managed. Where possible the patient herself should be involved in the management. In this way compliance with treatment strategies is maximised.

The diagnosis and management of oedema is often a challenge and usually a rewarding experience.

Further Reading

Dale W (1973) The swollen leg. Current Problems in Surgery. Yearbook Medical Publishers, pp 1–66
Macleod IB, Shaw Dunn J (1985) Lower Limb. In: Forrester JM, Passmore R, Robson JS (eds) (1986) A companion to medical studies: anatomy, biochemistry and physiology, 3rd edn. Blackwell Scientific Publications, Oxford, pp 20.41–20.43
Ruschhaupt WD (1983) Differential diagnosis of oedema of the lower extremities. Cardiovasc Clin 13:307–320
Schirger A (1982) Differential diagnosis and management of leg oedema in the elderly. Geriatrics 37:26–32

Chapter 10

Weight Loss

P. Finucane

Due to a reduction both in body fat and in lean muscle mass there is a gradual decrease in body weight with advancing age. This is scarcely noticeable in the individual unless his or her weight is recorded over a considerable period of time. The maintenance of body weight depends on the balance between energy expenditure and energy (food) intake. In the elderly, and especially in extreme old age, both a decrease in the basal metabolic rate and a decrease in the level of activity combine to lower energy expenditure. This is accompanied by a decrease in energy intake so that weight is maintained within a narrow range.

Spontaneous loss of weight in the elderly person is abnormal, especially if it is rapid, severe or continuous. Its importance is twofold. Firstly, it may be accompanied by clinical or sub-clinical nutrient deficiency states. Protein deficiency, for example, is associated with impaired immunological function and can lead to hypoproteinaemia and oedema, especially when the individual is stressed by intercurrent illnesses. Overt disease states can result from deficiency of minerals (e.g. iron and zinc) and vitamins (e.g. B vitamins, vitamin C and vitamin D). Secondly, weight loss is a powerful indicator of underlying disease. Physicians concerned with the care of elderly people increasingly recognise the importance of screening for disease. The sooner impending medical breakdown can be recognised, the earlier remedial action can be taken. The expectation is that this in turn will be translated into improved patient morbidity and mortality. Looking for weight loss is among the most simple and most valuable of screening tests.

A rapid loss of weight reflects the severity of the underlying disorder while its extent reflects the chronicity. The cause of weight loss can be attributed to one or more of the following:

Decreased ingestion of food

Decreased digestion and absorption

Increased energy requirements

The cause in a given patient is often multi-factorial. Pancreatic carcinoma, for example, can result in loss of appetite (decreasing food ingestion), pancreatic insufficiency (impairing food digestion) together with metabolic derangement (increasing energy requirements).

Decreased Ingestion of Food

In developing countries it is children who suffer most from malnutrition, whereas in developed countries, old people are most at risk. Studies from many developed countries have shown that while inadequate dietary intake is common, this seldom results in overt malnutrition. In Britain some 50% of old people have an inadequate diet while only 3% are clinically malnourished. The common causes of decreased food intake are summarised in Table 10.1.

Table 10.1 Causes of prolonged decreased food intake

Decreased appetite
Mouth diseases (neoplasia, oral surgery, xerostomia)
Neuromuscular pharyngeal/oesophageal disorders (stroke, Parkinson's disease, motor
  neurone disease, achalasia, oesophageal spasm, globus hystericus)
Structural pharyngeal/oesophageal lesions (carcinoma, benign stricture, pharyngeal pouch,
  oesophageal web and diverticulum)
Nausea and vomiting
General debility
Poverty, ignorance and isolation

Decreased Appetite

A physiological decrease in appetite occurs with advancing age due at least in part to blunting of taste and smell. True anorexia is a symptom experienced by people of all ages during the course of some acute or severe illnesses. The cause is generally multi-factorial. For example, with malignant disease, alteration in taste or smell perception, production of lactates or ketones, direct effects on the appetite centre, tumour toxins and psychological factors have all been implicated.

Those organic diseases which commonly cause anorexia can be divided into gastrointestinal, systemic or psychological disorders. Among the gastrointestinal causes are peptic ulceration, gastric carcinoma, post-gastrectomy syndrome, biliary disease, mesenteric ischaemia and regional enteritis. Systemic disease in the form of any infective process, malignancy, alcoholism, liver dysfunction, renal impairment and chronic pulmonary disease may similarly cause weight loss by appetite suppression. Drugs are another important cause, with amphetamines being particularly implicated. Cigarette smoking is often overlooked as a factor causing anorexia. Psychological disorders include anxiety and depression. Anorexia nervosa is uncommon among old people, though it does occur.

Mouth Disease

Mouth diseases are an uncommon cause of weight loss though neoplastic diseases of the tongue and gingiva tend to present late, at a stage when they can interfere with mastication. Radical surgical resection of such cancers can also lead to problems with mastication and contribute to weight loss. Inflammatory mouth disorders are painful and if not rapidly self-limiting, cause the sufferer to seek relief long before loss of weight occurs. Though almost 90% of people aged over 75 years are edentulous, this alone has not been found to cause malnutrition. However, being edentulous or having inadequate dentures can limit the range of foods which people can eat and interferes with digestion and the pleasure of eating. Salivary gland secretions decrease with age and xerostomia can occasionally interfere with mastication. Severe xerostomia is almost always associated with systemic disease (e.g. Sjogren's syndrome) and especially with the use of drugs with anticholinergic properties (e.g. anti-depressants).

Neuromuscular Disorders of the Pharynx and Oesophagus

The physiological decline in oesophageal and gastric motility that accompanies the ageing process is asymptomatic. The symptom of dysphagia can result from a variety of neurological and muscular diseases which involve the pharyngeal muscles, cricopharyngeus and oesophageal musculature. These disorders constitute an important cause of weight loss among old people. Some 30% of patients have dysphagia in the acute stage after suffering a stroke. This is most likely to occur when the brain-stem territory is involved. In Parkinson's disease, dysphagia is due to difficulty in initiating swallowing together with diminished oesophageal peristalsis. Dysphagia is an early symptom of motor neurone disease, especially when the predominant form is that of progressive bulbar palsy. Achalasia of the cardia is due to dysfunction of the vagus nerve with resultant smooth muscle atrophy, but is seldom found in elderly patients. Diffuse oesophageal spasm is a benign disorder of oesophageal motility which is associated with reflux oesophagitis and presents with dysphagia and chest pain. Globus hystericus is a psychiatric symptom commonly found with anxiety states in the elderly. Patients present with painful dysphagia and other manifestations of an anxiety state are generally seen.

Structural Lesions of the Pharynx and Oesophagus

Pharyngeal and oesophageal carcinoma most commonly present with dysphagia and weight loss. A variety of non-malignant disorders can have a similar presentation. These include a benign oesophageal stricture which follows chronic oesophagitis, an oesophageal web which is associated with iron deficiency anaemia, a pharyngeal pouch and an oesophageal diverticulum.

Nausea and Vomiting

These are discussed in more detail in Chapter 21. Again they can be attributed to gastrointestinal disease, systemic disease and psychological disorders. Iatrogenic causes are important. Opiate drugs and chemotherapeutic agents cause nausea and vomiting together with suppression of appetite.

General Debility

An ability to provide and prepare food for oneself is one of the most basic skills required for leading an independent existence. Loss of weight, therefore, is an early sign of impending inability to cope, due to physical or mental disability. Physical disability may take the form of such conditions as an arthropathy which prevents the person from shopping or from lighting a gas stove – problems which may be easily rectified once they are identified. Mental disability from depression and dementia is even more prevalent as a cause of inability to care for oneself.

Poverty, Ignorance and Isolation

Following retirement the prevalence of poverty increases with increasing age and it is estimated that some 2 million pensioners in Britain live on or below the poverty line. Not surprisingly, poverty is positively correlated with malnutrition and both are more prevalent in countries without welfare assistance. The less nutritious foods are cheaper, causing some people to turn to inadequate foods like bread and jam for sustenance. Others feel financially insecure and fear to spend available money on food. This is further compounded by ignorance of what constitutes an adequate and balanced diet. Widowers unskilled in domestic work are particularly vulnerable, as are those who are socially isolated, the preparation and eating of food being a social event.

The trend for food retail outlets to be concentrated in shopping centres places old people at another disadvantage. Often these are not readily accessible and demand a degree of mobility of the customer as well as visual and mental competence. Food is often packaged in quantities unsuitable for people living alone and without storage and refrigeration facilities. The local "corner shop" which offers personal attention is disappearing, no longer offers a wide range of foods and is relatively expensive.

Nutritional deficiency, however, is not confined to people with inadequate social supports and has been found in various institutions, even when regular meals are provided.

Decreased Digestion and Absorption of Ingested Food

The digestion and absorption of food is particularly dependent on the pancreas and small bowel. Dysfunction of these organs (Table 10.2) is an important cause of weight loss. In addition to weight loss, diarrhoea and steatorrhoea are common findings in all forms of malabsorption, and abdominal distension may be present.

The ability to absorb all elements of the diet can be impaired. Fat malabsorption is confirmed by finding increased quantities excreted in the stools. As stools must be collected for at least 3 consecutive days, during which a fat-rich diet must be consumed, this test may not be feasible for frail elderly people. A ^{14}C-labelled fat when given orally will lead to ^{14}C being excreted in the breath once the fat is absorbed and metabolised. Low levels are excreted when fat absorption is impaired.

This is an easier and more reliable test of fat malabsorption in the elderly person. A xylose absorption test will examine carbohydrate absorption.

Table 10.2. Causes of decreased food digestion and absorption

Pancreatic disease (chronic pancreatitis, carcinoma)
Coeliac disease
Bacterial overgrowth
Inflammatory bowel disease (enteritis, Crohn's disease)
Chronic mesenteric ischaemia
Short bowel syndrome
Congestive cardiac failure
Drugs (broad-spectrum antibiotics, cytotoxic drugs, laxatives, cholestyramine, colchicine)

Pancreatic Disease

Chronic pancreatitis is the commonest cause of steatorrhoea in elderly patients, accounting for some 50% of cases. When a cause is found, alcohol abuse is most often implicated, while undernutrition can be a cause as well as a consequence. The condition may be difficult to diagnose as well as treat. Persistent epigastric or central abdominal pain is suggestive, though the condition can be painless. Chronic diarrhoea and/or steatorrhoea is usually a feature. Non-insulin-dependent diabetes mellitus frequently complicates the picture; frank diabetes or an abnormal glucose tolerance test in a patient with steatorrhoea is highly suggestive of a pancreatic cause. Jaundice is rare. A plain radiograph of the abdomen may show pancreatic calcification and ultrasonography may show structural abnormalities. A pancreatogram can be obtained by endoscopic retrograde choledochopancreatography (ERCP) and may show stones or abnormal dilatation of pancreatic ducts. Pancreatic function tests will show decreased concentrations of amylase and bicarbonate in pancreatic secretions. Treatment consists of analgesia to relieve abdominal pain. Medium-chain fat should replace long-chain fat in the diet, thereby decreasing steatorrhoea and improving nutrition. Pancreatic enzymes should be added to meals to further improve absorption. The addition of H_2 blockers will decrease gastric acid production and minimise enzyme degradation in the stomach. H_2 blockers also minimise the risk of further pancreatic damage.

Slow-growing pancreatic carcinoma is an uncommon cause of malabsorption. Jaundice and abdominal pain which radiates to the back are common features. Ultrasound examination, ERCP and CT scanning are the diagnostic tools of choice. Curative treatment is never feasible though palliative surgery will relieve the jaundice and accompanying pruritus, which is often the most distressing symptom.

Coeliac Disease

Some 5% of all patients with coeliac disease are first diagnosed when over 65 years of age and the condition can present even in extreme old age. The clinical features are often non-specific with weight loss, weakness and bone pain being found more often than steatorrhoea. Anaemia due to iron or folate deficiency is a frequent accompaniment. Diagnosis is by intestinal biopsy and the condition responds to a gluten-free diet. Elderly people often have difficulty in adapting to a new and re-strictive diet, so elimination of gluten from the diet is primarily undertaken for symptom control. With diet symptoms resolve rapidly, while the mucosal abnor-mality may take many months to revert to functional and morphological normal-ity. Nutrient deficiency should therefore be treated, and if a gluten-free diet is not prescribed, supplementation must be for life. Folic acid, calcium and vitamin D are the nutrients most likely to be deficient and supplementation often must be with large doses. As with younger sufferers, an association with dermatitis her-petiformis and with lymphoma of the small bowel is found in old people.

Bacterial Overgrowth

Bacterial overgrowth is among the commoner causes of malabsorption in the elderly. Anatomical abnormalities of the gut allow its contamination by bacteria which are abnormal either in their amount or type. Enteropathic *E. coli* and bacteroides are the commonest offending organisms. The anatomical gut abnor-malities can occur spontaneously (e.g. Crohn's disease or jejunal diverticula) or they may be iatrogenic (e.g. following a "Polya" gastrectomy or gastroenteros-tomy). Small bowel diverticula are found in about 10% of the elderly, but only in a tiny minority are these associated with malabsorption. Bacterial contamination can occur in a morphologically normal gut, especially if gut motility is impaired (e.g. following a vagotomy). Bacteria may colonise an achlorhydric stomach and subsequently spread to the small bowel. The abnormal bacteria degrade bile acids and lead primarily to fat malabsorption. The bacteria also utilise nutrients in the bowel lumen, leading particularly to vitamin B_{12} deficiency. Steatorrhoea and anaemia are therefore common clinical features in addition to weight loss. Bac-teria can produce folic acid, high levels of which are a clue to the diagnosis. Confir-mation depends on culturing pathogenic organisms from a small bowel aspirate. A ^{14}C bile salt breath test indirectly detects bacterial overgrowth. If conjugated bile salts whose amino acid is labelled with ^{14}C are administered orally, abnormal bacteria will deconjugate the bile salts in the small bowel. An abnormal amount of ^{14}C will subsequently be excreted as $^{14}CO_2$ in the breath. While the test is not de-manding on the patient, false negative results are obtained in some 25% of pa-tients. Underlying morphological abnormalities can be demonstrated by barium examination. Treatment is with a broad-spectrum antibiotic such as tetracycline or metronidazole. The condition is likely to recur if any bowel abnormality per-sists and life-long antibiotic therapy may then be required. Alternatively, surgical correction of the abnormality may be appropriate.

Inflammatory Bowel Disease

Inflammatory bowel disease can be of infective or non-infective aetiology. An in-fective cause is by far the commonest and a wide variety of viral, bacterial, fungal and protozoal organisms are enteropathic. Infection is usually acute, transient and self-limiting and weight loss results from dehydration due to vomiting and diarrhoea. However, a protracted course can lead to significant weight loss. This is especially likely to occur with bacterial organisms (e.g. *Campylobacter*, *Shigella*, *Salmonella* and the tubercle bacillus) and with protozoal organisms (e.g.

Giardia lamblia). *Giardia lamblia* occasionally colonise the small bowel and while not always pathogenic, can cause villous atrophy and severe malabsorption. Other parasitic infestations (e.g. ascariasis) compete with the host for nutrients rather than causing malabsorption and are seldom found in Western countries. Enteritis is discussed in more detail in Chap. 11.

Crohn's disease is a non-infective inflammatory disorder of the gastrointestinal tract which predominantly involves the small bowel. It has a bimodal age incidence, the second peak occurring in people aged 60 to 80 years. About half the cases involve the terminal ileum, as in the younger age group, but there are relatively more cases of distal colonic disease in older patients. The clinical features are similar in all age groups with abdominal pain, diarrhoea and anaemia commonly accompanying weight loss. Complications include peritonitis, intestinal obstruction and fistula formation (resulting in bacterial contamination). Diagnosis is most easily made by barium examination of the small bowel. Treatment is identical in all age groups (see Chap. 11). Steroids will suppress inflammation but should be reserved for acute flare-ups. There is doubt regarding the value of sulphasalazine in Crohn's disease confined to the small bowel.

Chronic Mesenteric Ischaemia

Atheromatous disease of the mesenteric vessels causes chronic abdominal pain which is exacerbated by food intake. While weight loss is most often due to decreased food intake in an effort to avoid pain, true malabsorption is probably an additional factor. There is almost always other co-existent vascular disease (in the coronary, cerebral or lower limb vessels). A bruit over a stenosed abdominal vessel may be audible. Mesenteric angiography will demonstrate the extent of the condition, though such investigation is not usually indicated as surgical correction is seldom feasible, the atheromatous disease being widespread. Nutritional supplementation should be given together with advice to take small, frequent meals and thereby avoid post-prandial pain.

Short Bowel Syndrome

Short bowel syndrome is an infrequent cause of malabsorption and results when small bowel resection (especially of the distal portion) has resulted from Crohn's disease or mesenteric ischaemia. Small frequent feeds should be given and as fat malabsorption is a particular problem a low fat diet with medium chain triglyceride is necessary.

Cardiac Failure

With therapeutic advances in heart failure, severe weight loss (cardiac cachexia) is largely of historical interest. However, lesser degrees of weight loss are masked by oedema and the true extent of weight loss is often not apparent until a diuresis has been induced. Congestion of the gastrointestinal tract causes nausea, vomiting and abdominal pain. There is probably an additional contribution to weight loss from malabsorption due to mucosal oedema.

Drugs

Many drugs have the potential to cause malabsorption by damaging the small intestine mucosa, binding bile salts, promoting bacterial overgrowth or by increasing or decreasing intestinal mobility. In practice, however, they appear to be of little clinical importance. Such agents include the broad-spectrum antibiotics, cytotoxic agents, laxatives, cholestyramine and colchicine.

Increased Energy Requirements

A variety of diseases have metabolic effects that result in a catabolic state, causing weight loss. Such diseases are listed in Table 10.3.

Table 10.3.   Causes of increased energy requirements

Malignant disease
Chronic infective illnesses (e.g. tuberculosis, lung abscess, bronchiectasis)
Hyperthyroidism
Diabetes mellitus

Malignant Disease

While weight loss is obvious in many patients with end-stage malignancy, significant loss has been documented in almost half of those sufferers without advanced disease. Wasting is an important feature as it has been shown that survival times are more than halved in undernourished cancerous patients when compared with similar people who are well nourished.

As already mentioned, the weight loss of malignant disease is usually due, at least in part, to decreased food intake and absorption. However, many tumours cause profound metabolic effects which contribute to cachexia. With some tumours, the degree of weight loss can be attributed to a large tumour bulk. The fact that some tumours can "consume" quantities of glucose sufficient to render the patient hypoglycaemic has been well documented. However, such tumours are uncommon and severe cachexia occurs in patients in whom the tumour bulk is small. This implies the presence of humoral agents with catabolic properties and such agents are being increasingly identified. In the case of non-pancreatic tumours causing hypoglycaemia, abnormal proteins with insulin-like activity have been found. Alteration in hepatic gluconeogenesis and glycogenolysis has been demonstrated with such cancers. Pancreatic tumours can secrete an array of peptides such as vaso-active intestinal peptide (VIP) which causes the Verner–Morrison syndrome. Cachectin, or tumour necrosis factor, is a polypeptide hormone secreted by macrophages in the presence of tumour. It has metabolic effects especially in relation to lipid metabolism which contribute to weight loss.

Unexplained weight loss in an individual suggests the presence of an occult carcinoma. The most likely sites are the gastrointestinal tract, pancreas and liver, though lymphoma is also a likely cause.

Infective Illnesses

The mechanisms whereby infective disease causes weight loss are very similar to the mechanisms in malignant disease. Again, many factors are involved and cachexia can be due to the parasite load or to humoral mechanisms. Cachectin is among the humoral factors implicated. Infections most likely to cause protein and fat catabolism include chronic sepsis as found with a lung abscess or bronchiectasis. Tuberculosis is an important cause, especially in the older person and in people from ethnic minority groups.

Hyperthyroidism

Hyperthyroidism in the elderly patient more often occurs in a multi-nodular goitre (Plummer's disease) or in a uni-nodular goitre than in a diffusely enlarged goitre (Graves' disease). The presentation in the older person may be atypical with symptoms often referable to a single system only. Thus, unexplained atrial fibrillation is found to be due to thyrotoxicosis in some 10% of patients. Symptoms of angina pectoris may appear or existing angina may become more symptomatic. Weight loss is common and may be associated with anorexia rather than the increase in appetite which characterises hyperthyroidism in younger patients. Diarrhoea is less often a feature and constipation is more prevalent. Tremor may be present, but can be mistaken for the "senile" tremor which is commonly seen in old people. Signs of dysthyroid eye disease are conspicuous by their absence. Anxiety and hyperactivity are again less commonly found in the elderly patient. Indeed "apathetic hyperthyroidism" is found almost exclusively in old age. This form of thyrotoxicosis more closely resembles hypothyroidism in so far as inactivity and depression are the outstanding features.

Radioactive iodine therapy is the treatment of choice for hyperthyroidism in elderly people as it is highly effective, easy to administer and free of serious side effects. As it may take 4 to 6 weeks for a euthyroid state to be achieved; antithyroid drugs may be required in the interim. Physicians increasingly favour giving a higher dose than that given to younger people to ensure rapid and sustained control. This results in a much higher incidence of iatrogenic hypothyroidism which is easily controlled with thyroxine. It is essential to follow up patients for life following radioactive iodine therapy so that hypothyroidism, should it arise, is detected and treated.

Diabetes Mellitus

Over 15% of people aged 65 years, and over 25% of those over 85 years, are known diabetics. There is a preponderance of female sufferers. Due to increased longevity, increasing obesity and improved medical surveillance, the prevalence of known diabetes among the old is steadily rising. Non-insulin-dependent diabetes predominates and this is often asymptomatic. When symptoms arise, they are often related to microvascular complications (e.g. peripheral and autonomic neuropathy). Obesity is by far the commonest nutritional disorder. Occasionally, however, diabetes in old age presents in the same aggressive manner that typifies insulin-dependent diabetes in a younger patient, with polyuria and polydipsia, lethargy, pruritus vulvae and weight loss. Diabetes mellitus is therefore an important differential diagnosis of weight loss in people of all ages and must always be considered. Weight loss when it occurs, is due to fat and water depletion.

Attempts to achieve tight metabolic control, thereby minimising the risk of long-term diabetic complications, are often inappropriate for the older patient, especially if such measures put the person at risk from life-threatening hypoglycaemia. Dietary modification is the cornerstone of treatment, with the addition of an oral hypoglycaemic agent when this alone fails to achieve adequate control. Dietary advice must be practical and relate to the patient's current habits, formed over a life-time. Sulphonylureas are considered relatively safe oral hypoglycaemic agents, but can cause life-threatening hypoglycaemia even when taken in small doses. A biguanide (i.e. metformin) is appropriate for obese patients and is less likely to cause hypoglycaemia than a sulphonamide but can cause lactic acidosis in patients with impaired renal, hepatic or cardiac function. Combinations of metformin and a sulphonylurea may improve diabetic control where either alone is unsatisfactory. When insulin is required, it is usually feasible to achieve adequate control with a single daily dose of a medium- or long-acting preparation.

Clinical Evaluation

An extreme degree of weight loss is all too obvious (Fig. 10.1). However, less obvious loss can often be neglected both by the patient and his doctor. The labels of marasmus and kwashiorkor can be applied to the elderly malnourished patient as they can be to malnourished children. With the former, inadequate intake of both protein and calories results in decreased protein and fat stores. Patients appear wasted, but serum protein and immune function are preserved. With kwashiorkor, on the other hand, protein deficiency is accompanied by adequate caloric intake. Such patients appear normal or possibly obese and their malnutrition is easily overlooked. Oedema results from low serum proteins, further increasing the impression of obesity. Impaired immune function puts these people at risk of sepsis, especially if they become stressed by intercurrent illness or surgery.

People are often aware of even minor degrees of weight loss. Many weigh themselves regularly or notice when clothes become ill-fitting. Rings worn on the fingers may become loose. Weight loss which is rapid is more likely to be noted and to be reported. However, with some, especially those living alone, even gross weight loss may be ignored, the problem being noticed by relatives or friends who have not seen the person for some time.

An adequate nutritional assessment can be obtained from the majority of patients within a few minutes. Leading questions should be asked regarding the frequency with which cooked meals, meat, vegetables and fresh fruit are eaten. An assessment of the amount taken at each meal should be made, though such information is often unreliable. The source of the food should be noted as people are more likely to eat when they themselves or their family prepare rather than what is provided in day centres or by Meals-on-Wheels.

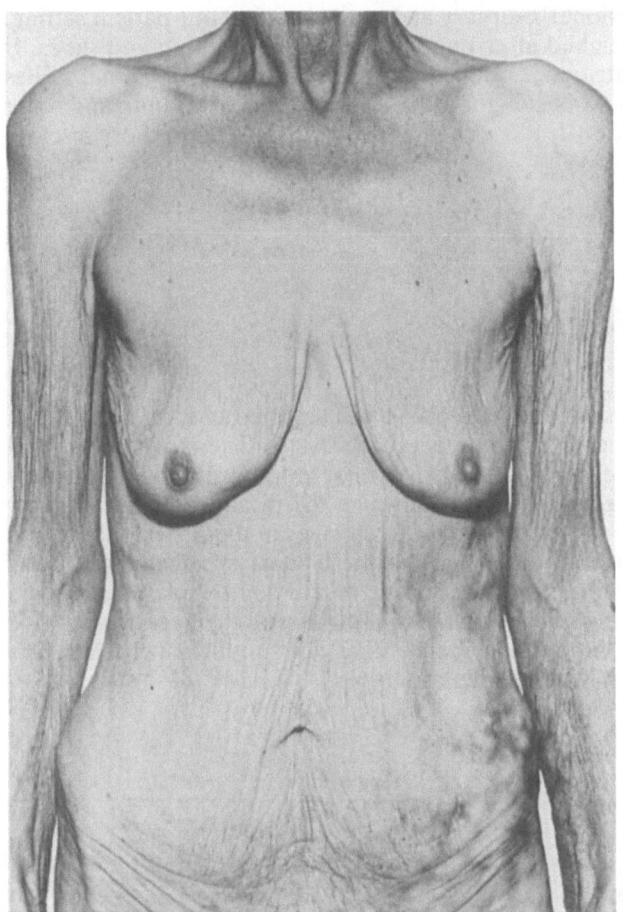

Fig. 10.1. Marasmus: protein and calorie malnutrition.

All aspects of the history are important. Other presenting complaints such as pain typical of peptic ulceration can immediately suggest the source of the weight loss. The past history, for example, may reveal that the patient had a gastrectomy years earlier. The social history should concern itself with the person's financial status and degree of social integration. The drug history should deal specifically with drugs known to cause weight loss, including nicotine and alcohol. The systems review must be thorough and seek associated symptoms of diseases causing weight loss. An assessment of the mental state and a functional assessment in relation to activities of daily living are also of importance.

Objective evidence of loss of weight is indicated by the presence of lax skinfolds, especially on the abdominal wall. Measurements of the body mass index (height/weight^2), mid-arm circumference and triceps skin-fold thickness indicate undernutrition, but are unsuitable for routine clinical use. The simplest and most valuable recording is that of serial weights and these should be recorded regularly both in the general practitioner's surgery and in the hospital out-patient setting. The patient should be weighed after removing all heavy clothing and shoes. If there are signs of undernutrition, evidence of hypoproteinaemia (oedema, ascites and pleural effusion) should be sought together with signs of vitamin and other nutrient deficiencies. Obviously a search must be made for signs of those diseases resulting in weight loss.

Management of Weight Loss

In the first instance the cause of weight loss must be identified and, where possible, underlying factors reversed. This alone is not always sufficient and nutritional supplementation may be required as a short-term or long-term measure. As with all forms of treatment the benefits must outweigh the disadvantages and many people, but especially the old, are resistant to changes in dietary habits formed over many years. Such procedures as naso-gastric feeding are even more likely to be resisted. Particular problems arise with nutritional supplementation in cancerous patients as there is a fear that the tumour as well as the patient may be fed, although the limited available evidence does not support such fears. The available forms of nutritional supplementation are:

Oral supplementation
Enteral nutrition
Parenteral nutrition

Oral Supplementation

The advice required by the individual patient depends on the particular deficiency present. Thus the patient may need calories, protein, vitamins, minerals or a combination of these. With regard to protein and calorie supplementation, various commercial preparations are available and come in all shapes and sizes. Usually, however, meals can be prepared from "ordinary foodstuffs". Food may need to be given in semi-liquid form when a patient has dysphagia. The advice and follow-up of a dietician may be invaluable. Follow-up is often essential in the case of vitamin and mineral supplementation as there is a potential risk of toxicity if it continues after the deficiency has been corrected. As already mentioned it may be necessary to continue supplementation for life (as in the case of coeliac disease where a gluten-free diet is not prescribed).

Enteral Nutrition

Enteral nutrition is primarily used in the convalescent phase of acute illness and is usually carried out in hospital, though home enteral nutrition is feasible. It is used either to provide total nutrition or for nutritional supplementation and can only

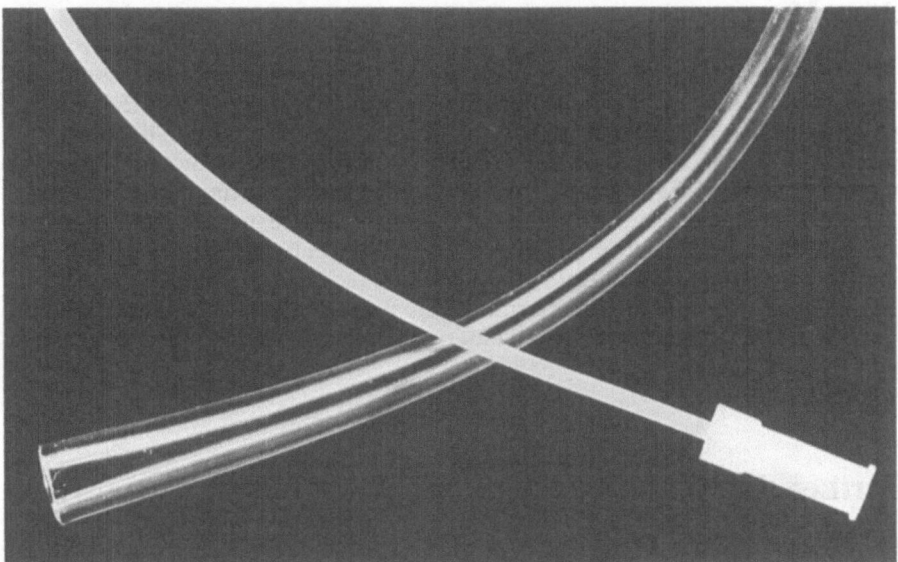

Fig. 10.2.   A fine bore naso-gastric tube and a wider bore Rhyle's tube.

be used when the gastrointestinal tract is functioning normally. Fine bore naso-gastric tubes have become increasingly popular as they are less obtrusive and less likely to cause complications than the wide bore Rhyle's tube (Fig. 10.2). These are generally easy to insert and cause little discomfort. Food is given in liquid form. Several proprietary preparations are available or specific formulations can be made up for an individual patient following dietetic assessment. Liquid whole protein preparations are cheaper than oligopeptides and amino acids, but the latter are more readily absorbed by a diseased bowel. Complications include aspiration (with or without the tube being correctly sited), gastric retention and diarrhoea. The latter is the most common problem and can be overcome by giving dilute feeds initially and thereafter by gradually increasing the concentration of the feeds. Continuous feeding through the tube rather than giving bolus feeds also lessens the tendency to diarrhoea. This is particularly convenient when used at night while the patient is asleep.

Parenteral Nutrition

Parenteral nutrition is used when the gastrointestinal tract is not functioning normally. Its main role is in the early stages following abdominal surgery, though ambulatory home parenteral nutrition is feasible for people with long-term bowel dysfunction. A catheter is inserted into a large vein, usually the superior vena cava. Complications result from catheter sepsis, catheter fracture, venous thrombosis, air embolism, fluid overload and malpositioning of the catheter.

Other Measures

It is probable that improvement in the financial status of elderly people would lead
to improved nutrition. Financial benefits are available for people in Britain who
have medical problems requiring special diets (e.g. peptic ulcer and diabetes mellitus). The improvement of services such as Meals-on-Wheels and improving the
nutritional content of the meals provided should also lead to improved nutritional
status. Increased provision of day centres where meals are provided and improved
access to such centres are other areas where improvement of services is possible.
Some people would benefit from better cooking facilities at home.

Preventive medicine has an enormous role to play in the field of nutrition but,
sadly, provision of dietary advice to elderly people and their carers is a neglected
field.

Further Reading

Hellemans J, Vantrappen G (eds) (1984) Gastro-intestinal tract disorders in the elderly. Churchill
    Livingstone, Edinburgh
Young EA (ed) (1986) Nutrition, ageing and health. Alan R Liss, New York

Chapter 11

Constipation and Diarrhoea

Jane Bradshaw

A normal bowel action has been defined as the passage of stool between three times per day and three times per week. With a Western diet the stool weighs on average 100–200 g of which 60%–85% is water. An increase in the final volume of water in the stool of 100 ml or so is enough to produce looseness, whilst a reduction in water content produces hardness. Constipation may be defined as having a bowel action less frequently than three times per week and/or passing hard motions with a reduced water content. Diarrhoea similarly may be described as having a bowel action more frequently than three times per day and/or passing loose motions with an increased water content.

Constipation has long been recognised as a problem of old age. In the tenth century, Avicenna recommended "food with a laxative action" as being most appropriate for the elderly and advocated that they should, if necessary "get their bowels opened gently" with the aid of an "unctuous enema". An up-to-date indication of the prevalence of the problem can be obtained by the frequency with which laxatives are prescribed; one recent study reported that 73% of long-stay hospital patients were prescribed laxatives on a regular basis. Constipation refractory to oral bulking agents or softeners is a problem familiar to all who regularly treat old people.

Diarrhoea is a less common problem in old age, but may be more socially disabling if the individual becomes faecally incontinent as a result. Spurious diarrhoea, faecal impaction with overflow or excessive purgation may be the underlying cause, but a wide variety of other conditions, including malabsorption and inflammatory bowel disease may also be implicated. Acute diarrhoea may cause profound constitutional disturbance and electrolyte imbalance, resulting in dehydration and confusion in elderly patients.

Constipation

The underlying causes of constipation are listed in Table 11.1. While it is commonly attributable to local disorders, underlying systemic causes should not be forgotten.

Table 11.1. Causes of constipation in old people

Motility disorders (cathartic bowel, ignoring call to stool, immobility, low fibre diet, reduced fluid
    intake, irritable bowel syndrome)
Intestinal obstruction (hypokalaemia, carcinoma)
Endocrine disorders (myxoedema, diabetes mellitus)
Metabolic disorders (hypercalcaemia)
Drugs (digoxin, diuretics, antidepressants, anticholinergic agents, opiates)
Neurological disorders (autonomic neuropathy, multiple sclerosis, paraplegia, depression)

Motility Disorders

Motility disorders are of primary importance among old people. Many have been
brought up in the belief that a daily bowel action is essential to their general well-
being and this may have led to the regular use of purgatives (e.g. liquid paraffin,
phenolphthalein and senna). Long-standing purgative abuse inevitably leads to
the *cathartic bowel*, which is atonic and unable to evacuate without stimulation. In
some patients pigments are laid down in the rectal mucosa leading to melanosis
coli, visible on sigmoidoscopy and which, if necessary, can be confirmed by rectal
biopsy.

The majority of patients with a natural bowel action experience the need to defaecate in the early morning or after the first meal of the day. *Ignoring the call to
stool* because of immobility or inconvenience suppresses this gastro-colic reflex.
In time, this leads to blunting of the urge to defaecate following rectal filling and
tolerance of a full rectum.

Constipation is uncommon in those who take regular exercise. Activity and
exercise appear to promote intestinal transit and a regular bowel habit. *Immobility* on the other hand has a tendency to cause constipation even in those individuals with a previously normal bowel habit. Patients who become temporarily
immobile or bed-ridden as a result of injury or illness are particularly prone to
constipation. The relatively immobile patient who is restricted because of joint
disease, neurological disease or general frailty also suffers.

Elderly people with mobility problems may deliberately restrict *fluid intake* in
order to reduce the number of visits to the lavatory. As the stool has a high water
content, restricting fluid intake inevitably reduces its volume, resulting in smaller,
harder motions. *Diet* may also be deficient in fibre in the elderly, who may rely on
convenience food for ease of preparation and consequently neglect fresh fruit and
vegetables. Foods with a higher roughage content may be too difficult to eat with
dentures, whilst fruit and wholemeal bread may be avoided because of cost and
poorer keeping qualities than white bread or tinned produce.

Intestinal Obstruction

Severe *hypokalaemia* can lead to paralytic ileus (adynamic obstruction) with abdominal distension, absent or tinkling bowel sounds, constipation and the absence
of flatus. Hypokalaemia may develop gradually following prolonged diuretic
usage and inadequate potassium replacement or acutely in patients with diarrhoea
or vomiting. Other causes include intestinal fistulae, increased urinary loss,
anorexia nervosa and persistent purgative abuse. Patients with severe

hypokalaemia experience generalised muscular weakness and there may be other associated features such as depression of reflexes, cardiac and ECG abnormalities and mental confusion.

The diagnosis is confirmed by the presence of fluid levels on supine and decubitus X-ray films of the abdomen. Treatment consists of reversal of the underlying cause. Until the condition resolves, an adynamic bowel must be rested, using a "drip and suck" regime.

Colorectal Carcinoma

Colorectal carcinoma may present with either constipation or diarrhoea. Other features commonly seen in old age include abdominal pain, weight loss, anorexia, vomiting, anaemia and an abdominal mass. A small proportion of patients present with intestinal obstruction. Elderly people with a rectal tumour may have rectal bleeding, though tenesmus is uncommon.

If a carcinoma is suspected, faeces should be tested for occult blood and sigmoidoscopy (with biopsy of suspicious lesions) and barium enema should be performed. If surgical intervention is contemplated liver function tests and ultrasound scanning of the liver should be carried out to detect the presence of hepatic metastases. Abdominal ultrasound may also reveal enlarged para-aortic lymph nodes.

Patients who are referred to a geriatrician rather than to a surgeon are more likely to present with constipation, anorexia, vomiting or an abdominal mass and are less likely to have the classical symptoms of intestinal obstruction. Such patients present at a later stage and are less likely to be suitable for surgical intervention. Thus, only 32% of geriatric patients have a curative resection for colonic or rectal carcinoma, while almost half the patients are unfit for any kind of operation at the time of diagnosis. For patients with advanced disease but who are fit for surgery, palliative procedures such as defunctioning colostomy, by-pass or palliative resection may be considered to relieve or minimise future symptoms. The incidence of post-operative complications and mortality is high, necessitating careful pre-operative patient selection.

Endocrine Disorders

Endocrine disorders should not be overlooked in the elderly patient with bowel dysfunction. *Myxoedema* is the commonest endocrine cause of constipation in this age group. The classical facies of a pink and white complexion, puffiness, loss of the outer third of the eyebrows and sparse, dry hair are of little diagnostic value in older patients, but other features such as a hoarse voice, cold intolerance, tiredness, bradycardia and anaemia in an obese patient should arouse suspicion. Other symptoms such as depression, apathy and carpal tunnel syndrome may also point to the diagnosis. In view of the unreliability of clinical signs, thyroid function tests should be performed if there is the least suspicion of myxoedema.

Constipation in old people is sometimes attributed to *diabetes mellitus*, but as both conditions are common the relationship may be casual rather than causal. Long-standing diabetic patients may develop an autonomic neuropathy. Its distribution is often patchy, but if the autonomic innervation of the gastrointestinal tract is affected and gastrointestinal motility becomes impaired, constipation or diarrhoea may result. Other evidence of autonomic neuropathy includes the loss of control of sweating, a fixed heart rate and postural hypotension.

Primary *hyperparathyroidism* is being recognised with increasing frequency in old age, probably as a result of more frequent routine measurement of plasma calcium. Hypercalcaemia is frequently an incidental finding in an asymptomatic patient, but otherwise non-specific symptoms predominate in old people with constipation, muscle weakness, tiredness, general malaise and cerebral impairment being the commonest features. Other symptoms include polyuria, itching and headache. Less frequently, the elderly patient presents with the long-term complications of hypercalcaemia – hypertension, peptic ulceration, pancreatitis, renal stones and bone disease. In neoplastic disease the presentation is generally more abrupt and constipation is not a major feature.

Neurological Disorders

Constipation is common in patients with impaired mobility secondary to neurological disease such as stroke or Parkinson's disease (see Chap. 15). In such individuals it should be anticipated and actively treated. Patients with multiple sclerosis may also be subject to profound constipation.

Spinal cord lesions may present initially with sphincter disturbances – constipation and urinary retention. These may precede symptoms or signs in the lower limbs. If rectal examination reveals absent sphincter tone and an anaesthetic perineum, cord compression should be suspected. Spinal radiography, bone biochemistry and an urgent myelogram must be performed and if cord compression is confirmed, surgical intervention must be undertaken within 24 hours to avoid a permanent neurological deficit. It should not be assumed that cord compression in an elderly patient is due to metastatic disease, as a benign spinal tumour or a prolapsed intervertebral disc may be the cause.

Depression

Some elderly patients with depression present with somatic rather than psychiatric symptoms, and complaints of anorexia, weight loss and constipation are not uncommon. Numerous unnecessary investigations may be undertaken before depression is diagnosed. However, depression may be a feature of other disease such as myxoedema and primary hyperparathyroidism, which may also cause constipation.

Drugs

Many drugs cause constipation in the elderly. Diuretics will tend to reduce the volume of water in stool, resulting in smaller, harder motions, whilst drugs acting on the nervous system may also affect gastrointestinal motility and predispose to constipation. Aluminium-containing antacids and drugs containing codeine will constipate, whilst nearly all patients on opiates will require laxatives – an important point in the management of terminal care patients (see Chap. 26).

Diarrhoea

The principal causes of diarrhoea are given in Table 11.2. As with constipation the causes can be classified as primarily bowel disorders or systemic disorders. The primary bowel disorders may predominantly involve the small or the large bowel.

Table 11.2. Causes of diarrhoea in old people

Dietary indiscretion
Infection (viral, bacterial, protozoal)
Drug induced
Endocrine disorder (thyrotoxicosis, Addison's disease, diabetes)
Irritable bowel syndrome
Malabsorption (see Table 10.2)
Large bowel disease (diverticular disease, colorectal carcinoma, ulcerative colitis, Crohn's colitis, faecal impaction)
Surgical problems (gastrectomy, blind loops, intestinal fistulae)
Radiation

Note: Diverticular disease, colorectal carcinoma, ulcerative colitis, Crohn's colitis, ischaemic colitis and pseudomembranous colitis can cause bloody diarrhoea.

Infective Diarrhoea

Infective diarrhoea can be due to viral, bacterial or protozoal organisms. It is generally of acute onset and of limited duration, the majority of patients recovering within 48 hours. Bacterial infections (especially with *Shigella* and *Campylobacter*) may run a prolonged course. Patients with *Campylobacter* enteritis may experience severe abdominal pain mimicking acute appendicitis or other surgical emergencies. Stool samples should be sent for microscopic examination and culture. Blood cultures may be necessary in severely affected patients with possible septicaemia.

The majority of infections are self-limiting and require no specific treatment, but if diarrhoea and vomiting is prolonged, patients may require intravenous rehydration and correction of electrolyte disturbance. Antibiotics should be avoided as there is evidence that they may prolong the carrier state. Exceptions to this rule are severe cases of *Campylobacter* diarrhoea, which may require treatment with erythromycin or tetracycline, and extreme cases of shigellosis which may be treated with ampicillin or co-trimoxazole. In institutionalised patients attempts should be made to locate the source of infection. Infected patients should be barrier-nursed to reduce the risk of spread.

Irritable Bowel Syndrome

Patients typically complain of alternating diarrhoea and constipation with or without abdominal pain or distension. Not infrequently the patient may complain only of "bouts of diarrhoea" or "bouts of constipation" with a relatively normal bowel habit at other times. Motions may be described at times as "ribbons" or "rabbity pellets". Patients will usually describe having several bowel actions in the morning with no further bowel action until the next day. There is no accompanying weight loss.

The condition can usually be confidently diagnosed on the clinical history with the confirmatory evidence of a normal blood count and ESR. Further investigations are unnecessary unless the diagnosis is in doubt. With regard to management, dietary advice on increasing fibre and reducing refined sugars, explanation and reassurance may be all that is required. However many patients will continue to experience abdominal pain and require an antispasmodic. The most effective of these is mebeverine, but dicyclomine, mepenzolate or enteric-coated peppermint oil may be of benefit in some patients.

Malabsorption

The most common causes of malabsorption in the elderly are bacterial overgrowth, pancreatic insufficiency, coeliac disease and post-gastrectomy syndrome. These are discussed in Chapter 10. While classical steatorrhoea is often described, patients may complain merely of frequent, poorly formed stools. Wind and abdominal distension, due to gas-forming organisms acting on the undigested food in the bowel, frequently accompany the diarrhoea. Weight loss, bone pains and abdominal pain are also common. The elderly may present with non-specific features of generalised ill-health such as mental deterioration, "going off their legs" or chest infection.

The management of malabsorption-associated diarrhoea depends on the underlying cause. A gluten-free diet in coeliac disease and enzyme supplementation in pancreatic insufficiency will improve the problem. Steatorrhoea due to bacterial overgrowth responds well to metronidazole, though repeated courses or even life-long treatment may be required. Medium chain triglycerides may be useful in reducing steatorrhoea in biliary obstruction as these are transported unchanged across mucosal epithelial cells and do not require the presence of bile salts.

Diverticular Disease

Diverticular disease increases in prevalence with increasing age. In many elderly people it is asymptomatic and it may co-exist with other bowel diseases, causing diagnostic confusion. Symptomatic patients may present with episodic diarrhoea, abdominal pain, nausea, vomiting and constitutional upset. Pyrexia, tenderness of the sigmoid colon and a palpable mass may be evident when diverticulae become acutely inflamed (diverticulitis).

Diverticulosis is best treated by a high-fibre diet and oral bulking agents; some patients may, in addition, require an antispasmodic such as mebeverine. Diverticulitis may require antibiotic treatment, low residue diet and bed rest until the pyrexia and pain subsides. Thereafter, the management is as for diverticulosis.

Inflammatory Bowel Disease

Crohn's disease may affect any part of the gastrointestinal tract, from mouth to anus. Ulcerative colitis is predominantly a disease of the large bowel though the terminal part of the ileum may be involved in patients with pancolitis. It may be difficult to differentiate between colonic Crohn's disease, ulcerative colitis and ischaemic colitis at presentation, as bloody diarrhoea and abdominal pain are symptoms common to each condition.

Patients with Crohn's disease generally have lost weight and there may be associated features of an abdominal mass, perianal skin tags or fistulae, whilst the rectum may be normal on sigmoidoscopy; rectal bleeding is a less common finding. In ulcerative colitis, the rectum is always involved with the disease extending proximally to a variable extent. There may be a previous history of sacroileitis, iritis or pyoderma gangrenosum. The need to defaecate at night is an important diagnostic pointer to large bowel pathology. With ischaemic colitis, bleeding predominates and abdominal pain may become generalised. There is debate as to whether inflammatory bowel disease runs a more aggressive or benign course in old people. It is likely that whilst the disease itself is no more aggressive, the risk of death as a result of complications such as toxic megacolon, gangrene or bowel stricture is greater because of a higher operative mortality in the older patient. The activity of bowel inflammation should be monitored by sigmoidoscopy, haemoglobin, serum albumin and inflammatory indices (e.g. ESR and serum alpha$_1$ acid glycoprotein).

There are three major facets to the treatment of inflammatory bowel disease. Firstly, symptomatic control of diarrhoea, secondly, reduction of inflammation and induction of disease remission and thirdly, maintenance of remission. Codeine phosphate or loperamide are useful in controlling diarrhoea but will not affect the degree of disease activity. Corticosteroids are used to treat active inflammation in both Crohn's disease and ulcerative colitis. These may be given topically by retention enemas or orally for widespread disease or acute exacerbations. In the case of ulcerative colitis, remission is maintained by sulphasalazine (SZP). This drug is also useful in Crohn's colitis, though it is not effective in Crohn's disease of the small bowel. The elderly may be unable to tolerate the highest recommended dosage of 3 g/day and SZP should not be used if there is a history of sulphonamide or aspirin sensitivity. New preparations exist for delivering salicylate to the large bowel, e.g. mesalazine. These are effective, but should not be used in patients with known allergy to aspirin. Severe attacks require intravenous corticosteroids, bed rest, parenteral nutrition and close monitoring for the development of toxic megacolon or perforation. Small bowel Crohn's disease usually requires treatment with oral steroids, sometimes combined with azathioprine for its "steroid-sparing" effect.

The major indications for surgery in ulcerative colitis are panproctocolitis with severe unremitting symptoms or the development of toxic megacolon. The latter should be suspected in an ill colitic patient with increasing abdominal distension whose diarrhoea suddenly stops. Daily abdominal radiography may be required to monitor the diameter of the colon and the development of a toxic megacolon must be considered a surgical emergency. Fortunately, this is rarely seen in elderly patients.

Crohn's patients may require surgery for small bowel strictures leading to obstruction or fistulae. Elderly patients with colonic Crohn's disease rarely require operation.

Faecal Impaction with Overflow

This is probably the commonest reason for faecal soiling and faecal incontinence in old people and it should be suspected in all immobile or institutionalised patients. It is not uncommon for elderly patients who complain of diarrhoea to be administered constipating agents without a rectal examination being first performed to exclude faecal impaction. Urinary incontinence frequently co-exists and there may be a history of increasing confusion and loss of mobility. Plain radiographic examination of the abdomen may reveal the extent of faecal loading.

Villous Adenoma

Villous adenoma of the large bowel classically presents with watery diarrhoea and in old people, may lead to faecal incontinence. The tumour may be palpated on rectal examination and biopsied at sigmoidoscopy. Villous adenomata may be entirely benign or areas of malignant change may be found. It is important to distinguish between a villous adenoma and carcinoma as the former may be amenable to a lesser surgical procedure.

Drugs

Antibiotics are the most commonly offending agents, both in general practice and in hospital, with ampicillin and amoxycillin being most frequently implicated. Antibiotic-associated diarrhoea usually resolves spontaneously within a few days of withdrawing the offending drug, but if the diarrhoea is prolonged and the patient generally unwell, *pseudomembranous colitis* should be suspected. This may be caused by a variety of antibiotics (including lincomycin, clindamycin, ampicillin, tetracycline and chloramphenicol) which suppress normal bowel flora and allow the overgrowth of *Clostridium difficile*. A membrane is not always visible on sigmoidoscopy and stools should therefore be cultured for the clostridial organism. It is best treated with *oral* vancomycin 500 mg t.d.s. Patients require supportive treatment and close observation for signs of the development of toxic megacolon.

Excessive purgative consumption should also be considered in the older patient with diarrhoea. Magnesium, a common constituent of antacid preparations, has a laxative effect.

Endocrine Disorders

Diarrhoea is rarely seen in elderly patients with thyrotoxicosis or Addison's disease. Diabetic patients with an autonomic neuropathy may experience either diarrhoea or constipation as a result of impaired gastrointestinal motility.

Clinical Evaluation

It is important to determine what people mean when they complain of disordered bowel habit. Some people consider themselves to be constipated unless they defaecate daily and what is diarrhoea to some may be considered normal by others. By constipation most patients mean the passage of hard motions and the need to strain at stool. They may complain of the sensation of incomplete evacuation and resort to manual evacuation of the bowel. The feeling of incomplete evacuation does not necessarily imply the retention of faecal masses within the rectum – continued straining may result in the anterior rectal mucosa bulging into the rectum, giving the sensation of a mass.

The frequency and timing of bowel action, stool consistency and need to strain at stool should be documented. It is important to note whether there has been a change in the frequency of defaecation. Enquiry should be made whether blood or mucus has been noted in the stool and patients should be asked whether they have experienced black motions (melaena) or very pale motions. They may describe the bulky, putty-coloured motions of steatorrhoea. These tend to be loose or liquid stools which characteristically float and are difficult to flush away. Symptoms (e.g. pain) accompanying defaecation should be noted. The site and timing of pain in relation to defaecation should be ascertained.

Other aspects of the history are also important, none more so than the drug history. Many substances can disrupt bowel habit (see below). In addition to prescribed medication, enquire about "over the counter" preparations. An assessment of the person's psyche is an important part of the history taking. Depressive illnesses, anxiety and obsessive neurosis often present with symptoms of bowel dysfunction. Symptoms of systemic disorders which can affect bowel habit (e.g. thyroid dysfunction) should also be sought.

An abdominal and rectal examination is obviously mandatory. Remember that faecal impaction is the commonest cause of faecal incontinence in old age. On rectal examination, the anal tone and sphincter competence should be assessed. Proctoscopy and sigmoidoscopy can usually be performed in the out-patients department or general practitioner's surgery as prior preparation is often unnecessary. General medical examination may reveal an underlying cause of bowel dysfunction.

Management

The general principles of management of constipation and diarrhoea may be applied whatever the underlying condition. Where possible, however, any underlying cause or exacerbating factor should be identified and reversed.

Constipation

Mild degrees of constipation are best treated by increasing the fibre content of the diet and ensuring an adequate fluid intake. Elderly people are often reluctant to alter their dietary habits and it may not be possible to do more than persuade them to take a bran-containing breakfast cereal or bran-enriched porridge and wholemeal bread. Extra fibre can be given by prescribing ispaghula, methylcellulose or sterculia granules. These are effective bulking agents, but palatability may limit compliance. Lactulose, however, is well-tolerated in the elderly. It is an inert disaccharide which osmotically draws water into the stool, softening it and increasing bulk. It may lead to by-passing of retained faecal masses if these are not otherwise dealt with.

Hard stools may be softened by dioctyl sodium sulphosuccinate which may also promote bowel evacuation.

Institutionalised and poorly mobile patients may achieve adequate stool consistency by these methods, but effective defaecation may not occur, leading to a rectum full of soft faeces and seepage. The treatment of choice here is bisacodyl, either as a suppository or in tablet form. This stimulates intestinal motility and defaecation. Other stimulant laxatives (e.g. senna, cascara), should not be used as these eventually lead to an atonic colon and hypokalaemia.

Faecal loading and faecal impaction require more intensive measures. Regular phosphate enemas should be administered until the bowel is clear and oral bulking agents should be given on a regular basis thereafter. If the patient remains unable to evacuate the bowel it may be necessary to give regular phosphate enemas once or twice a week (see Chap. 12). Golytely (polyethylene glycol and sodium sulphate) is recommended as a pre-operative preparation for colonoscopy and has been used successfully in a trial of treatment of faecal impaction in the elderly.

People with chronic laxative abuse may have recurrent hospital admissions for subacute obstruction and hypokalaemia. Once the acute problem has been dealt with by intravenous administration of potassium-containing solutions and bowel clearance, regular oral potassium supplements may be required to prevent the hypokalaemia recurring. The urea and electrolytes should be monitored to ensure that the plasma potassium remains within normal limits.

In some cases (e.g. myxoedema), the constipation may improve when the underlying condition is treated, whilst in others, the constipation must be adequately controlled to prevent the patient's general condition worsening (e.g. hypercalcaemia). In patients with multiple sclerosis or paraplegia little benefit is obtained from bulking agents and it is better to achieve regular evacuation by means of stool softeners (dioctyl) and phosphate enemas, once or twice a week.

Diarrhoea

Acute diarrhoea may result in dehydration and confusion in elderly patients. Sodium or potassium loss may be excessive and early correction of electrolytes and adequate fluid replacement is essential. In infective diarrhoea water and electrolyte depletion is due to selective blocking of sodium absorption pathways in the small bowel by toxins which spare glucose-coupled sodium absorption. Oral glucose and electrolyte solutions may therefore be of use in promoting sodium and water absorption via this glucose-dependent pathway. Such solutions should also contain potassium and suitable bases, such as chloride and bicarbonate. If adequate rehydration cannot be achieved orally, intravenous rehydration and electrolyte correction will be required, but strict monitoring of fluid balance must be observed to avoid fluid overload and hyponatraemia.

There are four categories of antidiarrhoeal agents available for symptom control:

agents that absorb water (e.g. ispaghula, methylcellulose, sterculia)

agents that adsorb toxins (kaolin, chalk, activated charcoal)

agents that alter electrolyte transport or secretion (e.g. glucose–electrolyte solutions, loperamide, morphine, sulphasalazine)

agents altering intestinal motility (codeine phosphate, diphenoxylate–atropine, loperamide)

Codeine phosphate or loperamide are the drugs of choice in acute diarrhoea. Adsorbants such as kaolin are of little proven benefit. Diphenoxylate-atropine is less effective than either codeine phosphate or loperamide and may cause undesirable side effects in old people. Drugs altering intestinal motility may increase the abdominal pain of patients with irritable bowel or diverticular disease. Such patients are best treated with ispaghula, methylcellulose or sterculia.

Beware of prescribing for symptomatic control without adequate investigation and diagnosis. Low grade inflammatory bowel disease or villous adenoma may be missed and it is important to remember that elderly patients with diarrhoea may have faecal impaction with overflow, particularly if institutionalised or immobile. Constipating agents should never be prescribed until this diagnosis has been excluded by rectal and abdominal examination.

Further Reading

Bradshaw MJ, Edwards RTM (1986) Autonomic neuropathy – pathophysiology and management. Q J Med 60:643–657

Bradshaw MJ, Harvey RF (1982) Antidiarrhoeal agents: clinical pharmacology and therapeutic use. Drugs 24:440–451

Edwards RTM, Bransom CJ, Crosby DL, Pathy MSJ (1983) Colorectal carcinoma in the elderly: a geriatric and surgical practice compared. Age Ageing 12:256–262

Montgomery RD, Haboubi NY, Mike NH, Chesner IM, Asquith P (1986) Causes of malabsorption in the elderly. Age Ageing 15:235–240

Primrose WR, Capewell AE, Simpson GK, Smith RG (1987) Prescribing patterns observed in registered nursing homes and long-stay geriatric wards. Age Ageing 16:25–28

Chapter 12

Incontinence

Gladys M. Tinker

Urinary Incontinence

Urinary incontinence, though common in all age groups, is particularly prevalent in old age. Because of the associated social stigma, very few with the problem will admit to its presence when questioned directly. As a result the true prevalence rate is unknown, though studies in old people have suggested an overall prevalence of 20%, with the extent in hospital populations varying from 12.9% to 48%.

While urinary incontinence is not in itself a fatal condition, it can cause such feelings of embarrassment, degradation and low self-esteem in an old person that withdrawal from social contact and progressive isolation results. To the professional, dealing with incontinence often produces a feeling of frustration and despair and consequently is not approached with the same enthusiasm as the more socially acceptable disorders. Some cases of incontinence in the elderly can be cured. Very many can be improved. Virtually all can be managed better than they are when the patient first seeks professional help.

Bladder Function

Contraction of its sphincters together with relaxation of its smooth muscle coat allows the bladder to store urine. As the normal bladder fills, the detrusor muscle relaxes, so that the increasing volume can be accommodated without a rise in intra-vesical pressure. When the bladder approaches its capacity, the intra-vesical pressure begins to rise. Stretch receptors in the bladder wall are then activated and afferent stimuli are sent via the pelvic parasympathetic nerves to the spinal cord segments S2, S3 and S4. Following synapse, efferent fibres (also travelling in the pelvic parasympathetic nerves) innervate the detrusor muscle and cause it to contract. The bladder outlet is controlled primarily by the sympathetic nervous system and voiding occurs when detrusor contraction is accompanied by sphincter relaxation.

Such reflex emptying of the full bladder is seen in infants. Continence is gained when the brain becomes aware that the bladder is full and inhibits its reflex emptying. This is termed "cortical inhibition" and its development results in continence being achieved by 90% of children by the age of 5 years. Cortical inhibition can suppress the reflex arc for a finite time only. The interval between the initial sensation of the desire to void and the ultimate involuntary emptying by the reflex arc is crucial, this being the period of time within which the person has to find a socially acceptable place to void. This time diminishes with advancing age. Also with advancing age, bladder capacity decreases and the volume of residual urine in the bladder following micturition increases. These physiological factors predispose to urinary incontinence.

Another way in which the child learns to achieve continence involves emptying the bladder before it feels full. Throughout adult life most of us prematurely empty our bladders before car journeys, lectures or other activities when we anticipate a period during which micturition may be inappropriate. This skill may be forgotten by old people and may need to be relearnt.

Table 12.1 Causes of urinary incontinence in old people

Non-neurological disorders
Faecal impaction
Drug therapy
Impaired mobility
Urinary tract infection
Atrophic urethritis
Urethral obstruction
Pelvic floor incompetence
Psychological disorders
Endocrine disorders

Neurological disorders
Uninhibited bladder:
   central neurological disorders
   detrusor instability
Reflex neurogenic bladder
Autonomous neurogenic bladder
Atonic bladder

Normal bladder control is threatened by any disruption of the normal reflex arc or by loss of cortical inhibition. Such disruption can be due to local mechanical factors or to local or central neurological disorders. The main causes of urinary incontinence are listed in Table 12.1. The cause is often multi-factorial and some factors (e.g. drug therapy) can cause incontinence by more than one mechanism.

Non-neurological Disorders

Faecal Impaction

Faecal impaction can result in urinary retention with overflow incontinence. It is a common cause of urinary incontinence, especially when the problem is of short duration, and must never be overlooked as it is easily treated (see Chap. 11). Older people are notoriously unreliable in their history of bowel habit and it is a good policy to regard all incontinent elderly people as being impacted with faeces unless proven otherwise. While it can occur in any old person, impaction is particularly likely to occur in those people requiring institutional care, where it results from a combination of factors including a poor intake of food and fluid, impaired mobility and drug therapy.

Drug Therapy

Current prescribing patterns are such that urinary incontinence is much more frequently induced or exacerbated by drug therapy than it is improved by it. *Diuretics* are particularly implicated and are frequently used inappropriately. Not all oedema is due to cardiac failure, postural oedema being particularly common in immobile old people (see Chap. 9). Often patients with a past history of cardiac failure can have their diuretic therapy withdrawn or reduced so long as they are carefully monitored for recurrence of failure. Incontinence is more often associated with the use of potent, short-acting loop diuretics so less potent thiazide drugs should be used when possible. For some people, however, a brisk but short diuresis in the morning may be preferable as they may then be free of incontinence for the rest of the day. Diuretics should be chosen not only for their clinical need, but also by taking into account the patient's tendency to incontinence and the pattern of his or her daily activities.

Impaired Mobility (see Chap. 15)

For many people, their degree of continence is directly proportional to their level of mobility and to the proximity of a suitable place to void. In the field of rehabilitation it is well established that as mobility and independence improve, so does urinary continence. It is worth stating that a hospital environment often promotes incontinence rather than continence. Toilets may be far from the patient's bed and inadequately signposted. The use of inappropriate furniture such as "geriatric" chairs and cot sides practically guarantees incontinence and for this and other reasons should seldom if ever be advocated. In the home, difficulties in rising from low chairs and in reaching the lavatory in time are important causes of incontinence.

Urinary Tract Infection

Urinary tract infection is an undisputed cause of incontinence at any age and particularly in old people. Indeed, acute infection frequently has incontinence as its sole presenting feature. A residual pool of urine following micturition predisposes to infection, as does urinary tract disease (e.g. prostatic hyperplasia, bladder calculi) and the presence of an indwelling urinary catheter. When a temporary urinary catheter is removed, the urine should always be examined for the presence of infection which, if present, may result in continuing incontinence. There is no definite correlation between asymptomatic chronic bacteriuria and incontinence of urine.

Atrophic Urethritis

In a female patient, post-menopausal oestrogen deficiency affects the urethra and trigone of the bladder in a similar way to the vagina. Resulting urethritis and trigonitis can contribute to incontinence. Treatment is with a short course of either local or systemic oestrogen preparations. Local application of oestrogen has fewer side effects but may be unacceptable to some people.

Urethral Obstruction

Urethral obstruction of insidious onset results in urinary retention with overflow incontinence. This is predominantly a male problem resulting from benign prostatic hyperplasia or from prostatic carcinoma. Enuresis and continuous dribbling of urine during the day is the predominant complaint. In addition to overflow incontinence there is usually a degree of urge incontinence due to detrusor instability. The co-existence of detrusor instability is of practical importance as prostatic resection will relieve the obstruction but may not improve the detrusor instability. This is the reason why many incontinent patients with prostatic obstruction fail to regain continence following prostatectomy. Post-micturition dribbling is a third form of urinary incontinence found with prostatic obstruction.

Other causes of urethral obstruction include a urethral stricture and, in females, a large uterine prolapse, uterine fibroids and carcinoma and ovarian tumours. While these conditions are relatively uncommon causes of incontinence, they are important as they are potentially treatable.

Pelvic Floor Incompetence

Pelvic floor incompetence results in poor control of bladder neck closure and manifests itself predominantly as stress incontinence. Involuntary voiding usually occurs only on coughing or sneezing, though the problem can be so severe that leakage occurs even on standing from a sitting position. Minimal stress incontinence can trigger a full evacuation of the bladder. It is mainly a female problem resulting from peripartum damage and post-menopausal oestrogen deficiency, though age-related muscle weakness and bladder neck surgery are predisposing factors in both sexes. Stress incontinence may be distinguished from other forms of incontinence by the fact that it is less of a problem at night than during the day.

Psychological Disorders

Acute *anxiety* causes frequency of micturition in most people and in old people can result in incontinence. This is particularly noticeable when the elderly person moves to a new environment (such as hospital) where the surroundings are both unfamiliar and frightening.

It has been suggested that for some people, incontinence is an expression of *attention seeking* behaviour. The old person who is disabled and wet will be toileted, washed and changed by his carers, providing him with human contact which he may otherwise be denied. In hospital, such behaviour may manifest itself by frequent requests for a commode or help with toileting.

When elderly people feel aggrieved, there may be few ways in which they can express their *anger* and *frustration*. Such a situation may arise when elderly people are institutionalised. Many feel rejected by their relatives, find their new surroundings restrictive and feel that they have lost control of their destiny. One of the few ways in which they can express their sense of grievance is by incontinence.

The sensation of touch on the skin of the perineum is a factor in normal bladder control and anaesthesia of this area increases bladder volume before spontaneous voiding occurs. We are toilet-trained to the point where sensation of a toilet seat on the perineum promotes evacuation of the bladder. This *conditioned reflex* is disturbed by the use of bed pans or urinals. Similarly, the transport of patients to and from the toilet on a chair with a toilet seat rather than a flat seat may stimulate premature evacuation of the bladder.

Endocrine Disorders

Endocrine disorders such as diabetes mellitus and hypercalcaemia cause polyuria and hence predispose to urinary incontinence.

Neurological Disorders

There are four main types of neurogenic bladder as described below. Apart from an uninhibited neurogenic bladder they are uncommon causes of incontinence in old age. The sites of the lesions causing the problems are indicated in Fig. 12.1.

Uninhibited Neurogenic Bladder

Uninhibited neurogenic bladder occurs when normal cortical inhibition of bladder contraction is impaired to the point where, as soon as there is a desire to void, the bladder empties automatically and incontinently. The disorder complicates

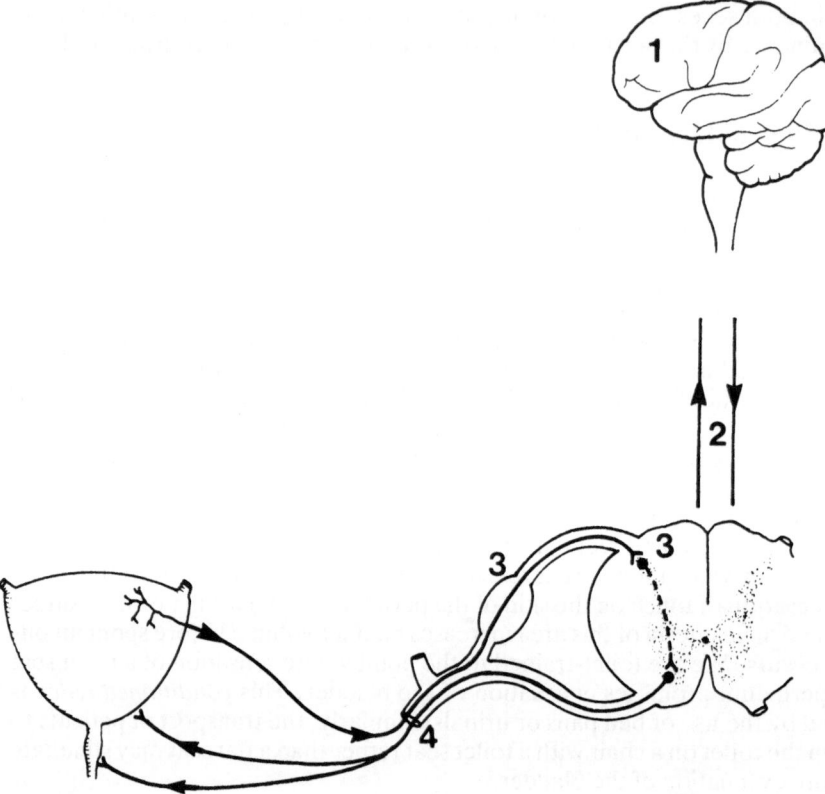

Fig. 12.1. The sites of lesions with the various forms of neurogenic bladder: 1, uninhibited neurogenic bladder; 2, reflex neurogenic bladder; 3, atonic bladder; 4, autonomous neurogenic bladder.

many forms of cerebral dysfunction including the dementing disorders and Parkinson's disease. In particular it results from focal frontal lobe disorders due to stroke or tumour.

Even in a person who is normally continent, the onset of an acute event can reduce cortical inhibition to a critical degree where continence is lost. This explains the frequency with which an *acute confusional state* is accompanied by incontinence. The incontinence generally resolves along with the acute confusion.

Drugs, especially hypnotics, sedative agents and alcohol also reduce cortical inhibition and are therefore an important cause of incontinence. Where there is a risk of incontinence, these drugs should be used only when absolutely necessary and it should be understood that recipients may require much closer supervision and regular toileting if incontinence is not to result.

The terms *detrusor instability* or *unstable bladder* describe a situation in which cortical inhibition is poorly developed. As a result the bladder contracts and voids on minimal stimuli, even when it contains only small volumes of urine. Provocative stimuli include standing, coughing and laughing, so that the history is easily confused with that of stress incontinence. There may be a congenital predisposition to the disorder and there is often a history of enuresis in childhood. While it may be regarded as a form of uninhibited bladder, no central nervous disorder may be found. The condition is often associated with local disease such as prostatic obstruction or urethral stricture. In addition to urge incontinence, patients may complain of urinary frequency and nocturia. The diagnosis can only be made with confidence by cystometry. In practice, however, the vast majority of patients with urge incontinence have detrusor instability.

Reflex Neurogenic Bladder

This results from a spinal cord lesion above the level of the reflex arc at S2, S3 and S4 and is most often seen in paraplegic patients. The reflex arc is maintained. The bladder fills normally and when its capacity is reached, it empties reflexly and incontinently. Younger patients can exert some degree of bladder control by stroking or tickling the skin over the perineum (supplied by S2, 3 and 4) thus stimulating the reflex arc and evacuating the bladder. Such voiding techniques are very rarely achieved by old people.

Atonic Bladder

Atonic bladder is caused by a lesion of the posterior nerve root or posterior horn cell as occurs in diabetes mellitus, disseminated sclerosis, tabes dorsalis and subacute combined cord degeneration. It results in loss of bladder sensation with chronic distension and overflow incontinence. This along with retention due to benign prostatic hypertrophy is one of the few common causes of a distended bladder in an elderly incontinent patient.

Autonomous Neurogenic Bladder

Damage to the cauda equina from tumour or trauma destroys the normal reflex arc and thereby bladder sensation. The bladder distends painlessly and overflow incontinence results.

Clinical Assessment

A full history must be taken along with a history of past and present episodes of incontinence. This includes details of awareness of bladder filling and the interval between awareness and involuntary emptying. The time pattern of incontinence should be explored. Is it predominantly during the day or at night? Is there any relationship to factors which raise intra-abdominal pressure (e.g. coughing, sneezing, standing). A full history of drug therapy and bowel habit must be obtained. An assessment of mental function will identify those with dementia, those who are anxious or depressed and those who are using incontinence as a manipulative measure.

Physical examination should include a comprehensive CNS assessment, a rectal examination and a vaginal examination in females. There is never an excuse for omitting a rectal examination in an elderly patient with urinary incontinence. Vaginal examination in most screening assessments will be limited to a gentle one finger examination looking for senile vaginitis, but a full bi-manual examination must be done if pelvic pathology is suspected.

Further Evaluation

A midstream specimen of urine (MSU) should be examined for evidence of acute infection. A blood sugar estimation is essential as diabetic patients may have an atonic bladder with overflow incontinence. The polyuria of uncontrolled diabetes further promotes incontinence.

Charting

By documenting the frequency of incontinence on a regular basis a pattern may be demonstrated around which treatment can be based. This may allow the carer to gauge when an episode is due and to abort it by premature toileting. The charting process is in itself a therapeutic tool as once interest is shown in the problem it often improves. Where feasible, the patient should be encouraged to involve herself in the charting process. It should be noted that if while charting, the elderly person is found to be incontinent, she must also then be toileted as well as washed and changed as incontinent voiding often results in ineffective emptying, with residual urine being left in the bladder.

Cystometry

Cystometry is undoubtedly of benefit for many younger patients, though its role in the assessment of old people is debatable. It involves measurement of bladder pressure, volume, the response to increased abdominal pressure, the volume at which there is awareness of bladder fullness and the volume at which involuntary emptying of the bladder occurs. The procedure can be carried out in combination with a micturating cystogram when, as well as obtaining urodynamic measurements, radiological imaging of the bladder demonstrates the anatomy, any gross pathology and movement of the bladder neck during micturition. Cystometry is primarily of use in identifying the uninhibited neurogenic bladder, although it is questionable whether the investigation is warranted when the treatment of this condition is so limited.

Management

For those patients in whom incontinence is of recent onset the most rewarding management strategies will be geared towards relieving faecal impaction, rationalising drug therapy and improving patient mobility. Any pelvic pathology, urinary tract infection or atrophic urethritis should be treated.

Pelvic floor exercises are important at all ages in the female. When performed prophylactically they reduce the risk of genuine stress incontinence and also reduce the possibility of minimal stress incontinence triggering the emptying of an unstable bladder. A simple programme of pelvic floor exercises suitable for old people involves frequently starting and stopping the urinary flow during micturition.

In the case of urge incontinence the period between the sensation of bladder fullness and involuntary voiding is brief and in recognition of this, the immediate environment must be adapted. Obstacles such as cot sides, "geriatric" chairs and beds that are too high should be identified and removed. Proper footware and walking aids which are both appropriate and readily available encourage safe mobilisation.

Regular visits to the toilet on a 1- or 2-hourly basis may be required, at least initially. The aim should be to extend gradually the interval between visits. The carer should approach the problem in a positive manner and a sense of optimism should be conveyed to the patient. Again it is well worth trying to involve the patient in the therapeutic effort. Wherever possible the toilet should be used rather than a bedside commode or bed pan. Within an institution, adequate signposting of the toilet and mapping the route to it in a simple pictorial fashion is of benefit. Toilets themselves may need to be modified by the provision of a raised toilet seat or a grab rail.

When the elderly person is found to be incontinent she should be encouraged to use the toilet to get rid of any residual urine in the bladder; the skin should then be carefully washed and dried and clothing must be changed. Whether the patient is at home or in an institution she must be provided with some means of calling for assistance should she require to use a commode or toilet. Where the patient has a communication problem it is particularly important that methods such as bells, buzzers or signals be employed. Attempts to improve mobility by walking the patient to the toilet once she expresses a wish to go are unwise. Continence may be lost on the way and it is far better if the patient is taken to the toilet quickly with continence intact and encouraged to walk back from it instead.

If a bedside commode is essential it should be stable and within easy reach of the person using it. The more severely disabled may benefit from a two-legged commode attached to the side of the bed (Fig. 12.2). Difficulty in getting out of bed even to use such a commode may be overcome by the use of a slipper pan.

Limiting fluid intake in the late evening may diminish nocturnal incontinence, but it is important that the overall fluid intake is maintained to prevent dehydration and possible urinary tract infection.

Clothing within an institution should be as normal as possible and preferably be the patient's own. There is no evidence that the ill-termed "geriatric" dresses with slits at the back do anything to improve the management of incontinence. They

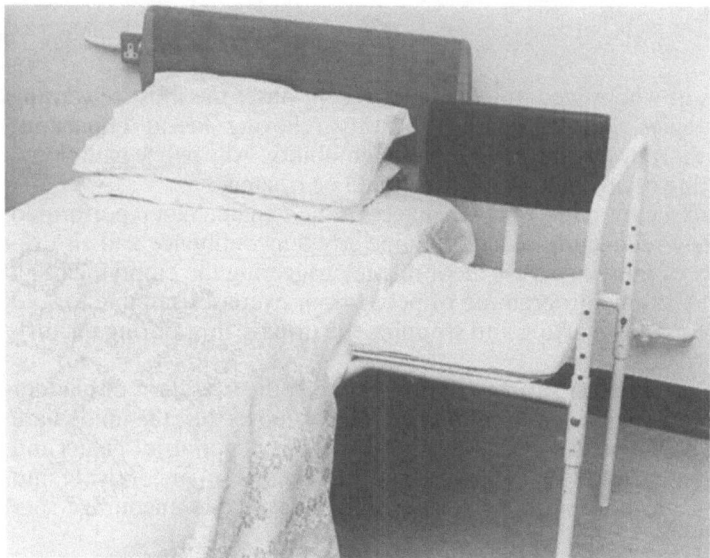

Fig. 12.2.   A two-legged commode.

certainly add to the degradation and lowered self-esteem that often precipitates
the incontinence in the first place.

Drugs

As yet drug therapy for incontinence is not very successful. Drugs with anti-
cholinergic properties (e.g. emepronium bromide, propantheline bromide and
imipramine) have been used in the past. Side effects frequently result and these
drugs are contraindicated in patients with glaucoma and prostatism. Emepronium
bromide also caused oral and oesophageal ulceration and is no longer licensed.

Flavoxate hydrochloride is a quaternary ammonium compound which has a
direct anti-spasmodic action on smooth muscle fibres and is sometimes effective
in incontinence due to detrusor instability. Recently terodiline, which has part
calcium antagonist and part anti-cholinergic properties has been introduced and
is proving to be a useful adjuvant to therapy. Oxybutynin has been used for many
years in the United States but is unlicensed in Britain. Unwanted effects seem to
occur more often with oxybutynin than with terodiline.

Incontinence Aids

Protective pads and pants should be used only where there is intractable incontinence. While an attempt is being made to regain continence, underpants and all
other clothing should be as normal as possible. Where protective clothing has to
be introduced pads which will absorb an adequate volume of urine should be
selected. The pants themselves should look as normal as possible so as to promote

dignity and self-respect. They should fit well and be in plentiful supply. Treating the older person like a baby by forcing them to wear a nappy will only exacerbate the incontinence. The choice of incontinence pads and pants should not be made solely on the basis of financial considerations and it is important for geriatric physicians and other concerned professionals to be involved in the selection of suitable materials. Incontinence sheets may be of benefit in the home care of the incontinent patient and, where available, a domiciliary laundry service bringing a supply of clean sheets to the home on a regular basis can prove invaluable.

The male patient may tolerate a condom or sheath catheter which drains into a leg bag, although most of these are designed for the younger male and adhesive tape may be needed to secure them to the shrunken penis of an elderly patient. The latex from which they are made, but more frequently the adhesive tape used to secure them, may cause skin excoriation. Better fitting devices which cause less skin reaction are becoming increasingly available. Irrespective of the type of device in use, scrupulous hygiene of the penile area must be observed so as to prevent excoriation and balanitis.

It may be appropriate, particularly in the home situation, to consider an indwelling catheter. This should be silicone based and attached either to a leg bag or to a bag supported by a waistband. Female patients should be fitted with a short catheter which is more comfortable, discreet and less likely to become kinked (Fig. 12.3). Again clothing should be as normal as possible and there is no reason why catheters should be seen protruding from the front of trousers or urine bags seen dangling on the floor.

The investigation and management of an elderly person with urinary incontinence is a challenge which should be faced enthusiastically by all members of the multidisciplinary team. If it is approached by professionals in a positive yet sympathetic manner the results are often quite dramatic.

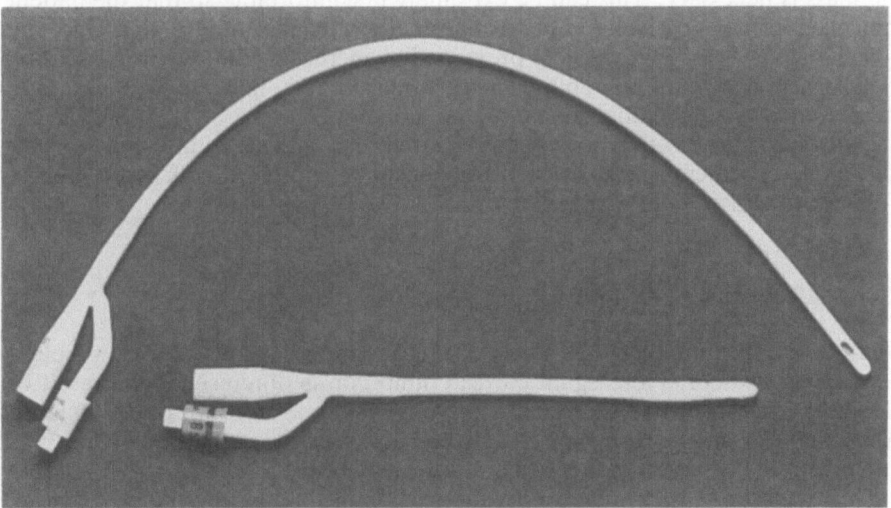

Fig. 12.3. A female catheter is much shorter than its male equivalent.

Faecal Incontinence

Faecal incontinence is far less prevalent than urinary incontinence among old people. Both for patients and their carers, however, it is a much more unpleasant problem to deal with and is much less likely to be tolerated in the community. Fortunately, with proper assessment and management, the problem can almost always be resolved.

Faecal incontinence is due either to gastrointestinal disorders including faecal impaction or to neurological disease. Both occur with equal frequency in established incontinence. With incontinence of recent onset faecal impaction is the most common cause, a point which cannot be overemphasised.

Faecal Impaction

Faecal impaction is due to chronic constipation (see Chap. 11) and results in the production of a faecal mass with a low water content and which is therefore stony hard. This results in partial obstruction of the colon and rectum with stimulation of mucus secretion. Liquid faeces mixed with mucus bypass the inspissated faecal mass resulting in the involuntary passing of a liquid stool with frequent staining of underclothes. This stool is often mistaken for diarrhoea with resultant inappropriate therapy. A rectal examination will point to the correct diagnosis. In addition to finding a hard mass in the rectum, the tone of the anal sphincter is usually reduced. Sometimes the faecal mass is high in the descending colon and cannot be palpated per rectum. An X-ray examination of the abdomen may then demonstrate the faecal loading and possibly partial bowel obstruction.

The rectum should be evacuated by whatever means are necessary. Usually this is accomplished by daily enemas which should be continued until no response is obtained. Occasionally the condition is so advanced that manual evacuation of the mass is necessary. This can be extremely uncomfortable so that the patient may need sedation or even a general anaesthetic when it is undertaken. Once the bowel is clear recurrence must be prevented by increasing dietary fibre and fluid intake, increasing patient mobility and by using a regular laxative. Bulk laxatives are preferable to stimulant laxatives in this situation.

Other gastrointestinal disorders such as carcinoma of the rectum, ischaemic colitis and diabetic neuropathy cause diarrhoea and can present with incontinence. They are described in more detail in Chapter 11.

Neurogenic Incontinence

Neurogenic incontinence has a similar pathophysiology to the uninhibited neurogenic bladder. Here again cortical inhibition is diminished as a result of global or focal insults to the central nervous system as occurs, for example, in Alzheimer's disease and stroke respectively. The rectum responds to the passage into it of a small amount of faeces by reflex evacuation.

The condition is best managed by inducing constipation and then evacuating bowel contents by means of regular enemas. Codeine phosphate is the most widely used constipating agent. Enemas then need to be given as infrequently as once or twice weekly. For a person living at home, enemas can be administered by the community nurse. This manoeuvre obviously does not improve control by the patient, but the infrequent and planned evacuation of the bowel is a satisfactory solution for most people and for their carers.

Evaluation and Management

The management of faecal incontinence starts with making a diagnosis of the underlying cause. Rectal examination is mandatory as without it faecal impaction will be missed. If other bowel pathology is suspected, a sigmoidoscopy and barium enema may be warranted. Thereafter, treatment depends on the underlying cause as outlined above. The problem can usually be managed without the need for incontinence aids. Pads and pants are available however, and they may provide patients and carers alike with additional security.

Further Reading

Brocklehurst JC (1972) Bowel management in the neurologically disabled: the problem in old age. Proc R Soc Med 65:66–67

Willington FL (1976) Incontinence in the elderly. Academic Press, London

Chapter 13

Visual Impairment

Lyn Beck and D. Jones

Visual impairment is a particular problem in old age with some 70% of those on the blind register being aged over 70 years. Blindness limits independence and is as common a cause of old people being housebound as is stroke, heart disease or lung disorders. Clearly, a lesser degree of visual loss will impair quality of life.

Visual impairment at any age may be due to one of three main causes:

Defective focusing of light (refractive error)
Defective transmission of light (opacities in the media)
Defective reception of light (retinal or neurological disease)

With age, physiological changes occur in the eye which may affect vision. The ciliary muscle becomes weaker and the lens less pliable. The resulting decrease in the accommodative power of the lens (presbyopia) impairs focusing on near objects so that reading glasses may be required. The lens increases in size as new fibres continue to be laid down on its outside, causing the anterior chamber to become increasingly shallow. The vitreous gel degenerates and retracts away from the retina (syneresis), causing symptoms of floaters and flashing lights. The resting pupil diameter decreases allowing less light into the eye, a phenomenon known as senile miosis. Finally, a decrease in tear secretion may cause blurring of vision.

Clinical Evaluation

In assessing the cause of visual impairment a careful and detailed history is essential. This should differentiate between unilateral or bilateral visual loss, sudden or gradual onset and whether or not the loss was painful. Long-standing visual loss can be mistaken for acute loss when it is suddenly discovered on covering the healthy eye.

Visual acuity should be checked for each eye using a Snellen chart and with the patient's normal distance glasses worn. If the patient is bed-bound, reading print may be used with the patient wearing his reading glasses. If the acuity is found to be impaired, it should be retested using a pin hole aperture (a hole made in a piece of card will suffice). This eliminates any refractive error.

A thin beam pen-torch should be used to check the colour of the globe of the eye (red or white), to look at the cornea (hazy or clear), to assess the depth of the anterior chamber (the space between the iris and cornea) and test the pupillary reactions. The Marcus Gunn test will elicit a defect in the afferent visual pathway: a light is moved from one eye to the other several times when, normally, both pupils should react briskly to light both directly and consensually. A loss of the direct pupillary reaction to light indicates a complete break in the afferent pathway on that side. Should the pupil dilate rather than remain constricted when the light is transferred into that eye (indicating that the direct pupillary response to light is weaker than the consensual response), a relative afferent pupillary defect (RAPD) is present. This indicates a defect somewhere between the photoreceptors and the mid-brain on the affected side and is a useful test of retinal and optic nerve integrity in the presence of a cataract. The intraocular pressure may be estimated by digital pressure or more accurately measured by applanation tonometry.

Table 13.1.   Causes of visual impairment in old people

Sudden loss	Gradual loss
White eye	
Retinal detachment	Cataract[a]
Vascular disorders	Chronic simple glaucoma[a]
Central retinal vein occlusion	Maculopathy[a]
Central retinal artery occlusion	
Ischaemic optic neuropathy	
Vitreous haemorrhage	
Age-related macular disease	
Red eye	
Angle closure glaucoma	
Acute iritis	
Diabetic eye	
Vitreous haemorrhage	Maculopathy
Vascular occlusion (venous)	Traction detachment
	Cataract

[a] These diseases are frequently bilateral and may co-exist.

The ophthalmoscope is first of all used to assess the red reflex in the pupillary area. This is done by holding the instrument at a distance of approximately 2 feet (60 cm) from the eye or at the normal distance with plus lenses. In the normal eye a red glow emanating from the retina is visible in the pupillary area. In the presence of lens or vitreous opacities black areas may be seen against the red glow. A dense cataract or vitreous haemorrhage will obscure the red glow completely. After assessing the red reflex the fundus is then examined in detail by first looking at the disc, then all four quadrants of the retina and lastly the macula. If the eye is not inflamed, it is almost always permissible to use a weak mydriatic.

The causes of visual loss can be classified according to the speed of onset and whether the affected eye is white or red (see Table 13.1).

Sudden Loss of Vision in the White Eye

A sudden loss of vision in the white eye is due either to retinal detachment or to a vascular problem (see Table 13.1).

Retinal Detachment

Retinal detachment occurs when the neuroretina separates from the underlying retinal pigment epithelium. There are two main types: rhegmatogenous (Gr. *rhegma*, a hole) and non-rhegmatogenous. Rhegmatogenous detachments are due to holes or tears in the retina and are by far the commoner, affecting 1 in 10 000 of the population each year. The commonest type of tear in the elderly is seen in the supero-temporal quadrant and usually follows a posterior vitreous detachment. With age the vitreous collapses away from the retina and as it does so may exert tractional forces resulting in a tear. Other predisposing factors include high myopia, areas of retinal degeneration, previous trauma and cataract surgery. Once a hole or tear is present, fluid may accumulate and lift off the neuroretina. Non-rhegmatogenous detachments usually occur secondary to a variety of exudative, haemorrhagic or tractional pathologies, including tumours and diabetes.

Symptoms of retinal detachment include the sudden onset of floaters, flashes of light, a shadow in the field of vision and impaired acuity. The extent of visual impairment found on examination depends on the degree of macular involvement. If the macula is totally detached the loss of acuity is profound. A RAPD in the affected eye may be present and fundoscopy reveals the presence of a detachment in the area diagonally opposite to the visual field defect. The affected retina appears blue/grey and the blood vessels appear darker than normal.

In the early stages, if a retinal hole or tear is found without an associated detachment, the tear may be sealed by welding around it using the argon laser or a freezing cryo-probe. Once a detachment has occurred, complex surgery is required to reposition the retina. The visual prognosis depends on the extent and duration of macular involvement. Since floaters and flashing lights can presage a retinal tear, careful fundal examination at this stage is imperative.

Retinal Vein Occlusion

Retinal vein occlusion increases in frequency with age, predisposing factors including systemic hypertension, chronic simple glaucoma, diabetes and hyperviscosity states. Both central retinal vein and branch vein occlusions occur, the latter being three times the more common. With central vein occlusion sudden painless blurring of vision is often first noticed on waking from sleep. The visual loss is severe, a RAPD is found and fundoscopy reveals disc swelling, tortuous dilated veins, scattered haemorrhages and sometimes cotton wool spots ("pizza pie" retina). With a branch vein occlusion obstruction usually occurs at the arteriovenous crossing and 60% involve the supero-temporal vein. Symptoms depend on whether the macular area is involved.

It is not possible to restore vision in the affected eye following central retinal vein occlusion. Prophylaxis, especially with regard to the other eye, includes control of hypertension and any pre-existing glaucoma. Apart from systemic investigations to eliminate predisposing factors, patients are usually monitored for local complications. Once retinal haemorrhages have been absorbed, fluorescein angiograms are occasionally performed to ascertain the degree of retinal ischaemia. Laser retinal ablation is then undertaken if large ischaemic areas are noted following both central retinal vein and branch vein occlusions. This has been shown to decrease the likelihood of neovascular changes, which can result in vitreous haemorrhage or thrombotic glaucoma.

Retinal Artery Occlusion

Retinal artery occlusions are more dramatic but rarer than their venous counterparts and again may involve the central or branch vessels. They are caused by embolic or thrombotic vascular disease and by inflammatory disorders such as cranial (temporal) arteritis. In association with a central artery occlusion the visual loss is profound, sudden and painless. A RAPD is present and fundoscopy in the early stages shows thread-like arteries and fragmented "cattle-truck" blood columns. After a few hours the retina appears oedematous and milky apart from the cherry red spot of the macula, which is the thinnest part of the retina and so shows the healthy underlying choroid. Occasionally the embolic cause is visible.

Amaurosis fugax describes the transient loss of vision found with embolic disease, particularly resulting from carotid artery stenosis. Symptoms last for seconds or minutes and are often described as a shutter or curtain descending over part of the visual field.

Treatment of central retinal artery occlusion is usually ineffective, but if the cause is embolic and if the patient presents within an hour or two of the episode, attempts may be made to reduce the intra-ocular pressure rapidly by ocular massage, intravenous acetazolamide or paracentesis of the anterior chamber in the hope of dispersing the embolus. An ESR should be performed in all cases though a normal value does not exclude cranial arteritis. If there is anything to suggest that this is a possible cause, immediate high-dose steroid therapy must be given. In the case of amaurosis fugax, underlying isolated carotid stenosis may be amenable to surgical treatment. Low-dose aspirin has been found to be of value in reducing the frequency of these attacks.

Ischaemic Optic Neuropathy

Ischaemic optic neuropathy can be caused by a variety of conditions, the single most important being cranial arteritis with involvement of the ophthalmic artery. This affects 1% of the population aged over 60 years, with visual loss occurring in 50% of those affected. Visual loss is sudden and painless. The patient may have symptoms related to underlying polymyalgia rheumatica (see Chap. 6), with malaise and temporal headache. In addition to severe visual loss, a RAPD is present and the optic disc is pale, swollen and often surrounded by splinter haemorrhages. The temporal arteries may be swollen and tender. No treatment is available to restore vision to the affected eye. The ESR is usually elevated and often exceeds 100 mm/h. However, it may be normal and if cranial arteritis is suspected, regardless of the ESR, high-dose systemic steroid therapy is indicated in order to protect the unaffected eye in which the risk of blindness is 50%. Thus cranial arteritis constitutes an ophthalmological emergency.

Vitreous Haemorrhage

Vitreous haemorrhage results in visual loss, the extent of which depends on the severity of the haemorrhage. The commonest cause in a non-diabetic patient is a retinal tear, but haemorrhages also occur following previous retinal vascular occlusions with ischaemic or neovascular changes. Symptoms vary from seeing streaky floaters to sudden severe loss of vision. Examination shows a variable degree of reduced visual acuity in the presence of normal pupillary reactions. Fundoscopy reveals either vitreous floaters as black streaks against the normal red reflex or total absence of the red reflex if the haemorrhage is dense. Bed rest has been advocated to hasten resolution of the haemorrhage but this needs to be balanced against the risks of developing deep vein thromboses and other complications of immobility. Once the vitreous is clear further treatment will depend on the underlying cause.

Maculopathy of certain types can present as sudden visual impairment and will be discussed in more detail later (see p. 171).

Gradual Loss of Vision in the White Eye

The three commonest causes of gradual loss of vision in the elderly patient are:

Cataract

Maculopathy

Chronic simple glaucoma

All three tend to occur bilaterally, though the extent of involvement may be asymmetrical.

Cataract

Cataract is the term for any opacity in the lens. It is the reason why 20% of elderly people are registered blind and is the greatest single cause of remediable blindness in this age group. The commonest cause is ageing itself, as suggested by the term senile cataract, the incidence rising steadily with age. Metabolic factors also play a part and senile-type lens opacities occur 10–15 years earlier in diabetic patients. Symptoms depend largely upon the position of the opacity within the lens. Cuneiform cataracts (Fig. 13.1a) are spoke-shaped peripheral opacities which cause blurred images, especially when the pupil is semi-dilated, due to diffraction effects, so that patients may experience maximal difficulty when driving at night. Nuclear cataracts often present with changes in refraction as they increase the

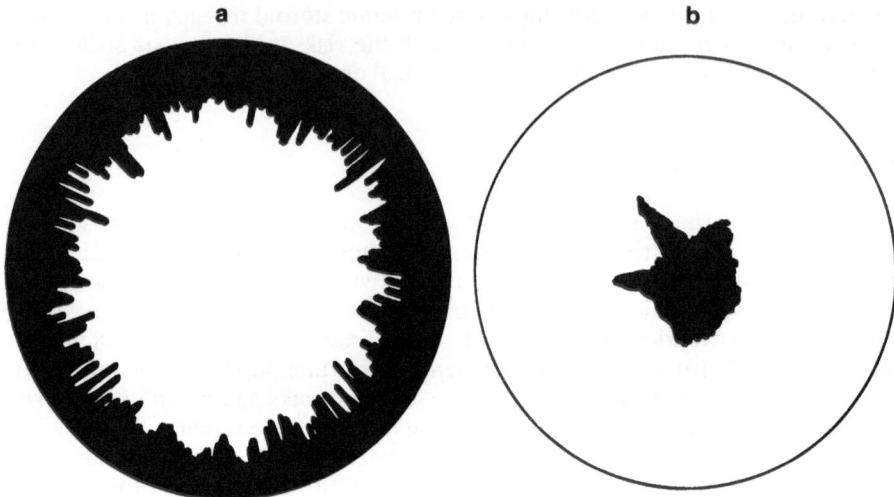

Fig. 13.1.   **a** A cuneiform lens opacity. **b** A posterior sub-capsular lens opacity.

converging power of the lens; this can allow some patients to read once more without glasses, although the image may be dimmed. Central lens opacities particularly of the posterior sub-capsular type (Fig. 13.1b), are situated on the visual axis and therefore cause much distortion in bright light or when reading (i.e. when the pupil is miosed). Occasionally people with cataract can experience monocular diplopia or polyopia or "haloes", but these are usually far less pronounced than those seen in angle closure glaucoma.

The visual acuity varies with the density and position of the cataract in the lens. Pupillary reactions are normal and light projection (the ability to identify the position of a light source) accurate in all four quadrants. Colour perception (tested with coloured light) is also normal. Early cataracts can be seen as black opacities against the red fundus reflex but dense cataracts will preclude any fundus view.

As a temporary measure with nuclear cataracts, the visual acuity may be improved by refraction and central opacities may seem less obtrusive if the pupil is kept dilated. However the definitive treatment is surgical and this is undertaken when it is considered that the cataracts are impinging upon the patient's quality of life. The technology now available allows the removal of a cataract at any stage of its development, "ripeness" (the term often used for mature, completely opaque cataracts) not being a prerequisite. Technique may vary between an intracapsular extraction where the whole lens is removed inside its capsule, or an extracapsular extraction where the posterior capsule and a rim of anterior capsule are left in situ. The latter method has a lower incidence of post-operative complications such as retinal detachment and macular oedema. Occasionally, using the extracapsular technique, a secondary thickening of the capsule can occur which subsequently may require opening via a surgical needling or a laser capsulotomy. Removal of a cataract renders the patient aphakic and the usual high hypermetropia (long-sightedness) that results requires correction. This can be accomplished either with glasses, contact lenses or intraocular lens implants. Glasses have the disadvantages of being of high power, heavy, subject to optical distortion peripherally and of causing distance misjudgements because of their magnifying effects. Elderly people often have difficulty in handling contact lenses. Nowadays, the corrective treatment of choice is often an intraocular lens, which has enormous optical advantages for patients. These can be inserted secondarily after an initial cataract extraction or, more commonly, as a primary procedure during an extracapsular extraction.

Maculopathy

The macula is the area of the retina responsible for fixation, all fine detail and colour vision. It is situated approximately 1½ disc diameters temporal to the optic disc and is viewed by asking the patient to look directly at the ophthalmoscopic light. Macular disorders account for 45% of conditions for which the elderly are registered blind. They classically result in a central field defect; the patient sees surroundings but the direct object of gaze appears blurred. He may complain of being unable to see details on faces, notice distortion of straight lines (metamorphopsia) and experience difficulty especially with reading. Age-related macular degeneration (or senile macular degeneration) is the commonest cause of visual loss in persons over the age of 65. The atrophic (dry) form is the commonest, but accounts for only 20% of severe visual loss with the neovascular (wet) form accounting for the remaining 80%.

There are several types of dry age-related macular degeneration, classified according to the underlying pathology. They all cause a gradual distortion and decrease in central visual acuity. Ophthalmoscopically, pigment changes or pale yellow drusen (colloid bodies) are seen which are often misdiagnosed as hard exudates. The condition is untreatable.

Wet age-related macular degeneration occurs when vessels grow forward from the choroid under or through Bruch's membrane causing elevation of the retina and distortion of the retinal photoreceptors. This is perceived as metamorphopsia. The symptoms are usually of sudden onset. Ophthalmoscopically, these are seen as a greyish elevated area close to or under the macula. Untreated, the vessels inevitably break through the retina and bleed, ultimately healing as a fibrous disciform scar (disciform maculopathy). The key investigation is a fluorescein angiogram which clearly demonstrates the new vessel frond. If the leading edge is sufficiently far away from the fovea (the centre of the macula) it can be treated by laser ablation. As a rule, the worse the visual acuity at presentation, the less likely it is that laser treatment will be feasible. All patients need to be referred as a matter of urgency. Disciform maculopathy is usually a bilateral condition and there is an ascending 3%–7% chance per year of the second eye being involved. Education of at-risk patients is therefore essential and early self-referral is strongly encouraged. It is important to reassure the patient that they will not go completely blind as the peripheral field of vision remains intact and navigational vision is retained. In almost all cases, reading vision can be helped by good lighting and magnification aids.

Chronic Simple Glaucoma

Chronic simple glaucoma is characterised by increased intraocular pressure with cupping of the optic discs and visual field loss. The field loss is due to ischaemic optic atrophy caused by the elevated intraocular pressure. Patients with the condition have open angles (i.e. the pathway to the drainage angle is normal) and it is the drainage meshwork itself which is faulty. The overall incidence is 0.47% and this rises dramatically with age, accounting for blindness in 15% of those elderly people on the blind register. There is a familial tendency and underlying diseases such as hypertension and diabetes mellitus make the optic discs more susceptible to injury.

In its early stages the disease is asymptomatic and thus the damage may be considerable before a diagnosis is made. Patients experience painless insidious visual field loss and until this encroaches on the central area it often remains unnoticed. By the time that central involvement attracts the patient's attention the disease is far advanced and total loss of vision in that eye may occur. On examination the visual acuity remains normal until the disease is far advanced. A RAPD may be found in a severely affected eye. Fundoscopy reveals a cupped disc with a cup/disc ratio of greater than 0.5. An asymmetry between the right and left cup/disc ratio should be regarded as suspicious. Perimetry (visual field analysis) usually shows classic defects in an arcuate or quadrantic distribution (Fig. 13.2a, b) and applanation tonometry shows the intraocular pressure to be raised.

The aim of treatment is to lower the intraocular pressure to a level at which no further field loss will occur. Initial treatment is medical, usually with a topical beta-blocker (if there are no systemic contraindications), which decreases aqueous humour production. This has the advantage of having no visual side effects such as pupillary constriction. Second line treatment includes topical pilocarpine, which works by increasing aqueous output and can therefore be used in conjunction with beta-blockers. Pilocarpine has a side effect of pupillary constriction and may induce mild myopia. Adrenaline is another alternative which is sometimes used. Poor medical control may necessitate surgical intervention in the form of laser trabeculoplasty which aims to thermally scar the trabecular meshwork at in-

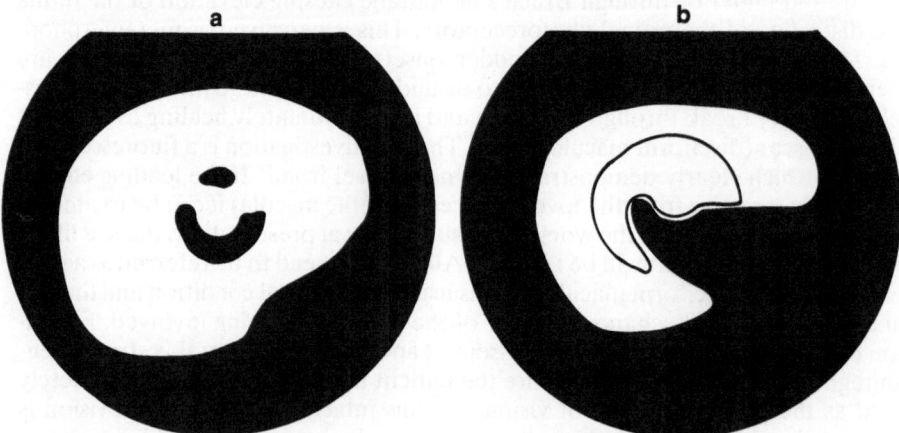

Fig. 13.2.   Visual field loss in chronic simple glaucoma. **a** An arcuate loss. **b** A quadrantic loss.

tervals, thus opening up the meshwork between scars and consequently increasing aqueous outflow. If intraocular pressure still remains too high, formal drainage surgery is indicated.

Because of the natural history of the disease, screening programmes for pre-symptomatic chronic simple glaucoma have been advocated. Problems arise in defining "normal" intraocular pressure, making mass screening programmes impractical, though selective screening of the older person in whom there is a family history of glaucoma may be valuable. The role of opticians in the diagnosis of this common condition is of great importance.

Visual Impairment in the Red Eye

This is less common than visual impairment in the white eye, the two major causes being:

Angle closure glaucoma
Acute iritis

Angle Closure Glaucoma

Angle closure glaucoma occurs in individuals with anatomically narrow angles and predominantly in hypermetropes. Aqueous humour, formed by the ciliary body, circulates through the pupil into the anterior chamber and drains from the eye through the trabecular meshwork in the angle into the canal of Schlemm. With age, the anterior chamber becomes progressively shallower due to the increase in size of the lens. In certain conditions (e.g. dim illumination), as the pupil dilates the peripheral iris bunches up in the angle, effectively narrowing it, preventing aqueous outflow and causing a sudden rise in intraocular pressure.

Symptoms consist of sudden onset of an aching pain in the eye, with severe headache, nausea and blurring of vision. Occasionally, prior to the onset of a full-blown attack, patients may experience sub-acute attacks of angle closure. These are characterised by seeing rainbow haloes around lights, blurring of vision due to the corneal oedema together with an aching pain in the eye. On examination, the eye is injected and there is a corneal haze. The anterior chamber is shallow and the pupil is semi-dilated and often fixed. The eye is stony hard on digital palpation and the visual acuity is reduced.

If left untreated permanent and severe visual loss can occur. The raised pressure needs to be rapidly reduced with a combination of osmotic diuretics (oral glycerol or intravenous mannitol if the patient is vomiting), intravenous acetazolamide to decrease aqueous formation, with frequent local instillation of pilocarpine drops to open the closed angle.

When the eye is less inflamed and tension lowered, further attacks of angle closure should be prevented by performing a peripheral iridectomy either surgically or with a laser. As the other eye is usually anatomically predisposed to the development of glaucoma a prophylactic iridectomy is electively performed.

Acute Iritis

This inflammatory condition of the iris is far commoner than angle closure glaucoma and the aetiology is usually idiopathic.

Symptoms consist of aching pain in the eye, blurring of vision and photophobia. On examination, there is ciliary injection with an occasional corneal haze and a variable reduction in visual acuity is found. The anterior chamber is of normal depth and the intraocular pressure may be normal or elevated. The pupil is often small and sometimes irregular due to the inflamed iris adhering to the lens (posterior synechiae). The diagnosis is confirmed by slit lamp examination, which will reveal the presence of flare (proteinaceous transudate) and inflammatory cells in the anterior chamber. In severe cases these cells precipitate to form a level of pus (hypopyon).

The condition is treated with a combination of topic mydriatics and topical steroids.

Diabetic Eye Disease

Retinopathy is one of the microvascular complications of diabetes mellitus and is responsible for some 15% of all new cases of blindness registered in Britain each year. Half of all people with diabetes of 10 years' duration have retinopathy and after 15 years almost all diabetics have some degree of retinopathy.

There are two types of diabetic retinopathy: background (non-proliferative) type and proliferative type. Background retinopathy is 10 times more common than proliferative retinopathy in diabetics of all ages and is even more prevalent in the older non-insulin-dependent diabetic than in the younger insulin-dependent patient. While proliferative retinopathy carries a tenfold greater threat to sight, it must be remembered that background disease can also cause severe visual disturbance, including blindness.

Background retinopathy consists of retinal vein dilatation and microaneurysms, hard exudates (due to lipid deposition), dot and blot haemorrhages and cotton wool spots (due to nerve fibre layer infarcts). Visual loss can occur if the macula is involved. Three types of diabetic maculopathy are recognised:

Exudative, where hard exudates deposited from leaking retinal vessels impinge on the macula

Ischaemic maculopathy

Cystoid macular oedema

Exudative maculopathy is the most easily recognised clinically, whereas the other two types often require fluorescein angiography to confirm their presence. Of these maculopathies, the only one amenable to treatment by laser ablation of the leaking vessels is the exudative type.

Proliferative retinopathy occurs more commonly, but not exclusively, in insulin-dependent diabetics, affecting 50% of these after 20 years of the disease. New vessels grow on the optic nerve head and elsewhere in the retina as a response to a vascular proliferative factor released by the ischaemic retina. These new vessels are abnormal in structure and bleed easily, causing visual loss through vitreous haemorrhage. There is a fibro-glial element to the neovascular response and this can give rise to tractional retinal detachments in severe cases.

Left untreated, 70% of patients with proliferative changes would be blind within 5 years. Laser therapy can prevent blindness in 80% of cases. The aim is to pan-ablate the peripheral retina with an argon laser, so reducing the oxygen demand. The ischaemic stimulus for neovascular proliferation is thus removed and regression of the new vessels occurs.

Management of Visual Impairment

A variety of low vision aids are available for those elderly people with residual impairment following medical and surgical treatment. Hand-held magnifying glasses are useful for those with mild or moderate impairment and a fixed focus magnifying lens can be used for reading material placed on a table. Some lenses have built-in illumination which is essential for optimal results. An array of spectacles with magnifying lenses (for reading purposes) or with telescopic lenses (for distant vision) are available but elderly people often have difficulty in adapting to them. In order to be accepted, such aids must be comfortable to use and be of perceived benefit to the patient. An array of blind aids are provided by various voluntary organisations in Britain and in other developed countries.

Legal Aspects of Blindness in the Elderly

The statutory definition for the purposes of registration as a blind person under the National Assistance Act 1948 is that the person is "so blind as to be unable to perform any work for which eyesight is essential". It is important to note that visual problems only are considered and that other bodily and mental infirmities are ignored. Many registered blind people have some vision, though the acuity must be less than 6/60 on the Snellen test. If visual acuity is better than this, a person may still be entitled to registration should the visual field be contracted. Some people who do not qualify for registration as blind may, if they are substantially and permanently handicapped by defective vision, be registered as partially sighted.

Registration can only be undertaken by a consultant ophthalmologist who notifies the area health authority, who in turn notify the social services department and the patient's general practitioner. The certifying ophthalmologist indicates whether the person is blind or partially sighted. The decision can be appealed against and an independent referee's opinion sought. For those registered as partially sighted, they can be re-referred and re-examined should their vision subsequently deteriorate.

Social Aspects of Blindness in the Elderly

People who are registered as blind have access to specialised social workers for the blind and to mobility officers for the blind. Together with the services to which all old people are entitled (see Chap. 28), they can be provided with a white cane and "talking book" service free of charge.

Financial benefits for those registered as blind with a local authority include a blind pension, a higher supplementary pension, higher tax allowances and a lower rent for council tenants. An income tax concession in the form of a Blind Person's Allowance is also available.

Further Reading

Blach RK (1983) Treatment of diabetic retinopathy In: Rose FC (ed) The eye in general medicine. Chapman and Hall, London

Epstein DL (ed) (1986) Chandler and Grant's Glaucoma, 3rd edn. Lea and Febiger, Philadelphia

ffytche TJ (1976) Macular disease. In: Rose FC (ed) Medical opthalmology. Chapman and Hall, London

Chapter 14

Hearing Problems

Carol Comlay and S. D. G. Stephens

Dr. Johnson described deafness as the greatest human calamity. While this may appear to be an overstatement, the society in which we live depends upon verbal communication for the exchange of ideas, information and friendship. Such communication may be denied the person with impaired hearing.

Verbal communication is a two-way process and hearing loss in one person has implications for both the listener and speaker. The hearing-impaired person fears failure while the hearing person has a fear of being misunderstood. The resulting strain of conversation with the need for regular repetition can cause great embarrassment for both. The necessity to speak in a loud voice highlights the handicap and makes intimate conversation often impossible. Misunderstandings and inappropriate answers increase such embarrassment.

Straining to understand what is being said is tiring and the effort involved may cause frustration and irritability. It may prove easier for the hearing-impaired person to withdraw from conversation. This in time may lead to varying degrees of social isolation and to feelings of social rejection. Some people attempt to overcome their handicap by monopolising conversation. While this minimises the risk of being unable to respond appropriately to questions, such behaviour is not always socially acceptable and may itself lead to rejection. For others, an inability to understand what is being said leads to feelings of paranoia. Deafness also places people at an increased risk from accidents, when warning sounds are either not heard or are imprecisely located.

Some 60% of people aged over 70 years have significantly impaired hearing. Thereafter the prevalence of deafness rises sharply with age to a point where 84% of those aged over 85 years have a significant deficit. Recent prevalence figures are almost twice those of previous estimates, suggesting that in the past a large proportion of significant hearing loss has gone undetected and therefore untreated. As the number of elderly people in the general population increases, the number with impaired hearing will also increase.

Age-related physiological changes result in a degree of hearing impairment in many old people (see Chap. 1). However, significantly impaired hearing is frequently and erroneously considered to be an inevitable accompaniment of old age. *Presbyacusis* is the term used to describe hearing loss in individuals over the age of 65 years in whom underlying causes have been excluded. Sometimes, however, the label of presbyacusis is loosely applied and is used to avoid undertaking detailed investigation for potentially treatable underlying causes. All patients with hearing problems should be assessed for remediable disorders.

Hearing loss among individual old people is often attributable to a variety of interacting diseases and insults. In the authors' experience, 32% of people aged over 65 years have more than a single identifiable cause while 8% have more than three identifiable causes. Table 14.1 lists the causes of impaired hearing among old people and indicates their prevalence. This information is drawn from the experience of one of the authors in various parts of Britain. In most cases, the hearing problem is located either in the middle ear (conductive hearing loss) or in the inner ear (sensory or cochlear hearing loss). In a number of elderly individuals there may also be disorders of the cochlear (VIIIth cranial) nerve.

Table 14.1. Causes and prevalence of hearing loss in old age

Conductive hearing loss		Sensorineural hearing loss	
Otitis media	(21%)	Vascular disorders	(27%)
Otosclerosis	(4%)	Noise/trauma	(15%)
		Genetic disorders	(8%)
		Metabolic disorders	(7%)
		Ototoxic damage	(3%)
		Unknown	(15%)

Conductive Hearing Loss

Amongst the causes of conductive hearing loss, chronic otitis media and otosclerosis are the most significant in old people.

Chronic Otitis Media

Chronic otitis media is generally the sequel of acute otitis media in childhood or young adult life. In most cases the disease process is burnt out, leaving deranged function of the tympanic membrane, with fibrosis limiting the movement of the ossicles. In other cases there may be a persistent perforation of the tympanic membrane with or without active infection. Care has to be taken in the fitting of hearing aids to any individual with a clean dry perforation as there is a risk of introducing a new infection, or aggravating a smouldering infection, when the external ear canal is blocked with an earmould. When active infection is present (chronic suppurative otitis media) this must be treated before an air conduction hearing aid is fitted.

In most Western countries the incidence of chronic suppurative otitis media dropped remarkably in the middle decades of this century for reasons that are not entirely understood. However, most elderly people presenting over the next few decades will have lived in times during which otitis media was common and therefore its prevalence can be expected to remain high into the next century.

Otosclerosis

Otosclerosis is an autosomal dominant condition of some 40% penetrance. It generally starts in the third and fourth decades. The hearing loss is caused by a thickening of the footplate of the stapes. Initially this is soft and spongy, but in the later stages of the disease the bone may become thick and sclerotic. In both stages the bony changes interfere with the transmission of sound through to the cochlea. Otosclerosis is generally bilateral, although unilateral involvement is not rare.

There is usually a relentless progression of the condition although the rate of progress slows with increasing age. In most patients the inner ear also becomes involved at later stages.

Patients with otosclerosis may be helped by stapedectomy in which the stapes is replaced by a metal or plastic piston, but fitting a hearing aid is the management of choice for most elderly patients.

Bone Disorders

Paget's disease (see Chap. 6) is the third most important cause of conductive hearing loss in old people. *Osteogenesis imperfecta* is a much rarer cause. In both conditions the otological changes are similar to those found in otosclerosis. *Trauma* can also result in a conductive hearing loss.

Sensorineural Hearing Loss

Most causes of sensorineural hearing loss affect the inner ear and so are generally referred to as sensory or cochlear. There is a wide range of aetiological factors which are generally indistinguishable audiometrically.

Genetic Disorders

While many hereditary syndromes include hearing loss, most genetic hearing loss is not accompanied by other abnormalities. Many different types of inheritance patterns occur and a late onset hearing loss, often becoming marked in the sixth decade, occurs not infrequently. Such conditions may be identified by taking an appropriate family history. This may also provide useful prognostic information as progression of the disease is often similar in the different generations affected.

Traumatic Hearing Loss

Traumatic hearing loss generally comes from acoustic trauma, noise trauma, physical trauma and from dysbarisms. The last are rare and will not be considered further.

Acoustic trauma implies a hearing loss caused by exposure to one or more high intensity sounds such as gunfire or bomb blast. Strictly speaking the latter, resulting in blast injury, should be considered separately as it generally results in middle ear damage as well as injury to the inner ear. Acoustic trauma generally results in a high frequency cochlear hearing loss with relatively good hearing at the low frequencies.

Noise trauma, resulting from long term exposure to high levels of noise, particularly in the workplace, results in a high frequency cochlear hearing loss often most marked in the 3–6 kHz range. As the hearing loss increases with continuing noise exposure it comes to affect both the highest and lower frequencies.

Physical trauma is generally due to head injury and may cause damage at almost any part of the auditory pathway. Frequently it affects several parts simultaneously: there may be damage to the ossicular chain, the inner ear, the cochlear nerve, brainstem or auditory cortex. Inner ear damage may resemble that caused by noise exposure or there may be a complete hearing loss with radiological evidence of a fracture passing through the temporal bone.

Ototoxic Damage

Ototoxic damage to the inner ear is an increasing problem in old people. Apart from the well known effects on hearing of drugs such as the aminoglycoside antibiotics, more relevant to the elderly are the loop diuretics frusemide and bumetanide, a variety of beta-blockers and NSAIDs. While most of the loop diuretics and NSAIDs generally cause a reversible hearing loss, it may become permanent. These drugs may also exacerbate related symptoms such as tinnitus.

Vascular Disorders

There is debate regarding the role of vascular disorders in the causation of hearing loss. Associated conditions include atheroma, atherosclerosis and hypertension, but whether the association is casual or causal is unknown. Many patients relate their hearing problems to episodes of myocardial infarction and ischaemia and hearing is significantly worse in individuals with such histories than in those without.

Metabolic Disorders

A variety of metabolic conditions have been implicated in the development of hearing loss in the elderly. These may be subdivided into endocrine and non-endocrine groups. Hypothyroidism and diabetes mellitus are the outstanding endocrine causes. Secretory otitis media with neural changes causing a flattish cochlear hearing loss occurs in myxoedema. With diabetes, however, the situation is less clear even though the subject has been studied extensively. The current weight of evidence suggests that diabetes enhances the "ageing process" in the outer ear and also causes some damage to the brainstem auditory pathways.

Dyslipidaemias are known to cause a non-specific high frequency hearing loss. Hyperuricaemia and uraemia have also been implicated, and part of the hearing loss in the latter may be reversible by appropriate treatment of the renal failure, at least in younger individuals.

Neoplasia

Neoplasia is an unusual cause of impaired hearing. The most common cause in this group is the acoustic neuroma (vestibulo-cochlear Schwannoma) which usually arises in the vestibular section of the VIIIth cranial nerve. In elderly patients such tumours generally grow very slowly. Metastases from primary carcinomas in the bronchus, breast, bone and liver may also occur in the cerebello-pontine angle and may be bilateral.

Ménière's Disorder

Ménière's disorder, while generally found in middle aged people, may also be present in elderly individuals. Classically it entails the triad of fluctuant low frequency cochlear hearing loss, tinnitus and vertigo, though often one or more of these components may be missing. A sensation of pressure in the ears is a common feature. Old people often have established Ménière's disorder in which the hearing loss may take a variety of forms, often affecting the high frequencies at least as much as the low frequencies.

Clinical Evaluation

In differentiating between the causes of hearing loss in the elderly the medical history is the single most important tool. From this the duration of the disorder, any precipitating factors, genetic factors and coincident systemic disease may be identified.

The problem of noise is worth considering in detail. Damaging levels of noise are usually associated with the patient having had to shout in order to communicate with nearby workmates and noticing dullness of hearing and temporary tinnitus at the end of a shift which was not present at the beginning. The same is true for acoustic trauma from military service, hunting and the like. Relevant physical trauma is usually associated with having been knocked unconscious, and history of boxing may be significant in this respect.

With regard to specific auditory symptoms, most patients with cochlear and cochlear nerve damage will complain particularly of difficulties in hearing speech against a background of noise. On the other hand many patients with conductive losses will often say that they hear better in noisy places: the phenomenon of *paracusis*.

Examination of the patient starts with general observation. Individuals with conductive hearing loss often speak softly. Those with severe sensorineural losses will tend to speak loudly. Examination of the external ear starts with the post-auricular region to look for scars of previous mastoid surgery. Next, using the largest speculum which will comfortably fit, the external meatus should be examined with an auriscope. Many patients will have a fair amount of wax in their ears which can generally be syringed unless there is a history of otorrhea or perforation. When the tympanic membrane can be seen, it should be noted whether it is normal and intact, perforated or scarred, thus giving information as to old otitis media. The mobility of the drum may be checked by a Valsalva's manoeuvre. The patient is asked to puff his cheeks out while holding his nose shut. This will reveal healed perforations or a hyper-mobile eardrum.

Tuning fork tests will give further differentiation between conductive and sensorineural losses. They are generally performed with a 512-Hz fork. The *Rinne test* compares the loudness of the fork by air conduction and by bone conduction and will detect a conduction component to the hearing loss. If bone conduction is louder (Rinne negative), this suggests a conductive hearing loss of at least 20 dB. The *Weber test* helps to confirm whether there is a conductive component to the hearing loss when it is unilateral or asymmetrical. It is not helpful when hearing loss is bilateral. If the Rinne test is positive (air conduction being louder than bone conduction) the *Bing test* may be performed. In this test, with the tuning fork on the mastoid, block off the ear canal; if the patient reports the sound as getting louder one can be sure that there is no significant conductive component to the hearing loss. A final useful tuning fork test is that for diplacusis binauralis. Hold the vibrating tuning fork alongside one ear and then alongside the other. A difference in the sound quality heard at the two ears is indicative of Ménière's disorder or of a retrocochlear lesion.

Further Investigation

A plethora of audiometric tests exists, but the four most useful are pure tone audiometry, acoustic immittance (impedance) test, tests of abnormal adaption (tone decay) and speech audiometry.

Pure tone audiometry measures the sensitivity of hearing over a wide range of frequencies. Most sensorineural hearing losses show worse hearing for the high frequencies than the low. In Ménière's disorder and certain other neurological conditions there is predominantly a low frequency hearing loss. Losses throughout the frequency scale often occur with certain metabolic disorders such as myxoedema. A measure of the conductive component of the hearing loss may be obtained by measuring the air–bone gap. This is the difference in thresholds obtained by air conduction and by placing a bone conduction vibrator in the mastoid.

In *acoustic immittance testing* the amount of sound absorbed by the ear is indirectly measured by a probe. The maximum sound absorption occurs when the pressure in the external ear canal is the same as that in the middle ear. Eustachian tube obstruction, for example, is detected by a shift in this peak of absorption, reflecting reduced middle ear pressure.

The change in the amount of sound absorbed with changes in pressure gives further information on middle ear function. Thus, with healed perforations or ossicular chain disruption there will be a large change in sound absorption with small pressure changes above or below the middle ear pressure. By contrast, in secretory otitis media, adhesive otitis media and some cases of otosclerosis, changes in the sound absorption will be reduced.

Other important information may be obtained from the acoustic stapedial reflex, whereby sound is reflexly damped down by the stapedial muscles. The afferent limb of the reflex involves the cochlear hair cells and cochlear nerve fibres. Excitation then passes via the cochlear nucleus to the facial nerve nuclei on both sides. Efferent fibres travel with the facial nerves to the stapedial muscles. Lesions in different parts of the auditory pathway may interfere with this reflex loop and by comparing the responses to ipsilateral and contralateral sound stimulation, much valuable information on the site of the auditory lesion may be obtained. Cochlear lesions may be separated from cochlear nerve disorders, brainstem disorders may be recognised and further evidence of conductive disorders may be obtained together with an indirect measurement of the hearing level.

The *auditory adaption test* measures "tone decay". Individuals with conductive or cochlear lesions will hear a loud, sustained tone for 30 seconds or more whereas those with cochlear nerve and brainstem lesions will hear the sound for only a few seconds.

Presenting words in *speech audiometry* and requiring the patient to repeat or recognise the word is of limited diagnostic value. In conductive hearing loss the speech discrimination is good. In cochlear hearing losses discrimination is good up to a loss of 30 dB and then gradually deteriorates. In hearing disorders of the cochlear nerve the discrimination is disproportionately bad when compared with the hearing loss.

Management

In their model, Goldstein and Stephens aim to bring the various techniques used in audiological rehabilitation together in a comprehensive procedural approach (Fig. 14.1). This model is useful when considering the appropriate management of elderly patients with a hearing impairment. However, this does not mean that every patient will pass through every level of the model.

If we look at the evaluation of the problem it is important to consider the patient's subjective feelings as to what his main difficulties are, as well as what we would objectively consider those difficulties to be.

Evaluation

With regard to the patient's *communication status,* answers must be sought to the following questions. What type of difficulties is the patient having due to his auditory impairment? Is he able to appreciate and to locate sounds which signal danger? Are there specific problems relating to home, leisure or employment? Are there any visual problems? The latter can affect the rehabilitative process by affecting the patient's ability to lip-read (speech-read). If glasses are worn, will they interfere with the fitting of hearing aids? When considering language it is important to consider the patient's native tongue: can management of the problem proceed in that language?

It is important to find out if the patient has received any previous rehabilitative help that may influence further management. Has he or she received any hearing

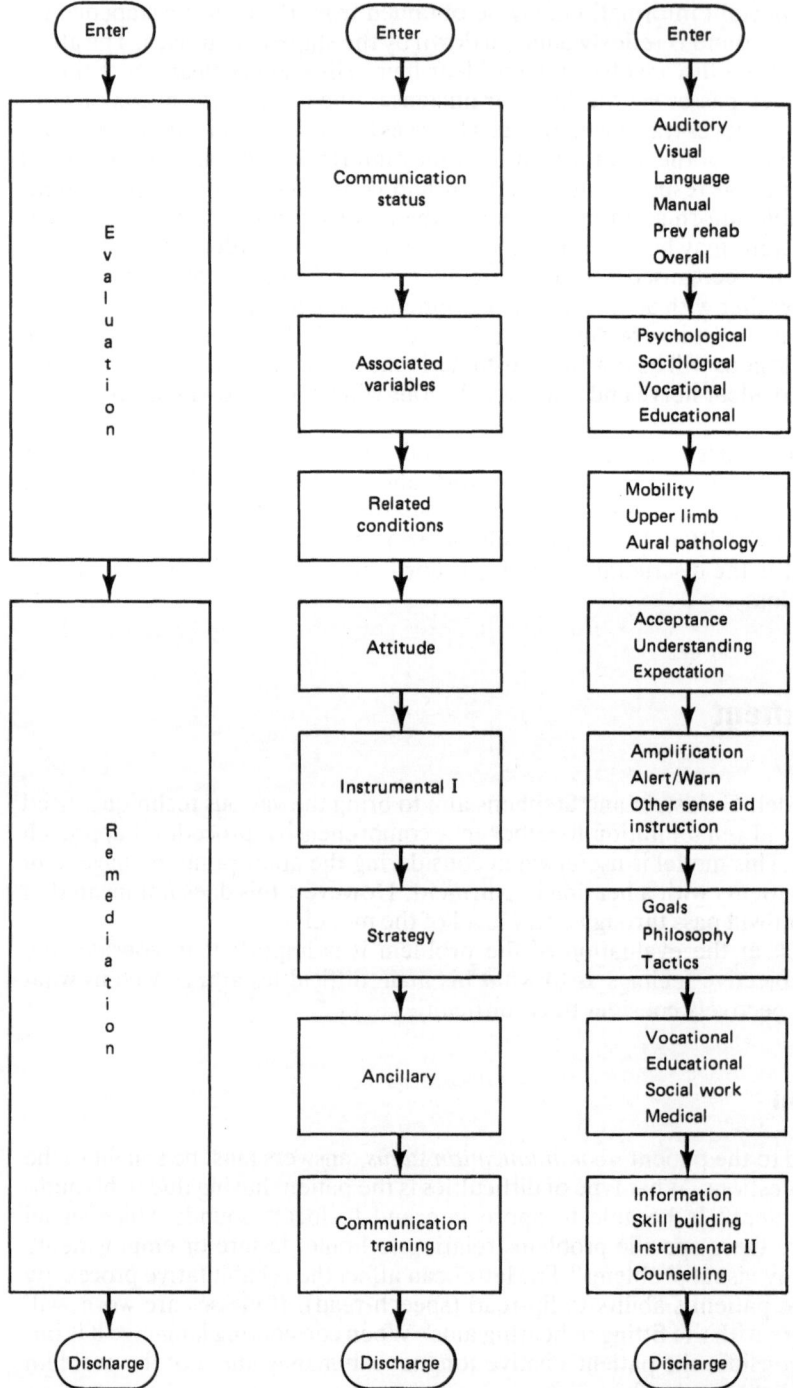

Fig. 14.1. A model for evaluation and remediation of impaired hearing (Goldstein and Stephens 1981).

aids and if so what problems, if any, were encountered? Enquiries should be made about any previous speech-reading tuition.

With regard to *associated variables*, it is important to find out the patient's attitude to his hearing disability and how this has affected his lifestyle and social activities. *Related conditions* is a term that covers other factors such as the patient's mobility. Is he fully mobile, chairbound or bed-bound? Would environmental aids be more appropriate than hearing aids? The upper limb function is important when considering the handling of the fine controls of hearing aids. Tactile sensitivity and manipulative skills may be affected by arthritis or cerebrovascular accidents, which can be a deciding factor in the decision between binaural or monaural hearing aid fitting. Does the patient have an ear condition such as tinnitus, vertigo or chronic otitis which can influence the type of hearing aid system used?

Remediation

The second half of Goldstein and Stephen's model (Fig. 14.1) deals with the remediation component of rehabilitation. It must be emphasised that hearing aids are but one component of the rehabilitation process.

The *attitude of the patient* is of paramount importance as the sequence and nature of treatment depends on it. Four main categories of patient can be identified. One group of patients will have a strongly positive view towards hearing aids and will be eager to proceed with rehabilitation. With another group, a positive attitude is counteracted by other influences such as an unfavourable past experience with rehabilitation or hearing aids. Yet another and smaller group will be negative towards the rehabilitation process although they may cooperate to some degree. They may feel stigmatised or degraded by having to use an aid and if one is fitted it is unlikely to be worn. It is preferable to try to modify attitudes initially and to defer fitting an aid until later. A fourth, small group of patients have a strongly negative attitude to hearing aids and other aspects of rehabilitation, rejecting them completely. They have usually been brought for assessment by a well-meaning relative or carer. They are unlikely to take part in the rehabilitation process and self-discharge from the programme is likely. With such patients, advice on environmental aids and communication tactics should be offered to family and friends and the opportunity for the patient to return for further guidance should be available.

In the past *instrumental remediation* has generally meant the fitting of hearing aids (Fig. 14.2). Recently, however, environmental aids have become more sophisticated and more widely available. These are particularly suitable for elderly people among whom wearable hearing aids may be of limited value.

Although they are also often valuable in suppressing tinnitus, amplification is the most basic function of hearing aids. While the aid makes it easier for the patient to hear sounds, it will not improve sound clarity. Sound distortion may already be present from a damaged auditory system and a hearing aid will amplify such distortion. Background noises (which are filtered by the normal ear) are also amplified. Most patients prefer an aid which is discreet such as the "in-the-canal" aid. However many old people do not have the manual dexterity to fit such an aid. Indeed many have difficulty in handling the more commonly used (and more sophisticated) "behind-the-ear" aids. Some, who have difficulty with the controls,

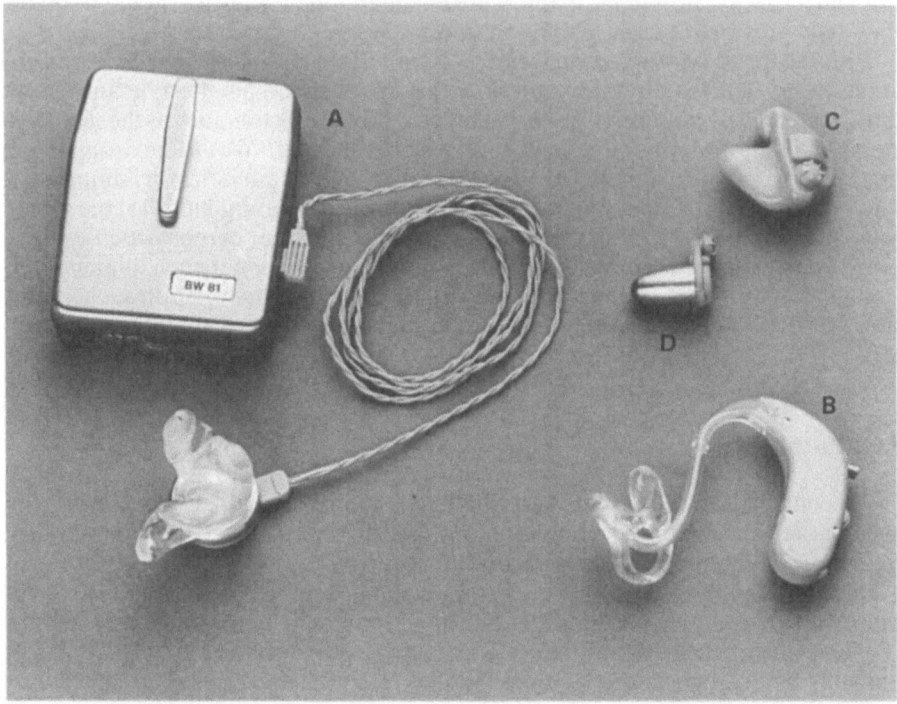

Fig. 14.2.   Hearing aids. **A** Body-worn aid with lead, receiver and earmould. **B** Post-aural aid with earmould. **C** In-the-ear aid. **D** In-the-canal instrument.

may need to be fitted with body-worn aids which generally have large simple controls.

Hearing aids, while never perfect, are of considerable help to most of their users. Modifications and alterations may be required once the aid has been in use for some time and the user has become familiar with it. One of the problems often encountered in old people is that of keeping the aid in position with an earmould. Simplification of the mould may be necessary to enable the patient to fit it in his ear and in certain cases stetoclips or "Walkman" headsets may be used instead.

Environmental aids are available to be used at home or at work, although they may also be used in public places such as hospitals, banks, shops, cinemas, theatres or railway stations. Such aids can be sub-divided into amplification systems and alerting/warning devices. They may be useful regardless of whether or not the patient is using a hearing aid and should generally be viewed as complementary to the aid rather than as an alternative.

Major problems often arise with television when the hearing-impaired individual needs to increase the sound volume to a degree where it disturbs others. In this case an additional external speaker can be positioned close to the hearing-impaired person's seat. Another approach entails the use of a small portable amplifier linked to the television and connected to lightweight headphones or a small insert receiver which is used by the patient. Electromagnetic (loop) systems create an electromagnetic field that picks up television sound and transmits it to the hearing aid user. Their major advantage is that the listener is able to hear the sound signal from the television without the interference of background noises from the room. A similar system can be used in theatres, cinemas and churches and other public places.

Telephone aids consist of either an additional amplifier in the handset or an electromagnetic system. Both systems can be usefully combined within the one telephone handset.

Alerting or warning systems are available to help overcome the problem of signal or noise discrimination (e.g. hearing the telephone ring while listening to the radio). The easiest ways to do this are to increase the loudness of the bell, put the bell closer to the individual, or a combination of the two. Alternatively, the bell may be coupled to a system in which a light on the telephone handset or lights in the house may be flashed on or off when the bell rings; a similar system is used for doorbells. Lights, louder bells and pillow vibrators may be used if the problem is with alarm clocks.

When planning the *remediation strategy*, the goals must be practical and relate to the nature of the hearing loss, together with the lifestyle, capabilities and attitude of the patient. Once such goals are defined, the individual must be given the opportunity to attain them. No single treatment strategy will work for all patients as the individual's personality and philosophy must be taken into account. The physical environment may need to be adapted and others may need to be made aware of the patient's needs and problems. This may involve teaching basic speech-reading tactics such as keeping background noise to a minimum, positioning the speaker so that he is facing the listener with the light on his face, speaking slowly and clearly and not obscuring the front of his mouth.

The rehabilitation process may require *ancillary help* from other specialists. The skills and advice provided by other members of the multidisciplinary team are described in Chapter 25 and the social services which people with a hearing handicap require are described in Chapter 28.

Communication training is the most important process in the remediation model (Fig. 14.1) and is the purpose and goal of the rehabilitation effort. Every patient must be considered as a candidate for this segment of rehabilitation. Some

Table 14.2. Factors producing variation in speech-reading ability

Visual acuity
Distance from speaker
Lighting
Conversational predictability
English competency
Motivation
Susceptibility to auditory distraction
Listening behaviour
Familiarity with speaker
Visibility of speaker's face and lips
Annunciation/accent
Communication tactics
Sensitivity to non-verbal cues
Perceptive ability
Individual's characteristics: shy/outgoing/dogmatic
Attitude towards hearing loss, hearing aid, speech-reading
Confidence in ability
Fatigue

may pass through very quickly while others may need repeated sessions. The patient should acquire sufficient information about how we hear, the nature and likely progression of hearing loss, how to use a hearing aid and basic hearing tactics. Skill building involves training in hearing tactics, how to fit, adjust and use a hearing aid and earmould. Also included in this category is basic training in speech-reading and the factors that can influence it (Table 14.2). Counselling entails receiving information about problems and experiences from the patient and discussing ways in which these can be dealt with. It is important to consider referral of patients in need of such support to a trained counsellor.

Communication training should be continued until the patient and therapist decide that as much has been achieved as can be reasonably hoped for. The patient is then discharged with the knowledge that he can return should any further problems occur.

Further Reading

Glendenning F (ed) (1982) Acquired hearing loss and elderly people. Beth Johnson Foundation, Keele, Staffs
Goldstein DP, Stephens SDG (1981) Audiological rehabilitation: management model 1. Audiology 20:432–452
Hinchcliffe R (ed) (1983) Hearing and balance in the elderly. Churchill Livingstone, Edinburgh
Salomon G (1986) Hearing problems and the elderly. Danish Medical Bulletin, special supplement series No. 3
Stephens SDG (1987) Audiological rehabilitation. In: Kerr AG, Groves J (eds) Scott Brown's Otolaryngology, 5th edn, vol 2, Adult audiology. Butterworth, London

Chapter 15

Impaired Mobility

Anne Freeman

Mobility is one of the basic necessities for an elderly person wishing to live an active and independent life. About a half of all retired people have a degree of impaired mobility. For many disability is slight and necessitates only a minor adjustment in life-style. However, there are some elderly people who are so severely handicapped by their immobility that they become confined to their house or even become bedridden. About 20% of patients admitted to a geriatric department will have been housebound for a significant length of time.

In order that immobile people can continue to live in the community some of the burden of care must fall on relatives, neighbours, friends and the community services. If medical treatment and rehabilitation fails to improve mobility and if there is inadequate support at home then the patient may be destined for long-term institutional care.

The incidence of impaired mobility increases with age and it is much more common in women (Fig. 15.1). Impaired mobility has many possible causes but locomotor and neurological disorders are the most important.

Locomotor Disorders (Table 15.1)

Foot Problems

Foot problems, which are very common in elderly people, include hallux valgus, deformed and overlapping toes, corns and onychogryphosis. They are discussed in more detail in Chapter 16. Almost a quarter of old people are unable to cut their own toe-nails. Ulcers on the feet, either due to ischaemia or diabetes mellitus (neuropathic ulcers), can cause difficulty with walking. Mobility can be further impaired by ill-fitting shoes and slippers. Some elderly patients need to be properly assessed for shoes or boots in the surgical appliances department.

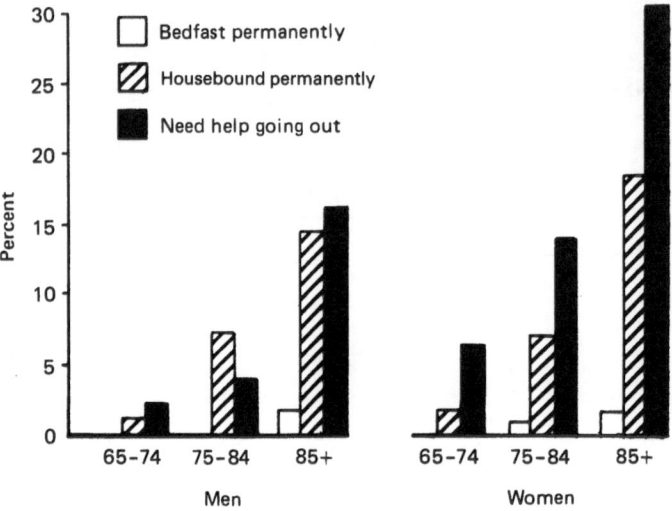

Fig. 15.1. Percentage of men and women with loss of mobility in each age group. (From Hunt A (1978) The elderly at home. HMSO, London.)

Table 15.1. Locomotor disorders causing immobility

Foot problems:	Deformities, corns, onychogryphosis, ischaemic ulcers, trophic ulcers
Bone disorders:	Fractures, osteoporosis, osteomalacia, Paget's disease, primary and secondary tumours
Joint disorders:	Osteoarthritis, rheumatoid arthritis, gout, pseudogout, septic arthritis
Muscle disorders:	Polymyalgia rheumatica, ischaemia, proximal myopathy
Miscellaneous:	Limb amputation

Bone Disorders

Fractures of the lower limb bones (especially the femoral neck) become more common with increasing age due to osteoporosis, osteomalacia, Paget's disease, secondary tumour deposits and the increased risk of falling. Patients usually present following a fall with pain in the hip and external rotation of the leg. Occasionally, however, the history is of increasing immobility and pain in the upper leg with no recent history of significant trauma. Radiographic examination may show an impacted and undisplaced fracture which can be treated conservatively with adequate analgesia and then mobilisation. However, for the majority of cases prompt surgical intervention is indicated (pin and plate insertion for intertrochanteric fractures and total hip replacement for the more proximal fractures). These patients should be able to weight-bear the day after their operation and then active rehabilitation should follow.

Osteoporosis, osteomalacia, Paget's disease and bone tumours are other bone disorders which impair mobility. They are discussed in Chapter 6. Osteoporosis can be a consequence as well as a cause of immobility.

Joint Disorders

Joint disorders are common accompaniments of old age. They include osteo-arthritis, rheumatoid arthritis, gout and pseudogout, septic arthritis and the seronegative arthroses. These also are discussed in Chapter 6.

Osteoarthritis affects mainly the weight-bearing joints such as the knees and hips, often causing great discomfort as well as immobility. All of the other arthritic conditions can also affect the lower limbs and impair mobility. Remember that elderly patients may have a combination of joint disorders such as, for example, co-existing rheumatoid arthritis and osteoarthritis.

Muscular Disorders

Muscular disorders causing impaired mobility include polymyalgia rheumatica (see Chap. 6), muscle ischaemia and proximal myopathy.

Peripheral arterial disease is a common finding in old age. It is usually chronic and is due to diffuse atheromatous narrowing of the arterial tree. It may present as intermittent claudication. On examination the legs are cool with absent peripheral pulses. There may be loss of hair and trophic ulcers. Radiological investigations (femoral arteriography or digital subtraction angiography) are essential in identifying the exact site and nature of the arterial narrowing.

Patients who smoke should be advised to stop and those with diabetes mellitus should be well-controlled to prevent further deterioration of the condition. Adequate foot care by a chiropodist and the prevention of both minor trauma and skin infection is important. Treatment with vasodilator drugs seldom improves the ischaemic limb. A localised stenosis can be treated surgically either by endar-terectomy or a by-pass graft. However, reconstructive vascular surgery has little to offer to a patient who has multiple diffuse narrowing from atheromatous plaques, though a lumbar sympathectomy can often give good pain relief and improve exercise tolerance.

With further arterial narrowing patients develop rest pain and finally gangrene (Fig. 15.2). Many of these patients will eventually require an amputation and the site of the operation (above or below the knee) must be carefully considered. It has to be proximal enough to allow the stump to heal while remembering that patients with a below-knee amputation do mobilise much quicker with an artificial limb because of the preservation of their own knee joint. Postoperatively the patient should be seen as soon as possible at a limb fitting centre to be measured for a prosthesis. In the meantime intensive physiotherapy can start, using a temporary pylon or a pneumatic post-amputation mobility (PPAM) aid (Fig. 15.3).

Patients occasionally present with a sudden occlusion to a large artery (e.g. a femoral embolus). The leg becomes cold with pallor, pain and paraesthesiae. An emergency embolectomy is then necessary in order to save the limb. Anticoagula-tion is the only hope for those patients who are too ill for surgery.

Proximal myopathy should be considered in any patient who gives a history of difficulty when climbing stairs or when getting up from a chair. The condition can be due to steroid therapy, thyroid dysfunction (hyper- or hypothyroidism), car-cinomatosis, osteomalacia, hypokalaemia and hypercalcaemia. The underlying cause must be identified and reversed.

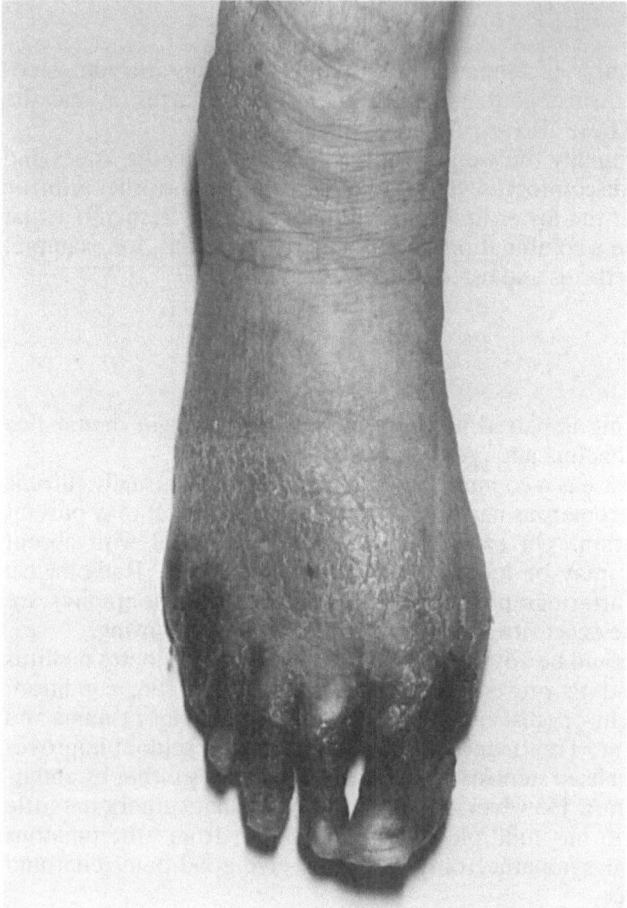

Fig. 15.2.   Gangrene of the foot in a patient with peripheral vascular disease.

Neurological Disorders (Table 15.2)

Cerebrovascular Disease

Cerebrovascular disease is the third commonest cause of death in the United Kingdom (after heart disease and cancer) and accounts for almost 20% of all medical and geriatric bed occupancy. It is the single most important cause of disability and yet it has been little researched. The most important risk factors are hypertension, diabetes mellitus, previous strokes, ischaemic heart disease and raised blood viscosity.

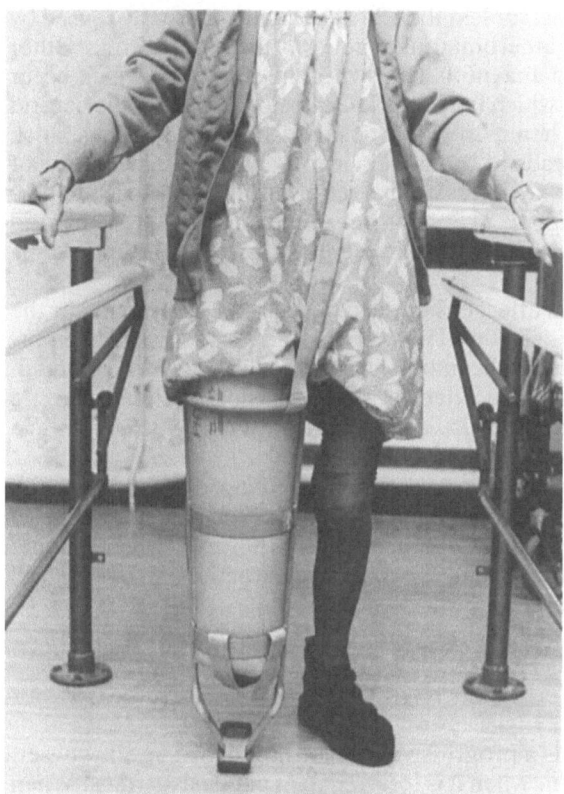

Fig. 15.3. Wearing a PPAM-aid shortly after a below-knee amputation. Temporary use of this aid allows partial weight bearing and early mobilisation.

Table 15.2. Neurological disorders causing immobility

Cerebrovascular disease
Parkinson's disease
Cervical myelopathy
Motor neurone disease
Peripheral neuropathy
Multiple sclerosis
Sub-acute combined degeneration of the cord
Cerebellar disease
Charcot–Marie–Tooth disease
Normal pressure hydrocephalus
Hemiballismus

A cerebrovascular accident is defined as a sudden ischaemic or haemorrhagic incident affecting the brain and usually resulting in neurological deficit. Strokes can be embolic or thrombotic (both causing cerebral infarction) or haemorrhagic. They can be conveniently divided into transient ischaemic attacks and completed strokes.

Transient ischaemic attacks last for less than 24 hours and are usually caused by small platelet emboli from an atheromatous plaque in the carotid tree. Other causes include hypotension and anaemia. The symptoms and signs which occur depend on the part of the brain which is affected. Occlusion of part of the carotid arterial system causes transient hemiparesis or sensory disturbance whilst a block in the vertebro-basilar artery leads to brain-stem symptoms of dizziness, loss of balance and visual disturbance. An occlusion in a retinal artery can cause temporary loss of vision (amaurosis fugax). Transient ischaemic episodes in the carotid arterial system carry a higher risk of a future completed stroke than those affecting the vertebro-basilar system.

A completed stroke may again affect either the carotid (most commonly) or the vertebro-basilar arterial system. The onset is generally sudden if due to a haemorrhage or an embolus whereas with a thrombotic stroke the onset is more gradual. Cerebral haemorrhage is strongly associated with hypertension and headache and unconsciousness occurs early in over 50% of cases. Loss of consciousness is less common with a cerebral thrombosis or embolus.

A hemiparesis of insidious onset (over weeks or months) suggests the possibility of a cerebral tumour. A short history of unilateral weakness and a fluctuating level of consciousness together with a history of a head injury (however trivial) should prompt the diagnosis of a subdural haematoma. In both situations a CT scan will be required to clarify the diagnosis.

Parkinson's Disease

Parkinson's disease (Fig. 15.4) is a progressive disease usually with a slow onset. The condition is usually idiopathic when it is referred to as paralysis agitans. When an underlying cause can be identified, drugs (e.g. neuroleptic agents) and poisons (e.g. heavy metals, carbon monoxide) are most often implicated. Parkinsonism resulting from an episode of encephalitis lethargica is now largely of historical interest. A Parkinson-like syndrome may occur with both Alzheimer's disease and multi-infarct dementia.

The disease is characterised by the triad of tremor, rigidity and bradykinesia. The tremor is most obvious in the hands and is classically "pill-rolling" in type. It is worst at rest and improves with purposeful activity. This serves to differentiate it from benign essential tremor which worsens with activity. The tremor is usually absent in the parkinsonism associated with Alzheimer's disease and multi-infarct dementia. The rigidity can be described as either lead-pipe or, more often, as cogwheel when there is associated tremor. The bradykinesia is demonstrated by a "mask-like" face (expressionless and unblinking) and a slow, shuffling, festinant gait with loss of the arm swing. Other features include difficulty in getting up from a chair or turning over in bed, micrographia, greasy skin, increased salivation and drooling (which is partly due to impaired swallowing) and a soft, monotonous voice. Postural hypotension and hypothermia can occur if there is damage to the autonomic nervous system (Shy–Drager syndrome).

Patients with Parkinson's disease usually experience increasing disability and decreasing mobility with time. The majority will benefit from physiotherapy, occupational therapy and speech therapy. Drug treatment is aimed at reducing the major symptoms. However, when the parkinsonism is secondary to Alzheimer's disease or multiple cerebral infarction there is a poor response to drug therapy.

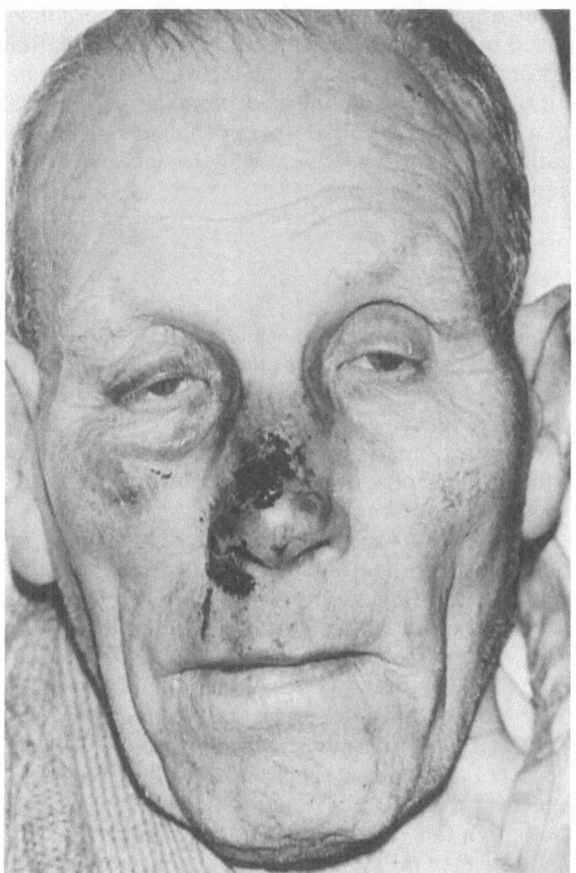

Fig. 15.4.   Facial injury following a fall in a patient with Parkinson's disease. This man also had profound postural hypotension.

Anti-cholinergic agents (e.g. benzhexol, benztropine and orphenadrine) are most effective in controlling rigidity and tremor. They can cause mental confusion and even psychosis so at least initially they should be used in small doses.

Levodopa (L-dopa) reduces bradykinesia and should be prescribed for all elderly patients whose mobility is significantly impaired. When given alone it tends to cause severe gastrointestinal side effects. It should therefore be combined with a decarboxylase inhibitor which, by blocking peripheral conversion of L-dopa to dopamine, will minimise side effects and allow larger doses to be tolerated. Small doses should be given initially and thereafter gradually increased until an acceptable degree of mobility is achieved. As the disease progresses so the dose of L-dopa may need to be increased. However, with large doses some patients experience dystonic movements which necessitate lowering the dose. An even greater problem is the "on–off" phenomenon seen in advanced disease. This is due to fluctuating levels of cerebral dopamine which when low may cause the patient to become totally immobile. The problem can be minimised by giving small doses of L-dopa frequently (sometimes as often as every hour).

Other effective drugs include the dopamine agonists bromocriptine, pergolide and lisuride. They are usually used in combination with L-dopa when the latter alone has failed to control symptoms. They may allow the dose of L-dopa to be lowered without loss of symptom control. Selegiline is a monoamine oxidase inhibitor and is most useful when combined with L-dopa in order to reduce the "on–off" phenomenon. Amantidine is an anti-viral agent which is largely free of side effects but is of sustained benefit to few patients.

Cervical Myelopathy

Cervical myelopathy is due to cervical cord compression which itself is usually secondary to cervical spondylosis or a prolapsed intervertebral disc. It often presents with stiffness and weakness in the limbs which gradually progresses over a period of months or years. Examination will reveal spasticity of the lower limbs with increased muscle tone, hyperreflexia and extensor plantar responses. Upper motor neurone signs are also found in the upper limbs, though if anterior horn cells are damaged, lower motor neurone signs will predominate in the area served by that spinal cord segment. Thus muscle wasting is a common clinical feature (Fig. 15.5) and tendon jerks may be absent. Sensory impairment from cord compression is common. Numbness and tingling in the fingers are often complained of and vibration and joint position sense are the modalities most likely to be impaired. Sphincter disturbance is usually only found in severe disease.

Radiographs of the cervical spine will show disc degeneration though this is present in 75% of all people over the age of 65 years. A cervical myelogram will confirm the diagnosis if this is in doubt. Treatment is either conservative or surgical. Neck immobilisation with a cervical collar may give symptomatic relief and possibly slow disease progression. Analgesia should be given for pain. Muscle spasticity can be reduced by dantrolene though this can sometimes exacerbate muscular weakness. Surgical management consists of either a laminectomy or fusion of the cervical spine. Disability from cervical myelopathy tends to fluctuate and so makes the evaluation of treatment difficult. However, there is no convincing evidence that surgical intervention offers better long-term results than conservative management. Such major surgery is therefore best avoided in the majority of elderly patients.

Motor Neurone Disease

Motor neurone disease most commonly presents between the ages of 50 and 70 years but is sometimes seen in the very old. Its course varies from a rapidly deteriorating illness to one which runs a prolonged course over 4 or 5 years. There are three main forms of the disorder which can be present alone or, more commonly, in combination.

With amyotrophic lateral sclerosis the pyramidal tracts are predominantly involved. The limbs (generally the lower limbs) are spastic and weak. Tendon jerks are brisk and the plantar responses may be extensor. Another form, progressive muscular atrophy, is due to degeneration of the anterior horn cells in the spinal column. It is characterised by muscle wasting, weakness and fasciculation. With the third form, progressive bulbar palsy, lower motor neurone lesions of the bul-

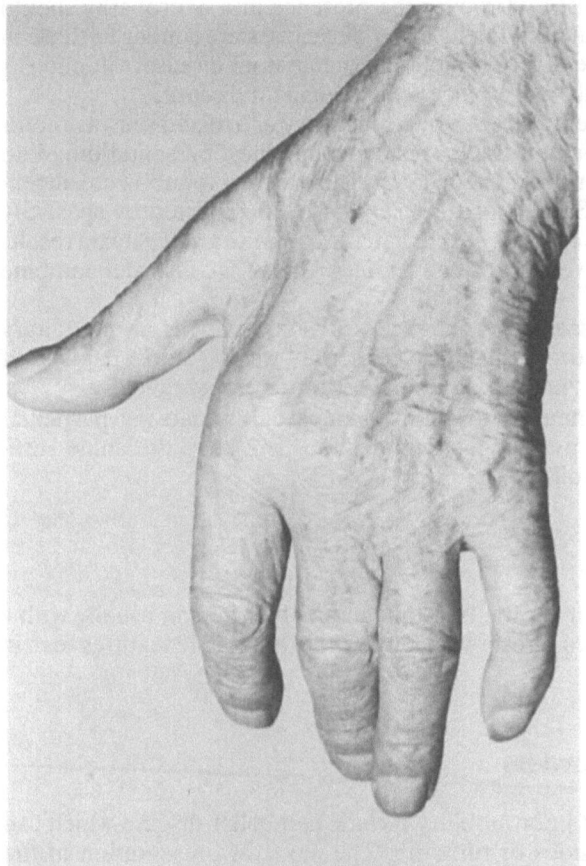

Fig. 15.5. Wasting of the small muscles of the hand in a patient with cervical myelopathy. (By permission of Dr. B. S. D. Sastry, University Hospital, Cardiff.)

bar muscles produce a wasted, fasciculating tongue with dysarthria and dysphagia due to palatal palsy. While a particular form of the disease is often predominant at presentation, with advanced disease elements of each are usually seen. There are no sensory signs.

The disease is relentless and there is no cure. Nutritional supplementation may be necessary when dysphagia limits food intake. Later on feeding through a naso-gastric or gastrostomy tube may be required. Parotid irradiation may decrease sialorrhoea if it distresses the patient. In the final stages the principles of terminal care apply (see Chap. 26) though pain is psychological rather than physical and death is usually due to pneumonia.

Peripheral Neuropathy

Peripheral neuropathy is common in old age. The ageing process itself can result in the loss of ankle jerks and impaired sensation (especially the modalities of vibration and joint position sense). However the presence of a neuropathy should always prompt a search for underlying disease. The causes are similar to those in younger patients and include diabetes mellitus, rheumatoid disease, vitamin B_{12} deficiency, drug (including alcohol) toxicity and malignant disease.

Elderly diabetics may develop either a purely sensory or a mixed sensori-motor neuropathy. Numbness or pain in the feet is the commonest presentation. With vitamin B_{12} deficiency the peripheral neuropathy can progress to sub-acute degeneration of the spinal cord. Spinal cord involvement is manifested by spasticity which initially affects the lower limbs but can later involve the arms. Ataxia results from posterior column involvement but all the elements of the disorder combine to impair mobility.

Charcot–Marie–Tooth disease (peroneal muscular atrophy) is an hereditary sensori-motor peripheral neuropathy characterised by wasting and weakness of distal muscles producing the "inverted champagne bottle" appearance.

Foot drop in peripheral neuropathy can impair mobility causing particular problems when climbing steps. A lightweight caliper will keep the ankle sufficiently flexed to improve mobility.

Multiple Sclerosis

Multiple sclerosis can present for the first time in an older person usually with a slowly progressive spastic paraparesis with few of the more classic features seen in the younger patient.

Other Neurological Disorders

Other neurological causes of poor mobility include cerebellar disease which can be secondary to vascular lesions or tumours. The mode of presentation of the ataxic symptoms will usually suggest the underlying cause.

Vascular and malignant lesions can also involve the spinal cord. Anterior spinal artery thrombosis causes a sudden paraplegia. Tumours involving the spinal cord are usually extrinsic rather than intrinsic and due to secondary deposits rather than primary tumours.

Normal pressure hydrocephalus is characterised by ataxia, incontinence and dementia of insidious onset. Despite its name the intra-cranial pressure is elevated and the condition can be improved by a ventriculo-peritoneal shunt.

Hemiballismus refers to unilateral, involuntary movements of the face and limbs and is usually due to a vascular lesion. The movements can be severe enough to impair mobility but are usually absent during sleep. Tetrabenazine is the drug of choice in controlling symptoms.

Non-locomotor and Non-neurological Disorders

A variety of non-locomotor and non-neurological disorders can either directly or indirectly impair mobility (Table 15.3). These conditions will largely have been described elsewhere in this book and so will be mentioned only with regard to their effect on mobility.

Table 15.3. Non-locomotor and non-neurological disorders causing immobility

Cardio-respiratory diseases
Impaired vision and hearing
Psychiatric disorders
Falls
Iatrogenic disease
Generalised weakness
Pain
Bedrest
Overprotection

Cardio-respiratory Diseases

Cardio-respiratory diseases such as angina pectoris, dyspnoea and lower limb oedema cause many elderly people to limit their activities. Again, immobility is a cause as well as a consequence of leg oedema and a vicious circle can result.

Impaired Vision and Hearing

Impaired vision and hearing are discussed in Chapters 13 and 14 respectively. Many blind, old people can remain mobile and independent when in familiar surroundings. Others, however, become anxious and lose confidence with the onset of either poor sight or poor hearing. This is more likely to happen when the handicap is of sudden onset or when they already had difficulty in coping due to existing disease.

Psychiatric Disorders

Psychiatric disorders causing immobility include depression, anxiety states, hysteria and dementia.

Depression (see Chap. 19) can present with weakness, tiredness, apathy and retardation (slowed thoughts and movements). The immobility is usually reversible with appropriate antidepressant treatment. Hysteria, presenting as hysterical paralysis, is very rare but can occur in an older patient usually in association with an underlying depression.

Senile dementia (see Chap. 18) can produce an immobility which may improve with physiotherapy. Alzheimer's disease can cause an extrapyramidal syndrome and multi-infarct dementia can result in a characteristic gait disturbance ("marche à petits pas"). Falls are more common in patients with dementia.

Falls

Falls are a cause as well as a consequence of immobility. They can cause bruising which, even when minor, can cause immobility due to discomfort on walking. The fear of falling and its consequences (timor cadendi) causes habitual fallers to lose their confidence and develop a phobic anxiety about walking. This usually occurs in people who have other features of an anxiety state. The careful use of tranquillisers and the availability of a telephone or an alarm call system often helps to alleviate these fears.

Iatrogenic Disease

Iatrogenic disease is common in old age and is most often drug induced. The most commonly offending drugs are listed in Table 15.4. Particular care must be taken in prescribing hypnotics and sedatives from which there is often a "hangover" effect on the following day. The excessive use of diuretics and laxatives can induce hypokalaemia which in turn can lead to weakness, proximal myopathy and cardiac arrhythmias.

Table 15.4.   Drugs causing immobility

Drugs	Mode of action
Hypnotics	Oversedation, hangover effect
Major tranquillisers	Parkinsonian features
Diuretics and laxatives	Hypokalaemia
Anti-convulsants	Osteomalacia
Laevodopa	Postural hypotension
Diuretics	Postural hypotension
Other anti-hypertensives	Postural hypotension
Antidepressants	Postural hypotension

Generalised Weakness

Generalised weakness may be due to a variety of disorders including myocardial infarction, infection, thyroid and adrenal disorders, electrolyte disturbance, osteomalacia and anaemia. It is also a common symptom of depression. The important point is that it should not be ignored but should prompt a search for the underlying cause. Anaemias and endocrine disorders are not uncommon in old people and are often found in patients with a longstanding history of increasing weakness and immobility.

Thyrotoxicosis usually presents with cardiac failure, loss of weight, anxiety or proximal myopathy. "Apathetic thyrotoxicosis" is also well recognised where the patient is lethargic rather than restless. Immobility can be a prominent feature of myxoedema due to general "slowing down" and the other classic features such as weight gain, mental confusion, cold intolerance, diffuse hair loss, puffy complexion, delayed ankle jerks and bradycardia may also be found.

Hypokalaemia can be caused by vomiting, diarrhoea, diuretic therapy and an inadequate dietary intake. Severe hypokalaemia can cause profound weakness and even complete paralysis which is reversed with replacement therapy. Hypomagnesaemia is probably under-recognised as a cause of generalised weakness as it is seldom looked for.

Cushing's syndrome causes weakness due to hypokalaemia and proximal myopathy whereas Addison's disease causes a generalised weakness. However, both are rare in the elderly population.

Pain

The locomotor causes of immobility almost invariably cause pain and the individual response to perceived pain is very variable. Stoics will endeavour to remain mobile despite severe pain whilst others "take to their beds" with only a minor discomfort and can then rapidly become totally immobile. Most people try to avoid those factors which precipitate pain and the elderly are no exception. Therefore, if movement causes severe pain they may avoid getting up and walking whenever possible.

Bedrest

Although bedrest may be indicated for some people (e.g. following a fracture or a myocardial infarction) immobility is a common outcome for an old person who stays in bed even for a few days. Often they will require hospitalisation to treat the resulting immobility rather than the original illness. Time in bed must be kept to the minimum and patients who require prolonged bedrest (e.g. for traction following a femoral fracture) should have regular passive or active movements to their limbs.

People who like to stay in bed should be discouraged from doing so and educated about the dangers of immobility. Any underlying cause should be reversed. For example, many old people stay in bed through boredom, depression or in an effort to keep warm in winter. In hospital, cot sides should always be used sparingly as they prevent patients from getting in and out of bed independently to go to the toilet. Patients who do have to be catheterised should have a discreet drainage bag strapped to their thigh. Dignity as well as mobility will thus be maximised.

Overprotection

Members of the patient's family can unwittingly cause immobility by overprotecting and "molly-coddling". It is often easier and quicker to do a job oneself than wait for an older person to do it. Families should try to encourage independence by allowing their elderly relatives to continue to do domestic tasks.

Similarly in hospital, nurses find that patients take a long time to get to the toilet usually because of the increased distance involved. However, they must avoid taking these patients in a wheelchair simply because it is a quicker alternative.

Some elderly people like to be cared for and attended to and are only too ready to surrender their independence to their carers, whether they are at home or in an institution. The carers occasionally welcome this dependence and encourage the person to adopt a "sick role". This unhealthy relationship should be discouraged for obvious reasons.

Complications of Immobility

The main complications are listed in Table 15.5. Contractures and fixed-flexion deformities should be preventable by regular active and passive movements of the limbs during a period of enforced immobility. However, once developed they can occasionally be corrected either by gradual extension exercises or by surgical tenotomy.

Pressure areas are common especially in the frail elderly and are always exacerbated by immobility. There are now many different types of mattresses and cushions available to help with the prevention of pressure sores and an occupational therapist can advise on the appropriate choice. Immobility aggravates venous stasis and further reduces venous return from the legs. Venous ulcers can occur, usually over the medial malleolus, and are often hard to treat. By comparison, arterial ulcers usually occur over the anterolateral aspect of the ankle and lower part of the shin.

Hypothermia can occur in patients who fall and are unable to get up without assistance. If they live alone they may spend many hours on the floor before they are found.

Table 15.5. Complications of immobility

Contractures and fixed-flexion deformities
Muscle wasting
Obesity
Pressure areas
Constipation
Urinary incontinence
Pneumonia
Venous thrombosis and pulmonary embolism
Hypothermia
Prolonged hospitalisation
Loss of confidence
Loneliness and social isolation
Dependency on others

Clinical Evaluation

All too often elderly people accept failing mobility as an inevitable accompaniment of growing old. Ageing itself does produce a minor degree of neuromuscular impairment but if an old person is having difficulty in coping with the activities of daily living then it is likely that there is an underlying disorder which needs to be investigated. Carers should be made aware of this and should ensure that the patient seeks appropriate medical attention.

Symptoms relating to immobility may often be vague and yet can be caused by significant underlying disease such as a myocardial infarction. Generalised weakness is an example and patients of all ages find it difficult to say exactly what they mean by it. The history and clinical examination should allow one to decide whether it is due to a neuromuscular or to a systemic disorder.

As impaired mobility is often not perceived by the patient as an active problem it may therefore not be reported. It follows that in assessing all elderly patients the clinician should enquire as to how mobile he or she is. Ask a woman where she shops, as a person who shops in the city centre can be assumed to be reasonably mobile. Asking about holidays is another good screening question as non-essential travel is generally foregone with the onset of mobility problems.

Once a history of impaired mobility is obtained one should enquire about its onset, duration and severity. Specific questions to elucidate any underlying causative factors should be asked. It is essential to know how the patient copes with her disability, so details about her housing and social supports must be sought. A drug history is important as drugs are an important cause of immobility. History-taking should also aim to reveal other problems which compound that of immobility, for example impaired hearing or vision.

Disorders of any system of the body can result in, or contribute to, impaired mobility. It follows that the physical examination must be thorough. A full neurological examination and an assessment of the locomotor system is essential. Remember to look for evidence of proximal myopathy by asking the patient to rise from a chair without using the upper limbs. The single most important procedure in the assessment of a person's mobility is getting them to stand and walk. Observe the gait and measure balance with Romberg's test.

Management

Rehabilitation

Rehabilitation is essential in order to maximise mobility or at least to minimise the complications of immobility. The principles of rehabilitation are described in Chapter 25. It is very important that the patient's carers become involved in the treatment plan.

Community Services

Community services can make all the difference between an immobile or partially immobile patient being able to live at home or having to live in institutional care. Remember that those caring for dependent people may themselves need support. The loneliness and social isolation experienced by many old people is an enormous problem and it is only partially solved by the provision of voluntary transport to day centres and luncheon clubs and other functions arranged by voluntary organisations. The statutory and voluntary services available are described in Chapter 28.

Financial Support

Financial support is available for patients of any age with severe physical or mental illness. The details of this kind of help are also described in Chapter 28.

Further Reading

Coni N, Davison W, Webster S (1988) Lecture notes on geriatrics, 3rd edn. Blackwell Scientific Publications, Oxford
Hall MRP, MacLennan WJ, Lye MDW (1986) Medical care of the elderly, 2nd edn. John Wiley & Sons, Chichester
Martin A (1981) Problems in geriatric medicine. MTP Press, Lancaster
Wilcock GK, Gray JAM, Pritchard PMM (1982) Geriatric problems in general practice. Oxford University Press, Oxford

Chapter 16

Foot Problems

D. F. Jessett

"It is rare indeed for an elderly person to have normal feet."

(Dixon 1976)

It is estimated that between 50% and 80% of the adult population have something wrong with their feet. By the mid-1970s, over 1 million people of pensionable age were receiving free chiropody services in Britain annually. This does not accurately reflect the extent of foot problems in the elderly as the demand for services is not fully met, with some people going untreated and others being treated privately. As the numbers of old people continue to rise, the need for chiropody services will continue to increase.

The foot is vulnerable, being that part of the body which is subjected to the heaviest loads. It is at the most distal point of the circulatory system, the most peripheral part of the nervous system and its temperature is lower than that of any other part of the body. While hands are almost always in view, feet and legs are covered with hosiery and thrust out of sight into footwear. Long, slim feet and short, broad feet represent extremes of configuration which standard-sized footwear does not easily fit. Patients whose feet are deformed by congenital or acquired disease may experience even greater difficulty in obtaining suitable footwear. In choosing footwear, fashion and style often have a higher priority than fit and usage, a reason why more women than men develop foot problems.

Many patients of all age groups do not regard disabilities in the feet in the same light as other disabilities. They expect to retain mobility even when, for example, a seriously infected toe or diabetic ulcer may require a period of complete rest. The general level of activity of some patients may be extremely limited due to the extent and severity of their chiropodial problems. Treatment is sometimes necessary not because of any significant foot pathology, but because failing eyesight, obesity, arthritis, postural hypotension or some other disorder makes it hazardous or impossible for the patient to cut their own toenails.

Major Acquired Disorders

Arthritis

Arthritis results in joint swelling and deformity and is most often due to rheumatoid arthritis, osteoarthritis or gout. These are discussed in more detail in Chapter 6. Osteoarthritis and gout mainly affect the first metatarso-phalangeal joint. With rheumatoid disease the forefoot is often extensively involved (Fig. 16.1). Bizarre deformities of the toes may result making it impossible for the patient to wear ordinary footwear. Other joints and soft tissues may also be involved and further compromise the function of the foot. Vasculitis may cause skin ulceration over prominent joints. Even patients who are unable to walk may continue to need treatment for thickened nails and plaques of callus.

Diabetes Mellitus

More diabetic patients are hospitalised because of foot problems than because of any other diabetic complication. The diabetic foot may be ischaemic, neuropathic or the site of sepsis. The combination of sensory neuropathy and poor eyesight

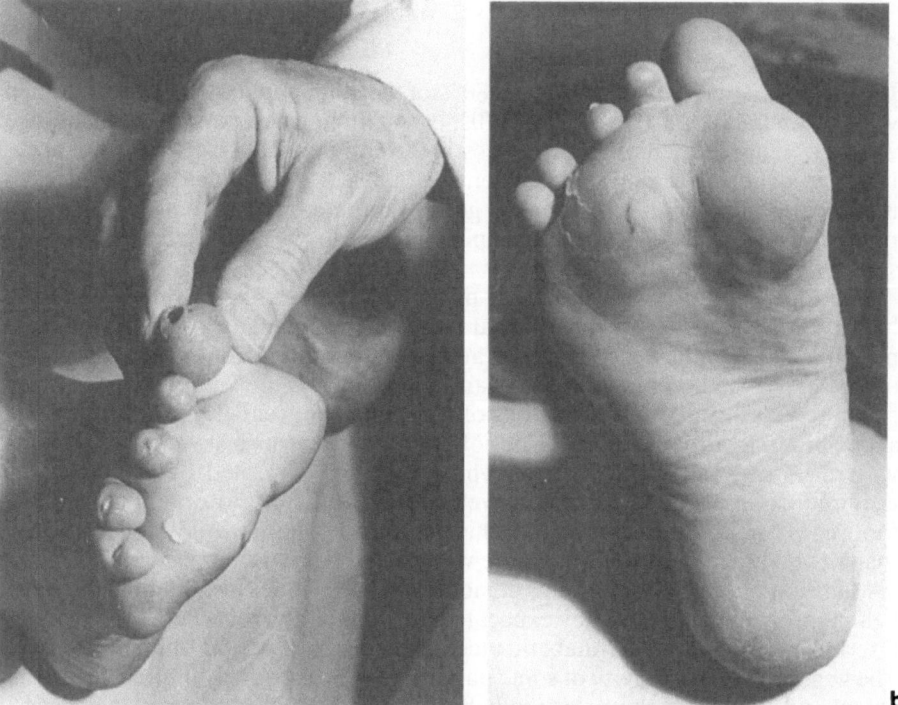

a   b

Fig. 16.1.   The foot in rheumatoid disease. **a** The metatarso-phalangeal joints are subluxed. There is a vasulitic lesion on the hallux and the nails are atrophic or absent. **b** There is a well-circumscribed plantar callus. The skin is atrophic and may ulcerate easily.

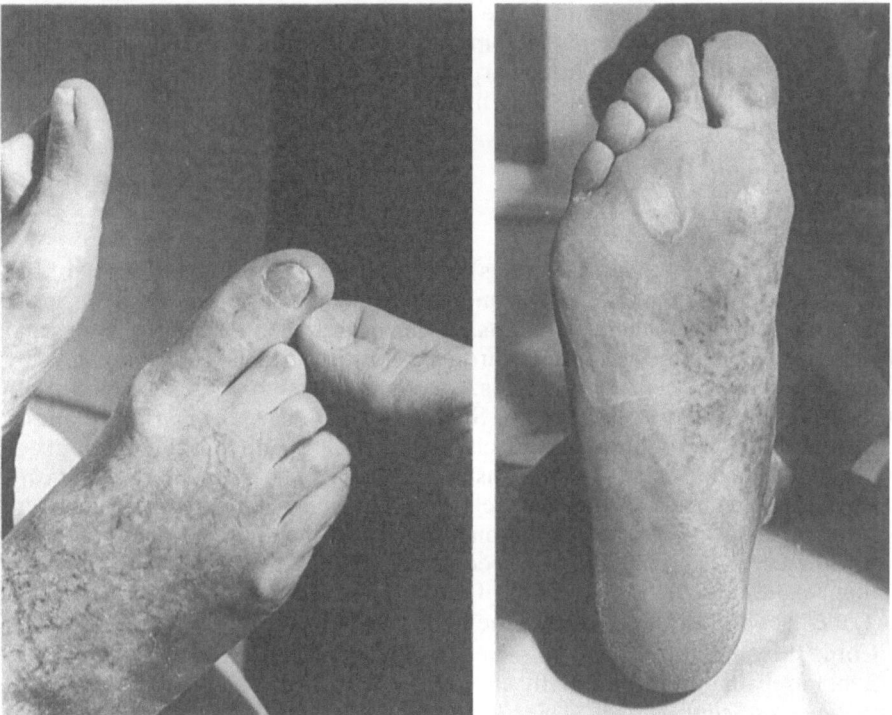

a   b

Fig. 16.2.   Superficial varices on **a** the dorsum and **b** the plantar aspect of the foot.

may, in the words of Bloom (1978), cause the elderly diabetic to be "divorced from his feet since he can neither feel them nor see them properly". Motor neuropathy may cause clawing of the toes with the development of callosities on the bony prominences thus formed. Autonomic neuropathy will disturb sweating patterns and cause changes in skin texture. Oedema is a further complication and when the foot is swollen, footwear may abrade the skin. Breaches in the skin admit pathogenic microorganisms which thrive in the sugar-rich environment and results in sepsis. This in turn may upset diabetic control and if untreated lead to gangrene and the need for amputation of part of the limb.

Vascular Disease

Oedema of the foot is most often due to varicose veins (see Chap. 9). Deposits of haemosiderin from leaking capillaries discolour the lower third of the leg and the dorsum of the foot. Varices are seen most commonly over the dorsum and plantar surfaces of the foot, and may extend as far as the toes (Fig. 16.2). They are subject to trauma and the resultant haemorrhage can be copious. The slowing of the blood flow caused by varicose veins slows the healing of wounds and alters the texture of skin and nails. Such skin tolerates the prolonged application of adhesive dressings badly. Varicose veins themselves can be treated by compression, by surgical excision or by sclerotherapy.

Arterial insufficiency may improve if a patient stops smoking. Surgical inter-vention in the form of sympathectomy or arterial by-pass grafting may be re-quired. Before the arrival of fitted carpets, walking on cold linoleum used to give relief to patients with rest pain. Pain, uncontrolled by analgesics, may presage the need for amputation.

Callus and Corns

A thickening of the epidermis (callus) is a normal response to intermittent but chronic pressure. In the foot it is common on the plantar surface around the heels, under the metatarso-phalangeal joints, on the dorsum and apices of the toes and the plantar aspect of the great toe. Chronic callosities are usually accompanied by atrophy of the subjacent dermis. This, together with microscopic changes in the sub-dermal tissues give rise to pain. Such lesions are almost invariably compli-cated by the inclusion of blood vessels, nerve endings and variable amounts of fibrous tissue (Fig. 16.1b). In some instances they may be bound to the joint cap-sules. Blood may be forced from vessels, creating small haemorrhagic spots in the corn or callus. Sometimes a haematoma may be formed and an ulcer may form below the corn. It has erroneously been stated that these ulcers, especially in a diabetic patient, develop as a result of the careless removal of callus, whereas in fact, the hyperkeratotic mass hides the underlying ulcer.

Corns (heloma durum) are characterised by the presence of a nucleus. This is 1–2 mm in diameter and is usually circular, though it may be much larger and is sometimes crescent shaped. The nucleus is harder than the callus in which it is embedded though both have a lamellar structure. It has been suggested that nuclear formation is due to parakeratosis and histologically it resembles psoriasis. Corns may occur wherever there is a bony prominence which provides a resistance to pressure on either the dorsum or the plantar aspect of the foot. The skin is sub-ject to intermittent stress: a combination of pressure, friction and shearing. Such stresses can also occur between adjacent toes, in the nail grooves and below the nail plate. Interdigital corns may become macerated by retained sweat, hence their name "soft corns" (heloma molle).

Neurovascular corns (heloma neurovasculare) signify a long-standing lesion. They are frequently the result of improper treatment which produces a haemor-rhage and poor aftercare. They develop readily on poorly nourished skin and on the site of broken chilblains. The junction of dorsal and plantar skin at the borders of the feet is also a common site for these exceedingly painful lesions. Corns may be complicated by the presence of a bursa in the subjacent tissue. Over-enthusias-tic enucleation can open a path to the bursa which may then become infected.

Where a corn or callus is situated over a joint, fibrosis can cause them to become bound down to the adjacent joint capsule. Chronic joint sepsis which is particu-larly intractable and resistant to antibiotics may result. Repeated healing and breakdown over a period of years may suggest underlying osteomyelitis.

Ulcers

Ulcers are secondary to a variety of causes ranging from circulatory insufficiency to diabetes and vasculitis. Those associated with diabetes commonly occur on the plantar aspect of the first metatarso-phalangeal joint though they may occur over any bony prominence, even being produced in bedridden patients by the weight of limbs or bed clothes. They may penetrate to involve deeper structures, including bone and sometimes need surgical treatment such as debridement and skin grafting. Vasculitic ulcers are superficial and once the underlying cause is treated, and pressure reduced by appropriate dressings, they heal rapidly.

Nails

Patients unable to care for their nails are often too ashamed to show them to another person or ask for help in cutting them. The discomfort of the thickened nails may prevent the patient from wearing anything but house slippers and they can easily become housebound.

Being appendages of the skin, nails reflect its state, becoming dry, hard, thickened and brittle with age. Past trauma may have produced a thickened nail (onychauxes) and the "Ram's horn" nail (onychogryphosis), which is thickened and deformed, can twist across the foot to penetrate the skin and produce infection (Fig. 16.3). The transverse curvature of the nail plate is often greatly increased (involution) and is also thickened (Fig. 16.4). This so-called ingrowing toenail is extremely painful. Attempts to dig out the corner frequently lead to infection (paronychia) and give only temporary relief. Paronychia when combined with poor circulation may have serious consequences.

Thickened nails are reduced in length and thickness by means of nail nippers, scalpel or an electrically driven bur. Callosities, corns or skin debris under the free edge of the nail or in the lateral grooves are then removed. Packing may be applied where the nail plate digs into surrounding soft tissue. Slivers of chamois leather or even a silicone such as Viscogel may also be used. Severely involuted nails may be treated by partial avulsion under local anaesthetic if the patient's gen-

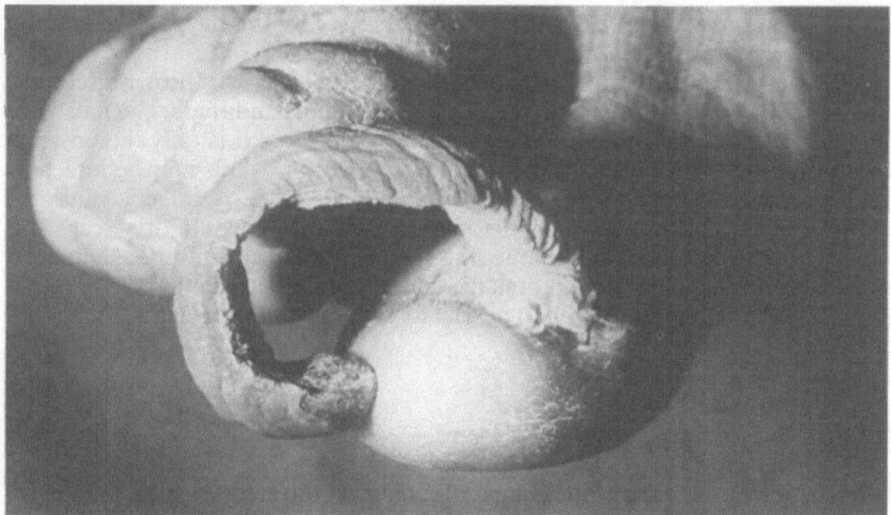

Fig. 16.3. Onychogryphosis.

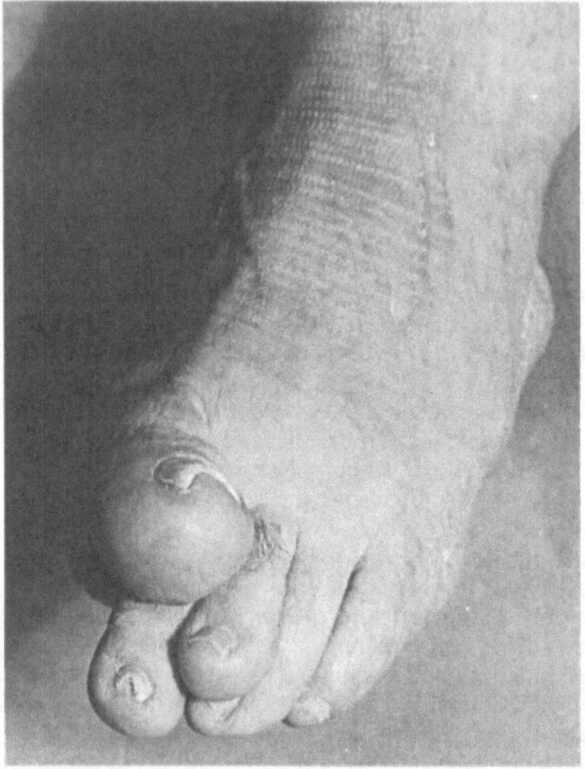

Fig. 16.4.   Involuted nail plate ("ingrowing toenail") of the hallux and second toe.

eral health permits. Solutions of local anaesthetic used for this purpose must never include adrenaline as gangrene may result.

Mycotic infections of the nail plate produce streaks of yellow or brown discoloration which may extend from the free edge to the lunula and under the nail fold. The nail plate becomes thickened and brittle. Very often it is only the unsightliness of the nail which disturbs the patient. One or more nails may be affected. The commonest infecting organism is *Trichophyton rubrum*. Infection may be confined to the nail, though the surrounding skin may become dry, scaly and itchy. Whilst mycotic infections of the skin respond well to anti-fungal agents such as miconazole nitrate, treatment of nails is disappointing. Reduction of the thickened nail and the application of an acrylic to give a smooth surface are the most satisfactory means of treatment.

Bursitis

Inflammation of the adventitious bursa situated over the medial aspect of the first metatarso-phalangeal joint is very common – a bunion. Bursitis may also affect the bursae superficial and deep to the Achilles tendon, the plantar aspect of the

heel and the lateral aspect of the fifth metatarso-phalangeal joint. In some instances the bursa may rupture and secondary infection can ensue. A sinus sometimes develops and chronic sub-acute bursitis results. The plantar calcaneal bursa
is particularly vulnerable in those instances where the sub-cutaneous fibro-fatty
plantar padding is deficient as a result of dehydration. Enforced rest through
debilitating illness can provoke this sequence of events.

In treating acute bursitis, inflammation should be reduced and stress on the
area relieved by means of padding and strapping. Often the bursitis becomes
chronic and requires long-term treatment, prolonged application of padding and
strapping or the wearing of a suitable shield. Plantar calcaneal bursitis may require shoe modification or the use of heel pads within the footwear. With atrophy
of the plantar padding, the patient feels as though he is walking on pebbles and is
relieved by an insole of Plastazote. This is washable, moulds easily to the shape of
the foot and can be obtained in a variety of densities. It is easily cut to shape to fit
within the shoe.

Scarring

However much care is taken in performing surgery on the foot, scars will sometimes occur on vital weight-bearing areas. The plantar metatarsal area is a common site. On a foot deficient in sub-cutaneous fibro-fatty padding, such scars
extending across the width of the foot can be disabling. Patients will require
chiropody treatment to reduce the callus and corns which develop within the scar
tissue.

Fissures

Fissuring of the skin is a feature of moist or dry skin. Between the toes moist fissures will follow the flexure lines. These may extend into dermis and bleed freely.
Any infection in this area can readily penetrate deep into the foot along the fascial
planes and may require surgical drainage.

Around the heel the fissure will be of the dry variety. These too may extend into
the dermis, bleed or become infected. The edges of dry fissures will be keratinised
and this prevents healing. These edges should be reduced with a sharp scalpel.
What callus remains may be painted with 12½% salicylic acid in collodion. This is
repeated at weekly intervals for 2 or 3 weeks. Thereafter, bland emollients will
help to maintain the skin in good condition and prevent further fissures from
developing.

The application of an antiseptic such as polynoxylin will help fissures to heal
rapidly, but they are best avoided by careful hygiene and frequent washing and
drying of the feet.

Clinical Evaluation

Inspection of the feet is part of any routine medical examination and is mandatory
in some patients (e.g. diabetics). Attention must be paid to joint deformity and

mobility, skin, nails, blood vessels and nerve supply. An appreciation of how foot problems have arisen is essential so that proper treatment can be planned and recurrence prevented, or at least the patient's discomfort minimised.

Because of its range of mobility, the forefoot has the greatest potential for deformity and some 80% of disorders treated by the chiropodist are situated here. Foot deformities can be congenital or acquired. If congenital, or acquired in childhood (e.g. due to poliomyelitis), normal development will not have occurred and the patient may have a lifetime of problems with secondary lesions such as collosities and corns. Acquired disorders arise from a multitude of causes and major alterations in the shape and function of the foot can result from insults such as trauma or following a stroke. The mobility of the whole foot is important in the causation of painful secondary lesions. Rigid feet usually have circumscribed callosities on the plantar aspect of prominent joints (e.g. the first and fifth metatarsophalangeals only) whereas mobile feet may have callus distributed over the plantar aspect of several such joints.

Inspection of the skin should include an assessment of skin colour, blistering or cracking of the skin, ulceration and signs of fungal and other infections. The areas between the toes are often affected and must be examined. Nails should be inspected for evidence of dystrophy or of ingrowing. Nail abnormalities may indicate systemic disorders. Cyanosis of the nail bed occurs in a variety of respiratory and cardiovascular disorders. Clubbing of the toenails may indicate pulmonary disease while other nail changes occur in psoriasis, iron deficiency, liver disease and many other conditions.

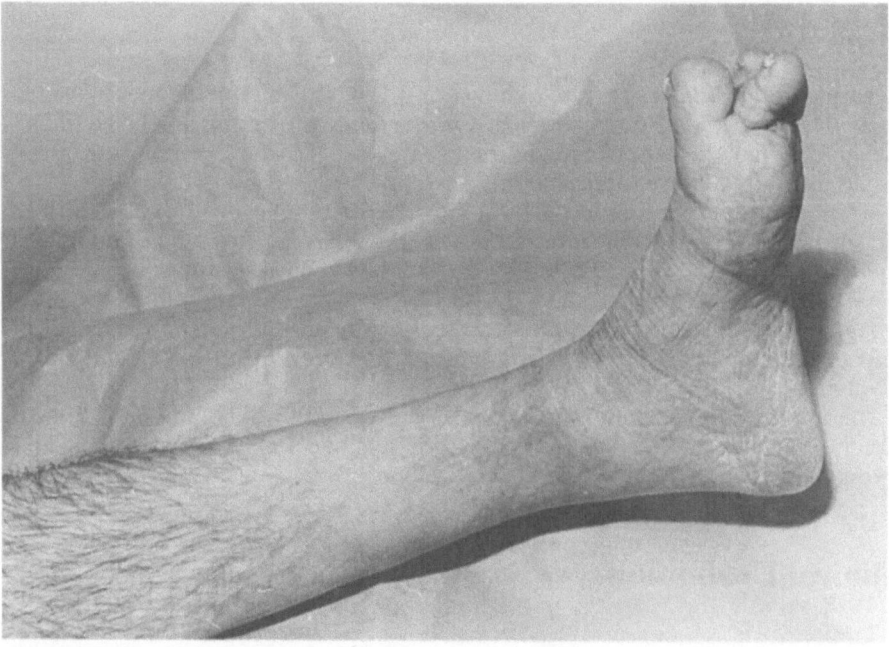

Fig. 16.5.   An ischaemic foot showing loss of hair, dry atrophic skin and nails. The plantar fibro-fatty padding is diminished in quantity and quality.

Claudication of the muscles of the foot on exercise is the commonest symptom associated with a diminished arterial blood supply. This can lead to rest pain which is usually worse at night when the body is warm. The dorsalis pedis and posterior tibial arteries should be routinely palpated and the pulse volume noted. If the pedal pulses are absent the popliteal and femoral pulses should be palpated in turn so that the level of the obstruction can be determined. With ischaemia a general atrophy of tissue occurs, hair is lost (Fig. 16.5), the texture of the skin becomes dry and inelastic and a temperature gradient is found, sometimes with a line of demarcation. The fibro-fatty pads below the heel and forefoot lack bulk and resilience. A red discoloration of the foot (ischaemic rubor) is found in advanced arterial disease. The capillary filling time gives a crude but useful index of foot ischaemia; it measures the time taken for the colour to return to an area of skin which has been blanched by finger pressure. Varicose veins should be looked for as should the sequelae of circulatory insufficiency, such as arterial or venous ulcers.

The sensory nerve supply to the foot should be assessed by checking cutaneous sensation. Motor nerve lesions produce muscle imbalance and lead to deformity such as clawed, retracted and hammer toes.

Note should be made of the state of general health and current medication. Patients taking anti-coagulants or steroids pose particular difficulties when having foot problems treated.

The patient's footwear should also be inspected as this can yield much diagnostic information (Fig. 16.6). Occult diabetes mellitus in male patients may be detected by urine splashes on the uppers of their footwear.

Management

As maintenance of mobility and independence are dependent on healthy feet, it follows that foot care is the concern of all those responsible for the well-being of old people. The chiropodist has particular skills in this area and is therefore

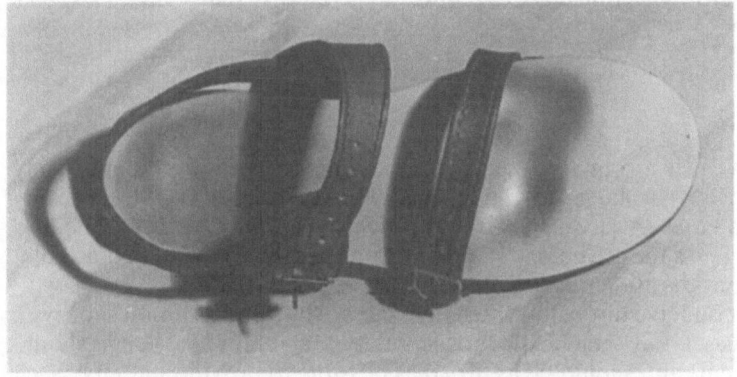

Fig. 16.6. Sandal worn by patient in Fig. 16.1. Note the deep depression produced by the overloaded metatarsal heads. There are no wear marks where the toes would ordinarily be.

an important member of the geriatric multidisciplinary team. Input from a chiropodist can be invaluable in the diabetic clinic for example. Here, regular inspection of the feet is a relatively cheap and effective way of monitoring an "at risk" group. In addition to treating existing disorders, incipient disorders can be identified and their progress arrested. An opportunity is also afforded to educate the diabetic patient about care of the feet and such patients should be encouraged to follow a daily routine of prophylactic measures.

Foot Care

The same advice regarding foot care can be given to elderly people as is given to diabetic patients since they share similar problems.

Feet should be washed daily in warm water and dried carefully, especially the area between the toes. The temperature of the water (including bath water) should not exceed 40°C and must be checked with a thermometer or by immersing one's elbow in it. Emollients should be applied to dry skin immediately after bathing.

Toenails should be trimmed straight across rather than cut back along the lateral grooves. They must not be picked or torn as this leaves rough edges which may penetrate the skin and become infected – a true ingrown toenail (onychocryptosis). Corns and callus should be treated by the chiropodist. Patent corn cures must not be applied as they contain salicylic acid which, if injudiciously used, can ulcerate the skin and can cause serious necrosis. Minor cuts and abrasions should be covered with clean gauze and reported to the chiropodist or doctor if healing does not occur. Any obvious change in skin colour must be reported to the chiropodist or doctor.

People should not sit too close to fires or heaters. Warm clothing should be worn especially during winter months. At night the bed may be warmed with a hot water bottle or an electric blanket; the bottle should be removed, however, or the blanket switched off, before entering bed. Loose-fitting bed socks may be worn.

Female patients should not use tight garters nor wear shoes with pointed toes; the former may reduce circulation to the leg and the latter will certainly impair circulation in the toes. Before putting on shoes the inside should be felt for roughness, nails or small stones which the foot may not feel due to neuropathy. Hosiery should be free of darns.

Footwear

Adequate footwear is a primary requirement in the successful treatment of any foot morbidity. Boots or shoes must be of an adequate width and depth, especially at the level of the toes. A lace-up shoe of the "Derby" style (Fig. 16.7) is near to the ideal as foot and shoe are held in the correct relationship. A lace is adjustable, an important consideration where a foot may swell with oedema. People with high-arched feet do have difficulty with a high lacing shoe and a slip-on shoe with an elasticated gusset may then be more acceptable. Maximum heel height should be 1½ inches (4 cm) and should be as broad as possible to provide stability. Such heels can be modified by the cobbler by floating them out on one side to further enhance stability.

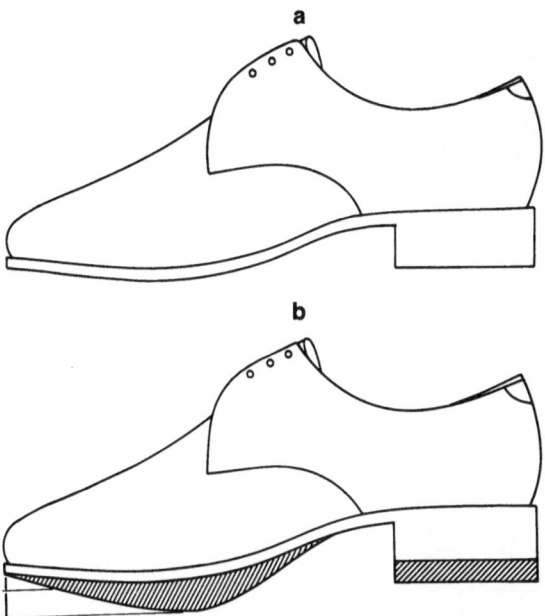

Fig. 16.7. **a** A "Derby" fronted lace-up shoe. The lacing comes high up on the instep and the front of the shoe is free of pattern and stitching (which can cause corns). **b** Shoe modified by the addition of a rocker sole. This aids walking where the hallux is rigid at the metatarso-phalangeal joint.

The upper of the shoe should be plain and made of leather. Patterns produced by stitching or overlapping pieces of leather seriously limit its "natural give" and prevent the shoe from moulding and accommodating minor foot deformities such as hammer toes and bunions. Soles and heels may be made from a variety of synthetic materials; rubber and polyvinyl chloride (PVC) are very acceptable. They should be thick so as to provide a surface which is shock-absorbing and insulating. Many modern shoes with moulded PVC soles are relatively waterproof too. These materials are light and hard-wearing and are readily modified. The addition of a rocker sole will limit flexion of the first metatarso-phalangeal joint (Fig. 16.7b). Such a modification can be carried out, to the order of a registered medical practitioner or chiropodist, by Somerset Orthopaedic Shoes, Merry Gardens, High Ham, Langport, Somerset TA10 9DB. The Bury Boot and Shoe Co., Bury, Lancs., have useful products for people with shoe fitting problems. Patients should be encouraged to keep footwear in good repair. A distorted shoe much worn over at the heel and outer border will quickly turn the foot over and may produce very serious injuries of the ankle and sub-talar joints.

Supports and Appliances

With many elderly patients correction of deformities is not possible and palliation is the chief aim. By the application of self-adhesive felts and foams of varying thickness and density, together with strappings, the chiropodist is able to further

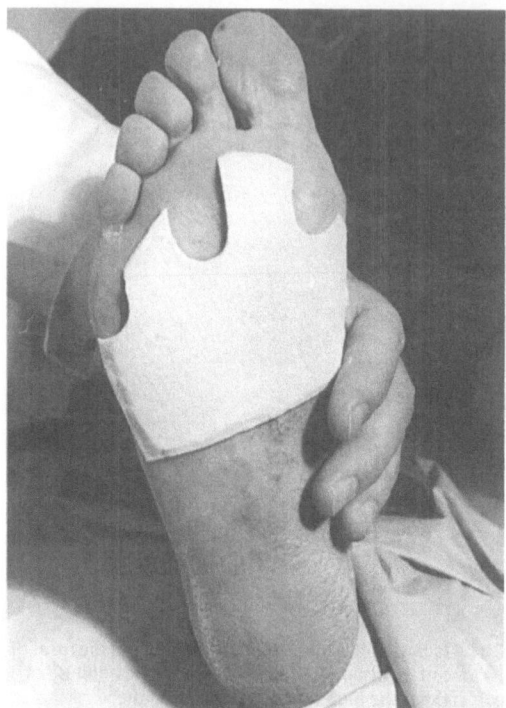

Fig. 16.8.   An adhesive pad used to relieve overload on parts of the foot.

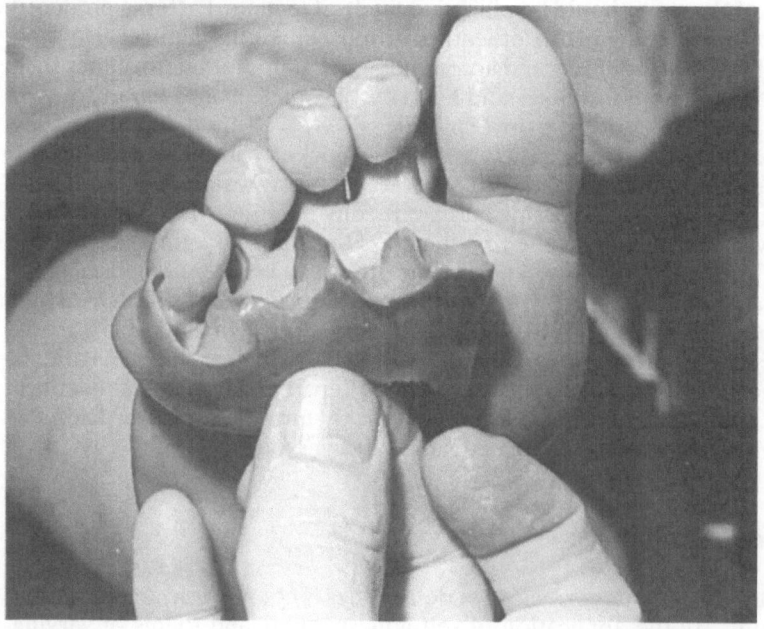

Fig. 16.9.   A multiple prop, designed to relieve stresses on the apex or dorsum of the toes.

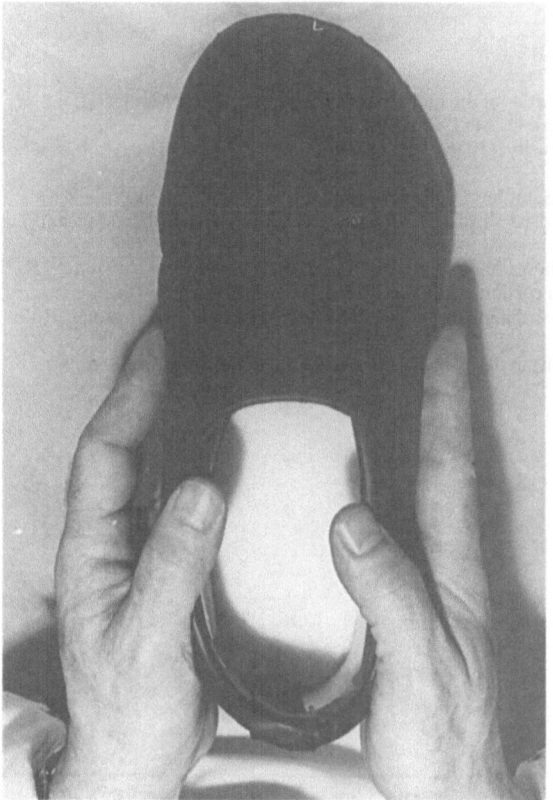

Fig. 16.10.   A space shoe.

reduce the effects of stress upon tissue (Fig. 16.8). Once the adhesive padding used in clinic has revealed the shape and bulk of materials that will achieve the desired affect, the pad may be fabricated in more durable materials to the individual requirements of the patient. The resulting appliance is aesthetically more pleasing because it can be kept cleaner than padding applied directly to the skin for long periods (Fig. 16.9).

Even with the use of modern hypo-allergenic adhesives, prolonged application of dressings is undesirable since the warmth and moisture caused by the occlusion of the skin may promote infection. The chief disadvantage of some of the appliances which may be fabricated by the chiropodist is the patient's inability to fit and remove them. If a relative or neighbour is not readily available to help the patient in this, then a space shoe is the only alternative. This is made from very light micro-cellular material and accommodates the most bizarre deformities (Fig. 16.10). Some patients resort to sandals, but these may not provide enough protection.

Further Reading

Beaven DW, Brooks SE (1984) A colour atlas of the nail in clinical diagnosis. Wolfe Medical, London
Bloom A (1978) Diabetes explained, 3rd edn. MTP Press, Lancaster
Department of Health and Social Security (1976) Prevention and health: everybody's business. HMSO, London
Jahss MH (1982) Disorders of the foot. Saunders, Philadelphia
Klenerman L (ed) (1982) The foot and its disorders, 2nd edn. Blackwell Scientific Publications, Oxford
Lake NC (1952) The foot, 4th edn. Bailliere Tindall and Cox, London
Marks R, Plewig G (eds) (1983) Stratum corneum. Springer-Verlag, Berlin Heidelberg New York
Neale D (1985) Common foot disorders: diagnosis and management. Churchill Livingstone, Edinburgh
Samman PD, Fenton DA (1986) The nails in disease, 4th edn. William Heinemann, London

Chapter 17

Falls and Syncope

D. Coakley

One of the most significant developments in the evolution of man was the achievement of an upright posture. The centre of gravity of the body lies in the neighbourhood of the second sacral vertebra and a plumb line through this point must fall within the base formed by the two feet if the erect body is to remain in equilibrium. If equilibrium is disturbed (e.g. by taking a step), corrective reflexes are immediately brought into play to prevent instability. Such corrective reflexes are controlled by a complex central mechanism involving the cerebral cortex, basal ganglion, cerebellum and brain stem. Sensory input is received from several sources including the eyes, ears, neck, skin and anti-gravity muscles.

An individual standing quietly in the erect position is never absolutely still but in constant movement known as *postural sway*. It is easy to measure and gives an objective assessment of the efficiency of postural control. In a series of classic experiments, Sheldon demonstrated that postural control is a skill acquired in childhood. This control does not vary significantly between the ages of 16 and 60, but begins to deteriorate in old age. These early observations were confirmed by Exton-Smith, who also noted that men had significantly better postural control than women.

Degenerative or disease changes in some central or peripheral areas will impair the stability of the individual and increase the likelihood of falls. In addition to walking, activities which demand rapid adjustments in the balance mechanism include rising from a chair, getting out of bed, stooping and turning suddenly. If falls occur during these routine movements it indicates a marked impairment of the balance control mechanisms. Falls which occur only after unexpected or accidental displacements suggest a less severe degree of impairment.

Falls may occur in patients with serious underlying illnesses, because of their increased frailty and general weakness. These have been described as *premonitory falls* and are associated with a bad prognosis. As many as 25% of patients die within a year of the fall. When several falls occur within a short period of time (clustering) it is associated with a particularly poor prognosis.

The incidence of falls is highest in the 80–84 age group and in any given age group females are more likely to fall than males. It is estimated that one-third of elderly people living at home will have at least one fall within a 12-month period.

Environmental or accidental falls account for about 45% of the total and tend to occur in active, healthy people. Spontaneous falls, on the other hand, result from sudden loss of balance and are mainly caused by pathological factors. They are therefore more common in frail, elderly people. However, dividing all falls into either spontaneous or environmental groups oversimplifies a complex situation. In many instances the aetiology of the fall will be mixed, with both environmental and pathological factors playing a role. It follows that all elderly individuals with a history of falls, whether environmental or spontaneous, should be carefully assessed.

The pathological factors which compromise postural control can be divided into two main groups: nervous system disorders (especially involving the special senses) and cardiovascular disorders which lead to ischaemia of the balance control mechanisms (Table 17.1). Musculo-skeletal problems which make it more difficult for the body to react swiftly to displacement also predispose the individual to falls.

Table 17.1.   Causes of spontaneous or non-accidental falls

Neurological disorders
Central: physiological age-related changes, cerebrovascular disease, Parkinson's disease, dementia, space-occupying lesion, epilepsy, transient ischaemic attack, drop attack
Peripheral: visual problems, vestibular problems, peripheral neuropathy, cervical spondylosis

Cardiovascular problems
Syncope (cough, urination, defaecation, vasovagal)
Cardiac arrhythmias
Aortic stenosis
Myocardial infarction
Carotid sinus hypersensitivity
Postural hypotension

Musculo-skeletal problems (see Tables 6.1, 6.2)

Drugs and alcohol

Serious underlying illness

Neurological Disorders

These can be either physiological or pathological and primarily involve central or peripheral mechanisms.

Physiological Age-Related Changes

Physiological age-related changes in the nervous system impair the mechanisms controlling balance. The reaction time (i.e. the time required for perceiving signals, selecting appropriate responses and executing them accurately) is prolonged in old people. Although peripheral mechanisms may contribute, the limits of speed of performance are determined largely by central processes. When walking, old people tend to compensate for neurophysiological changes which impair their balance by shortening their stride and by lowering the height of and broadening the base of their step.

Cerebrovascular Disease

Cerebrovascular disease is a common cause of falls in the elderly. Problems may result from a major infarct or haemorrhage, diffuse brain damage due to multiple infarction or small infarcts (lacunes) in strategic areas involved in balance control.

Space-Occupying Lesions

Space-occupying lesions such as tumours, haematomas, abscesses and cysts can all predispose to falls. Brain tumours are generally malignant, are often metastatic secondary deposits and are seldom amenable to surgical correction.

It should be remembered that a subdural haematoma may be the cause as well as the consequence of a fall. The most common presenting symptoms and signs include hemiparesis, personality or intellectual change, papilloedema, coma and unilateral pupillary dilatation. The symptoms and signs may fluctuate, but this does not happen in the majority of cases.

Parkinson's Disease

The extrapyramidal rigidity and abnormal gait found in Parkinson's disease (see Chap. 15) are risk factors for falls. These may also be associated with postural hypotension. Extrapyramidal rigidity and marked hypotension are found in the Shy–Drager syndrome.

Dementia

Patients with Alzheimer's disease (see Chap. 18) and indeed all confused patients are liable to unwise actions which may result in a fall. Demented patients may also have significant abnormalities of gait and balance, suggesting damage to the trans-cortical pathways participating in the integration of gait. Patients with multi-infarct dementia often have impaired balance due to damage to central areas. Vitamin B_{12} deficiency and tabes dorsalis should be remembered as rare causes of ataxia and dementia.

Epilepsy

Epilepsy increases in frequency with increasing age; the incidence doubles between the ages of 60 and 75 years. The commonest cause is cerebrovascular disease, though Alzheimer's disease, brain tumours, hypoglycaemia and other metabolic disorders are important causes. Idiopathic seizures do present for the first time in old age. The underlying cause of epilepsy can be confidently diagnosed in only half of patients, even when sophisticated diagnostic tools are used. It is likely that many of those with epilepsy of unknown aetiology have a smaller vascular lesion involving the cerebral cortex.

A patient is likely to describe an aura, loss of consciousness, self-injury (e.g. tongue biting) and incontinence. There may be an eyewitness account of involuntary movements and there may be a history of previous seizures. However, the presentation may simply be one of falls and it may remain undiagnosed for a long time, particularly if the patient is living alone.

While most physicians would not treat a single epileptic attack, recurring seizures require anti-convulsant therapy. Phenytoin and carbamazepine are the drugs of choice, the former having the advantage of once-daily dosage. As the required dose is often unpredictable, drug levels should be monitored. Adequate seizure control can usually be attained with a single drug in adequate dosage. The diagnosis of epilepsy has legal implications with regard to the patient's entitlement to drive (see Chap. 27).

Transient Ischaemic Attacks

Transient ischaemic attacks (TIAs) by definition, cause a neurological deficit lasting for less than 24 hours, though they may last for only a few seconds. The majority are due to emboli in either the carotid or the vertebro-basilar artery territory; other causes include cardiac dysrhythmias, hypertension and blood hyperviscosity states. While they do herald other (and possibly more severe) stroke events, patients with TIAs are more at risk from a fatal myocardial infarct than from a fatal stroke.

There is considerable controversy regarding the correct management of TIAs due to arterial emboli. Diseased carotid vessels can be studied using ultrasound or angiography. As the latter investigation is invasive, it should only be undertaken if surgical intervention is contemplated. Surgical intervention may take the form of endarterectomy or external–internal carotid artery anastomosis. Neither is of proven benefit. Regarding medical management, the use of aspirin, dipyridamole and anti-coagulants either alone or in various combinations is controversial. The optimum dosage of aspirin and dipyridamole is even disputed. Some studies suggest that aspirin is of use in men but not in women.

Drop Attacks

Drop attacks are sudden falls which occur without warning and which are not accompanied by neurological signs or loss of consciousness. It is usually not possible for the person who has fallen to get up without aid. Sometimes if the victim is able to press the soles of his feet against a wall, tone returns and he can rise unaided. The condition is characterised by a transient paralysis affecting the legs and some of the trunk muscles. The weakness may persist for many hours if the patient is not aided. It has been postulated that these attacks are due to brain stem ischaemia. However, there is no definite evidence to support this and it is likely that the aetiology of drop attacks is multi-factorial.

Visual Problems

Visual information becomes increasingly important with age, as degenerative and disease changes impair the other balance controlling mechanisms. Poor vision also places an individual at risk from environmental hazards. Falls have been shown to be much more common in those with poor vision. Lens opacities, retinal degeneration, glaucoma and hemianopia are among the conditions which should be considered (see Chap. 13).

Vestibular Problems

The vestibular system is not as important in man as it is in lower animals and does not play an essential part in either posture control or righting reactions under normal circumstances. However, patients with vestibular lesions become more dependent on vision to maintain their balance and as a consequence they are more likely to run into difficulties in the dark. Vertigo, especially where there is a rotatory sensation which persists when the eyes are closed, indicates a vestibular lesion. True vertigo is found in a minority of older patients who fall. Tinnitus is another pointer to vestibular pathology. Nystagmus and ataxia may be found on clinical examination during an attack. When a patient complains of "dizziness" she usually means a feeling of disequilibrium or disordered spatial orientation provoked by movement, rather than true vertigo.

Degenerative changes commonly affect the vestibule. The otoliths may become fragmented and they can create abnormal signal patterns in the hair cells. Distorted sensory input due to pathological changes in the vestibular system may be one of the reasons for the sense of disequilibrium which some elderly people experience.

Patients with peripheral vestibular lesions may be helped by agents such as cinnarizine, betahistine or prochlorperazine. All too often, however, these agents are inappropriately used as blanket therapy for patients with "dizziness", irrespective of the underlying cause.

Peripheral Neuropathy

Loss of proprioception and touch due to peripheral neuropathy will increase the likelihood of falls (Table 17.2). Autonomic neuropathy is one of the causes of postural hypotension.

Table 17.2. Common causes of polyneuropathy in old age

Diabetes mellitus
Neoplasia
Guillain–Barré Syndrome
Connective-tissue disorders
Pernicious anaemia
Drugs
Uraemia
Alcohol

From George and Twomey (1986) Age and Ageing 4: 248

Cervical Spondylosis

The ataxia and dizziness associated with cervical spondylosis occur particularly on head turning. They are thought to be due to an imbalance in the inflow of stimuli from damaged mechano-receptors in the apophyseal joints of the cervical spine. These mechano-receptors have a very significant influence on cervical and limb muscle tone and activity. The individual will become more dependent on visual input and therefore will be at particular risk in the dark. Cervical collars which immobilise the neck often accentuate the feeling of disequilibrium. A daily programme of gentle exercises to improve the range of neck movement will benefit some patients.

It has been claimed that cervical osteophytes cause vertebro-basilar ischaemia and falls by occluding the vertebral arteries. There is little evidence available to support this claim and it should be avoided as a diagnosis unless there is other evidence of brain stem ischaemia.

Cardiovascular Problems

Cardiac Syncope

Vasovagal episodes may result in a fall particularly in individuals who have an underlying problem such as anaemia. Syncope may also occur in association with coughing, urination and defaecation. Micturition syncope tends to occur in the early morning whereas defaecation syncope tends to happen at night. The syncope occurs after micturition or defaecation and is thought to be due to a combination of orthostatic hypotension and cardio-inhibitory reflexes. A fall with loss of consciousness suggests cardiac syncope or Stokes–Adams attacks. A cardiac basis for syncope should also be suspected if the incident is associated with palpitations, dyspnoea, cyanosis or chest discomfort. Facial flushing (due to reactive hyperaemia) may be observed after the episode. Myocardial infarction may present as syncope.

Tachyarrhythmias or bradyarrhythmias of sudden onset are an important cause of falls. The syncope usually occurs at the point of rhythm change. Dysrhythmias may be brought on by exercise, though effort-related syncope should also suggest the possibility of aortic stenosis. The finding of transient cardiac arrhythmias on a standard ECG or on a 24-hour ECG recording from a patient with falls should not lead one to assume that they are the cause. In recent years several studies have shown that transient cardiac arrhythmias (including ventricular arrhythmias) are commoner in the elderly than in the young and that they are asymptomatic in the majority of subjects. If clinical events coincide with ECG abnormalities, anti-arrhythmic therapy or a cardiac pacemaker may be indicated, depending on the arrhythmia present.

Carotid Sinus Hypersensitivity

Carotid sinus hypersensitivity is an unusual cause of syncope. Accidental massage of the carotid sinus will increase vagal tone, cause a bradyarrhythmia and syncope. The patient should not wear tight clothing around the neck and he should also be told to avoid sudden head movement. If this advice fails a permanent cardiac demand pacemaker may be necessary.

Postural Hypotension

Postural hypotension by definition is present when systolic blood pressure drops by 20 mmHg or more after standing for 2 minutes. However, the finding of a significant postural drop should not deter one from looking for other causes of falls as many patients with postural hypotension remain asymptomatic. Individuals who fall because of postural hypotension usually do so after rising from a lying or sitting position and walking a short distance. It is wise when assessing such an individual to ask them to walk about the room after getting up and then to re-check the blood pressure. A significant fall may then become apparent.

Postural hypotension may occur as a side effect of several drugs, including tricyclic antidepressants, anti-hypertensives, diuretics, tranquillisers and L-dopa. Management in the first instance consists of removing any underlying cause and of advising caution on changing position. The wearing of elastic stockings prevents venous pooling in the legs and promotes cardiac return. By raising the head of the bed at night, sodium retention by the kidney is enhanced and postural hypotension sometimes improves. Should these measures not relieve symptoms of postural hypotension, fludrocortisone may need to be introduced, beginning with 0.05 mg daily and then gradually increasing the dose.

Drugs

Drugs (Table 17.3) can cause falls through mechanisms other than postural hypotension. Sedatives and tranquillisers predispose to falls by making individuals excessively drowsy. Hypnotics with a long half-life should be avoided as night sedatives as they are more likely to cause problems on the following day. Tranquillisers also cause extrapyramidal rigidity and therefore increase the risk of falls. Hypoglycaemic episodes may result in falls in diabetic patients taking insulin or oral hypoglycaemic agents.

Table 17.3. Drugs associated with falls

Sedatives
Hypnotics
Tranquillisers
Antidepressants
Anti-hypertensives
Diuretics
Anti-convulsants
Levadopa
Oral hypoglycaemic agents
Alcohol

In recent years there has been a greater awareness of the problem of alcohol abuse in the elderly. Often it is very difficult to confirm the suspicion as some elderly secret drinkers manage to conceal their habit with great skill.

Musculo-skeletal Problems

Any condition which results in muscle weakness or which increases the rigidity of the body will make an individual more likely to fall. This would include patients with either osteoarthritis or rheumatoid arthritis (see Chap. 6). Osteoarthritis of the knees is often accompanied by wasting of the quadriceps muscles and daily exercises which strengthen the quadriceps will improve both mobility and stability. Osteomalacia causes proximal muscle weakness. Foot drop from whatever cause places the individual at a mechanical disadvantage. Increased muscular rigidity, as found in Parkinson's disease or following a stroke, impedes a person's ability to respond quickly to imbalance.

Foot pain or deformity are often overlooked when assessing patients who have fallen. Yet the feet are the structures which support the body in the upright position. Because of this, and also due to the stresses imposed by badly fitting shoes, the feet are among the foremost in showing the ravages of time. Painful calluses or ulcers and deformities such as hallux valgus and hallux rigidus, calcaneal spurs and metatarsalgia are all problems which may impair locomotion and therefore, predispose to falls (see Chap. 16).

Clinical Evaluation

In many cases the causes of falls can be diagnosed after a thorough history and physical examination. Exact details of the fall and the events surrounding it should be ascertained. When there have been recurring falls focus on the most memorable or the most recent one initially. Then enquire as to whether and in what way this differed from other falls. If the patient lost consciousness during the episode it suggests cardiac syncope. However, history of an aura, convulsive movements and incontinence would indicate epilepsy. Enquiries should be made as to whether the fall occurred on change of posture. A history of vertigo, tinnitus and deafness suggests an ear problem. When there is loss of consciousness or when the patient is unclear as to the events surrounding the fall an eye-witness account can be invaluable.

On examination of the cardiovascular system the pulse will give information on the presence of arrhythmias and signs of aortic stenosis. The blood pressure should be checked with the patient lying and standing. As already mentioned, a fall in blood pressure may only be found following a brief period of exercise. The carotid vessels should be auscultated for evidence of an atherosclerotic bruit and the heart examined for further evidence of aortic stenosis.

Visual acuity and fields should be tested carefully and nystagmus should be looked for. Examine for evidence of neurological dysfunction likely to impair mobility (see Chap. 15). It is essential to get the patient to walk; while he is doing so pay particular attention to the gait. Romberg's test should form an integral part of the neurological examination of all patients with falls. Examination of muscles, joints and feet must not be neglected.

Further Investigation

Several studies have shown that if the diagnosis is uncertain following clinical assessment, then further investigation is unlikely to be of help. However, an EEG, isotope brain scan and CT scan may be helpful if a neurological entity such as epilepsy or a space-occupying lesion is suspected. A radiograph of the cervical spine may reveal significant spondylosis, but it must be borne in mind that most elderly people have spondylotic changes in their necks. If eye or ear problems are identified following the clinical assessment, these patients should be referred to the appropriate specialist for further investigation and treatment of remediable lesions. Carotid doppler studies may give useful information if the falls are associated with a transient neurological deficit or if a bruit is heard in the neck. Twenty-four hour ECG monitoring should be carried out if an arrhythmia is thought to be contributing to the falls. A 24-hour ECG recording is most useful if falls or episodes of dizziness are frequent. It is less likely to yield relevant information if falls are episodic or infrequent. An echocardiogram will rule out conditions such as aortic stenosis or an atrial myxoma.

Complications of Falls

Loss of Confidence

Loss of confidence can be a major problem after a fall, causing the individual to be housebound and as a consequence socially isolated. Lack of sunlight and poor diet can lead to osteomalacia which in turn further impairs mobility and confidence. The patient may become extremely apprehensive when asked to walk, becoming very rigid, leaning backwards and grabbing desperately at people or objects for support. This, in itself, predisposes the individual to further falls. Inactivity may lead to immobility with all the attendant problems so aptly described by Asher in his famous essay "On the Dangers of Going to Bed".

Fractures

The risk of fractures is such that 25% of women will have at least one fracture by the age of 80. About 1% of falls result in a fracture of the proximal femur, which in turn is associated with a high morbidity and mortality. Old bones are easily broken because of osteoporosis and in some cases because of osteomalacia. Degenerative changes in pain-carrying nerve fibres and a higher central pain threshold mean that some patients may not complain of great discomfort. Consequently, a fracture should always be very high on the differential diagnosis if there is a sudden change in the mobility of an elderly person. Missing such a fracture can have disastrous results for the patient.

Subdural Haematomas

Subdural haematomas may follow minor trauma and can occur even where there is no evidence of direct head injury. They are caused by damage to veins traversing the subdural space and may be bilateral. The fall which caused the haematoma may be forgotten at the time of presentation. Certainly, if one suspects the possibility of a subdural haematoma, one should never be deterred from pursuing further investigations by the absence of a history of head injury. The author has experience of a 69-year-old patient who presented with ataxia and unilateral papilloedema. He vehemently denied any history of head injury. A CT scan confirmed a subdural haematoma. After evacuation of the haematoma the patient could then recall quite clearly that he had slipped on ice 6 weeks previously!

Other Complications

Falls may also lead to a number of other problems (Table 17.4) including burns, hypothermia, chest infections and decubitus ulcers.

Table 17.4. Complications of falls

Loss of confidence and mobility
Fracture
Subdural haematoma
Burns
Hypothermia
Chest infection
Pressure sores

Management

Treatment will depend on the underlying cause of the falls. Irrespective of the aetiology, many patients will have lost confidence and become less mobile. These problems must be treated promptly if further decline is to be prevented. If any programme is to be successful therapists must be empathetic, supportive and enthusiastic (see Chap. 25).

The patient should be made aware of the reasons for her falls and should be given commonsense advice about environmental hazards. If treatment is being carried out in a hospital or day hospital a home visit is essential so that hazards may be recognised and, where possible, corrected. Some form of alarm should be arranged if the patient is living on her own.

A physiotherapy programme should be devised to improve the patient's mobility and confidence. Back leaning may be a major problem in patients who experience a sensation of falling forwards when they stand up. A weighted apron is used to try and correct this tendency. Weights may also be placed on a walking frame.

Balance exercises form an important part of treatment. The programme should aim initially to achieve stability over a given base (e.g. sitting, standing). It should then concentrate on the ability to regain stability after disturbance, on movements of the trunk over a base and on changing from one position to another. Finally, the exercises should encourage the patient to balance over an unstable or moving base. Special attention should be given to improving the patient's gait. Patients with short and irregular step lengths should be identified. The patient's ability to lift the feet adequately during the swing-through phase of walking should be ascertained. As confidence improves emphasis must be placed on improving the speed of walking. Stair practice should also be incorporated. Instruction on how to get up after a fall should be an essential component of the programme.

Sticks and walking aids may improve a patient's sense of security. However, like the use of hypnotics, long-term dependence on walking aids should be avoided if possible as they induce their own problems. The Zimmer frame with its four legs converts the faller into a hexapod, replacing the proprioceptive information normally obtained through the subject's legs with that obtained through the legs of the frame. Isaacs has described the result of this as a "grotesque start–stop travesty of normal gait". These patients become extremely vulnerable if they do anything without the aid.

Accidental Falls and their Prevention

In the Home

Most falls at home occur indoors, mainly in the living room or on the stairs. The majority happen during the day. Most fractures of the neck of femur caused by accidental falls occur as a result of slips and trips. As might be expected the incidence of slipping is higher among the young elderly (65–74 years) whereas the older and more frail elderly are more likely to trip.

In the past much emphasis was placed on environmental factors, but now more attention is being paid to the health of fallers. However, certain factors such as loose mats, worn carpets, inadequate lighting and trailing wires predispose to falls. Attention should also be paid to the patient's footwear and he should be advised to wear well-fitting lace-up shoes.

In Hospital

Approximately 15% of elderly patients admitted to a geriatric department will have an accident as an inpatient. Ward furniture, particularly commodes, cotsides and "geriatric" chairs, have been implicated in as many as 40% of these accidents. Tinker observed that the brakes on beds, chairs and commodes are often ineffective and she emphasised the importance of regular maintenance. In contrast to the situation at home many falls in institutions occur at night and happen more frequently in the vicinity of the patient's bed or on the way to the toilet.

Hospital chairs should have arms to prevent sideways falls and there should be a range of sizes to suit different types of patient. Practitioners of Geriatric Medicine over the years have rightly placed great emphasis on the importance of encouraging independence. However, an over-zealous approach invites problems. For instance, patients recovering from stroke may not realise that their balance is still greatly impaired. The dangers of walking without supervision should be pointed out to these patients. Failure to do so may result in falls, which damage their confidence and which may result in a fracture. Relatively few falls occur in physiotherapy departments as physiotherapists are trained to anticipate and therefore prevent these problems. Regular exchange of information between therapists and nurses about the capabilities of the patients should heighten awareness and diminish the incidence of falls. Such an exchange of information is one of the hallmarks of good teamwork.

Education programmes for elderly people should contain information on falls. Stress should be placed on the importance of maintaining general health and fitness. Exercises which can be performed simply and which help to preserve muscle strength should be demonstrated. When a family doctor or health visitor calls at the home of an elderly person they should take advantage of the opportunity to look for hazards which are known to cause falls. Elderly people should also be advised about the dangers of open fires, particularly if they have a history of falls.

Unfortunately, advice is not always heeded and some elderly people will continue to take undue risks like the Old Countess of Desmond. She entered the annals of Ireland and Britain as an example of human longevity. Bacon in his "History of Life and Death" claimed that she reached the phenomenal age of 140 before her accidental death in 1614. Robert Sidney, Earl of Leicester, recorded the circumstances of the accident:

> She might have lived longer hade she not mette with a kind of violent death, for she must needs climb a nutt tree to gather nuts, soe falling down she hurt her thighe, which brought a fever, and that brought death.

Further Reading

Coakley D, Snell A (1980) Unrecognised fractures in old age. Practitioner 223:828–829

Isaacs B (1985) Falls. In: Exton Smith AN, Weksler ME (eds) Practical geriatric medicine. Churchill Livingstone, Edinburgh

Kataria MS (1985) Fits, faints and falls in old age. MTP Press, Lancaster

Overstall PW (1985) Falls. In: Pathy MSJ (ed) Principles and practice of geriatric medicine. John Wiley and Sons, Chichester

Pathy MSJ (1978) Defaecation syncope. Age Ageing 7:233–236

Sheldon H (1963) The effect of age on the control of sway. Gerontol Clin 5:129–138

Taylor I, Stout RW (1983) Is ambulatory electrocardiography a useful investigation in elderly people with "funny turns"? Age Ageing 12:211–216

Tinker G (1979) Accidents in a geriatric department. Age Ageing 8:196–197

Wagstaff P, Coakley D (1987) Physiotherapy and the elderly patient. Croom Helm, London

Chapter 18

Confusion

A. J. Bayer

Confusion is a widely accepted, but ill defined and often very loosely applied, term to describe symptoms of cognitive dysfunction and disturbed behaviour. In older patients it may be produced by almost any physical, psychological or social disturbance and is one of the most frequent reasons for referral to a geriatrician. It often replaces pain or fever as the main presenting symptom of physical illness and should always lead to a search for an underlying cause, which may then respond to appropriate treatment. Unfortunately it is often wrongly regarded as an inevitable result of ageing or is conveniently, but inappropriately, attributed to vague conditions such as hardening of the cerebral arteries, with the inference that nothing can be done to help the patient.

It is important to distinguish between acute and chronic confusion when making a prognosis and planning management. However, differential diagnosis is not always easy: about one third of hospitalised patients with chronic confusion have a superimposed acute confusional state and a small number of acutely confused patients may progress to chronic confusion. The doctor's responsibility is to obtain a detailed history, including one from a relative, friend or neighbour, to carefully examine the physical and mental state, to identify and treat reversible causes of confusion and to ensure that all available supportive measures are mobilised.

Acute Confusion

Acute confusion may be defined as a mental disorder of abrupt onset and relatively brief duration, characterised by concurrent disorders of cognition, attention and wakefulness ("clouding of consciousness") and disturbed psychomotor behaviour. The term is often used synonymously with delirium or toxic confusion, though strictly speaking these always imply the presence of an underlying physical condition and in 5%–20% of the acutely confused elderly no organic causative factor can be identified. The term "pseudo-delirium" has been proposed to describe such patients, in whom the aetiology is judged to be functional and usually associated with either social factors or affective, reactive or paranoid disorders. Studies of acute confusion suggest an incidence of 30%–50% among elderly hospitalised patients and it probably becomes commoner and lasts longer with increasing age. Though most cases resolve rapidly and completely, the mortality rate is about 25% within the first month, twice that of control patients. The presence of confusion also leads to longer hospital stays. The more severe the cognitive impairment on hospital admission, the poorer the outcome. Early detection and appropriate treatment improve prognosis and transition from acute to chronic confusion is then uncommon.

Causes

The aetiology of acute confusion is usually multifactorial, with physical causes interacting with psychological and environmental factors (Table 18.1). In the elderly patient the normal physiological changes of ageing, the impaired homeostatic mechanisms, the presence of chronic mental or physical disease, polypharmacy and poor vision and hearing are all predisposing factors. Very small alterations in physical or psychosocial state can lead to significant cognitive impairment and the ageing brain is particularly sensitive to the effects of hypoxia, dehydration and electrolyte disturbance. Systemic illnesses are more common causes than primary cerebral disorders. Pharmacokinetic and pharmacodynamic changes in old age (see Chap. 24), together with the often careless prescribing and widespread consumption of drugs by elderly patients, make drug intoxication probably the single most common cause of acute confusion. Abrupt withdrawal of drugs, notably alcohol and other centrally acting agents, may also precipitate a confusional state.

Table 18.1.   Causes of acute confusion

Physical disorders
Intracranial: cerebrovascular disease, trauma, infection, tumour, post-epilepsy
Extracranial: systemic infection, acute cardio-respiratory disease, metabolic problems, deficiency
    states, constipation, urinary retention, hypothermia

Drugs
Intoxication: sedatives, antidepressants, L-dopa, digoxin, hypotensives, opiates, corticosteroids, oral
    hypoglycaemics, cimetidine, diuretics, alcohol
Withdrawal: alcohol, benzodiazepines, antidepressants, barbiturates

Psychological
Acute and chronic pain, stress, sensory deficit, depression, anxiety, paranoid states

Environmental
Sensory deprivation or overload, unfamiliar environment

Clinical Features

The onset of acute confusion may occur over minutes or days. Symptoms fluctuate in intensity through the course of 24 hours and commonly become worse at night ("sundowning"), in darkness and on awakening, while so-called lucid intervals may be interspersed. The sleep–wake cycle is disturbed, with wakefulness characteristically reduced during the day and sleep fragmented and diminished at night. Attention and awareness of the environment are always disordered. Difficulty in sustaining concentration leads to only small parts of information being grasped and the ability to learn and to recall recent events is impaired. Long-term memory remains relatively intact, but distant memories may be recalled inappropriately and regarded by the patient as relevant to his current environment. This then leads to further distortion of already disorganised and usually impoverished thought processes. Ability to reason and solve problems and to plan actions logically is reduced and a poorly structured and changing paranoid delusional attitude is common. The complex hallucinations and dream-like thinking often experienced by younger delirious patients appear to occur less frequently in old age.

There is always some disorientation in time and, as the condition becomes more severe, also of place and person, though rarely of self. A tendency to mistake unfamiliar for known places and persons is then typical. Misperceptions of people, actions, sounds or objects may dominate the clinical picture and these relate closely to the patient's mood and level of arousal. Hushed conversations and ill-defined activity in a darkened hospital ward may provoke sudden fear or anger and lead to episodes of shouting or violence. A mood of apprehension and bewilderment tends to predominate, but may alternate with depression, apathy, irritability and rage, often in response to any change of environment. Symptoms of autonomic nervous system hyperarousal, disturbance of speech and incontinence of urine or faeces often occur. Characteristic of the most disturbed patients is plucking at sheets or clothing, a dislike of staying in bed and a desire to wander which can create particular difficulties in management.

Diagnosis

A history must be obtained from a close relative or neighbour and the characteristic rapid mode of onset, fluctuating severity and short duration of the present symptoms should be confirmed. Particular attention should be given to all drugs taken or discontinued in recent weeks. Care is needed to avoid the misinterpretation (as confusion) of isolated dysphasia or dyspraxia resulting from acute stroke. The mental state must formally be assessed – by using the Mini-Mental State Examination for example (Table 18.2) – and this can be repeated at regular intervals to monitor any change.

The search for an underlying medical cause should start immediately with a full physical examination, looking particularly for evidence of systemic disease, recent trauma and conditions leading to hypoxia. Choice of laboratory and radiological investigations should be guided by the findings of history and examination but might initially include full blood count, blood biochemistry, chest X-ray (CXR), ECG and MSU. Further tests are required if the diagnosis remains unclear. The EEG in severely delirious patients shows bilateral diffuse symmetrical slowing and is always abnormal, but this is rarely helpful diagnostically as similar changes occur in degenerative dementia, the major differential diagnosis.

Management

Although the only definitive treatment of acute confusion is to identify and reverse the underlying causal factors, there is also a need for supportive and

Table 18.2.   The Mini-Mental State Examination

Test	Maximum score
Orientation	
What is the . . . ?	
Year, Season, Date, Day, Month	5
Where are we . . . ?	
Ward, Hospital, District, Town, County (UK)	
Floor, Hospital, Town, County, State (USA)	5
Registration	
Examiner names three objects (lemon, key, balloon)	
then patient asked to repeat	
One point for each correct	3
Then repeat until patient learns all three	
Attention and calculation	
Subtract 7 from 100 then 7 from answer you get, etc.	
Stop after 5 answers (e.g. 93, 86, 85, 78, 71 scores 4)	5
(Alternative: spell WORLD backwards)	
Recall	
Ask for names of three objects learnt earlier	3
Language	
Point to a pencil and a watch and ask patient to name them	2
Ask patient to repeat "No ifs, ands or buts"	1
Ask patient to follow a three-stage command:	
"Take the paper in your right hand.	
Fold the paper in half.	
Put the paper on the floor"	3
Ask patient to read and obey a written command ("CLOSE YOUR EYES")	1
Ask patient to write a sentence of own choice	
Score if sensible and has a subject and verb	1
Copying	
Ask patient to copy a drawing (of two intersecting pentagons). Score if all	
sides and angles preserved and intersecting sides form a quadrangle.	1
Total score	30

After Folstein et al. (1975) J Psychiatr Res 12:189–198.

symptomatic care of the confusional state itself. A clear, reassuring and unhurried approach is required and very often repeated instructions and explanations are necessary. Those in contact with the patient should help orientation by always introducing themselves and giving a reminder of where the patient is and why. A single sitter, preferably a family member or friend, may be helpful. It is essential to provide a balanced sensory environment and, in hospital, a quiet, well-lit side room away from the noise and bustle of the general ward may be preferable. Personal clothing, family photographs and other familiar objects, a clock with the correct time, a calendar, daily newspapers and familiar television programmes may all help to keep contact with reality. Recovery can be helped by carefully planned stimulation and conversation, using known information from the patient's past to act as a bridge between patient and carer.

Bed rest should be minimised and particular attention given to adequate diet and fluid intake and to care of bowel and bladder. A minority of patients may require a short course of sedative drug treatment to reduce arousal, to control agitation and to help avoid injury. The dose should be carefully titrated to meet the needs of the moment. Haloperidol (0.5–10 mg) available as tablets, syrup, drops or injection is recommended, though thioridazine (25–100 mg) has fewer extra-pyramidal effects and chlormethiazole (384–768 mg) is widely used in alcohol withdrawal states. If disturbed sleep is the particular problem a short-acting hyp-notic such as temazepam (10–30 mg) or chlormethiazole may be suitable. It must be remembered that any sedative drug can paradoxically exacerbate confusion. There is no objective evidence to support the routine prophylactic or therapeutic value of vitamin supplements, and their use should be restricted to those with sus-pected nutritional deficiencies or alcohol withdrawal states.

Chronic Confusion

Chronic confusion in an elderly patient generally implies the presence of demen-tia. This is the acquired global impairment of higher cortical functions including: memory, the capacity to solve the problems of day-to-day living, the performance of learned perceptuo-motor skills, the correct use of social skills, all aspects of language and communication, and the control of emotional reactions in the absence of gross clouding of consciousness. The condition is often progressive though not necessarily irreversible. A distinction was formerly made between "presenile" and "senile" dementias but it is now recognised that such an arbitrary division was unjustified and unhelpful and should no longer be used.

The prevalence of dementia increases with age, though over the age of 85 years the rates may begin to fall off. About 10% of the population aged 65 years or over have dementia and half of these are severely disabled by the condition. Up to 20% of those aged over 80 years are severely demented. Demographic projections suggest a 50% increase in the number of those affected in developed countries over the next half-century, though the actual incidence rate for dementia may be dropping. Old people's homes and long-stay hospital wards contain a high propor-tion of patients with dementia, but many more are living at home where their problems are largely unrecognised by their general practitioners and other com-munity services. It should also always be remembered, however, that the great majority of old people are not mentally impaired.

Diagnosis

When assessing a chronically confused patient, the doctor must first confirm the presence of dementia by taking a careful history and objective testing of the men-tal state. It is desirable to reassess the patient after a few months to note any pro-gression of symptoms. Dementia must be distinguished from an acute confusional state, a focal disturbance of higher function and symptoms of a primary depressive illness ("pseudo-dementia"). Depressed elderly patients may present with pro-gressive cognitive changes almost indistinguishable from dementia, but their inconsistent performance on testing, their characteristic tendency to answer questions with "I don't know" and then often reply correctly when encouraged, help to suggest the correct diagnosis (see Chap. 19, Table 19.3).

A cause of the dementia should then be sought by considering particular features of the clinical history together with the results of physical examination and selective laboratory and radiological investigation. Initial emphasis must be on recognising those uncommon causes, present in about 5% of unselected patients, which may respond to medical or surgical intervention. Other reversible medical, emotional or environmental factors unnecessarily exacerbating confusion may also often be identified, of which inappropriate drug therapy (anti-cholinergics, sedatives, hypotensives, etc.) is the most common. Full blood count, blood biochemistry and thyroid function tests are indicated in all patients and vitamin B_{12} and folate level and serological tests for syphilis will be necessary in some. An ECG and CXR in selected patients will identify dysrhythmias, heart failure and bronchogenic carcinoma. Skull X-rays are seldom useful and CT scans are best reserved for those with recent onset of dementia or rapid deterioration, as well as those with unexpected or atypical neurological findings. An EEG has limited diagnostic value, but focal features act as a useful screen for detecting those likely to have CT abnormalities. The EEG is seldom normal in patients with organic mental disease.

The majority of elderly patients with dementia will be suffering from Alzheimer's disease, a diagnosis which can only be made with certainty at postmortem or by brain biopsy. Clinical diagnosis is thus largely one of exclusion. Vascular or multi-infarct dementia accounts for about 15% of cases and, as both Alzheimer's and vascular dementia are common, some patients have a mixture of the two conditions. About 10% of patients will have some other cause for their dementia.

Alzheimer's Disease

The symptoms of Alzheimer's disease are slowly progressive over several years. The onset is insidious, with a gradual impairment of intellect and memory for recent events, spatial disorientation, an unwillingness to attempt new activities and problems in adapting to change. In the early stages, depression and anxiety may be prominent, though this soon proceeds to apathy and it is rare for patients themselves to express great concern. There is a gradual deterioration in the ability to perform everyday activities and disorganisation of personality, with disinhibition and a coarsening of behaviour. Parietal lobe symptoms of aphasia, apraxia and agnosia are less prominent in the very old than in younger patients. In the later stages of the disease it is impossible to carry out household and personal hygiene tasks without help and supervision, with long-term survivors finally becoming incontinent, immobile and emaciated.

The disease is commoner among females and there is an increased risk, up to a factor of 4, among first-degree relatives. In younger patients particularly the condition may occasionally be familial and recently genetic markers for the condition have been identified. However, the cause of Alzheimer's disease remains unknown, with current interest centering on the role of aluminium, deposition of amyloid, immunological dysfunction, accumulation of free radicals, thyroid dysfunction and viral infection.

The characteristic neuropathological changes of the condition, senile plaque formation and neurofibrillary tangles, are found throughout the cerebral cortex and especially in the amygdala and hippocampus. The brain is shrunken in size,

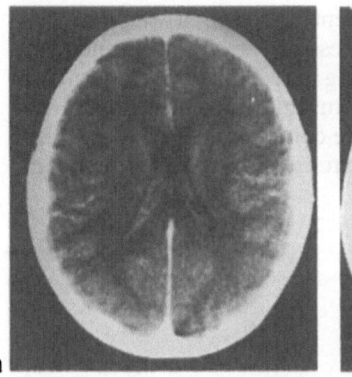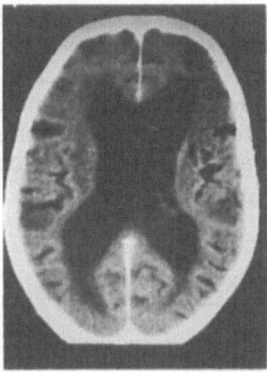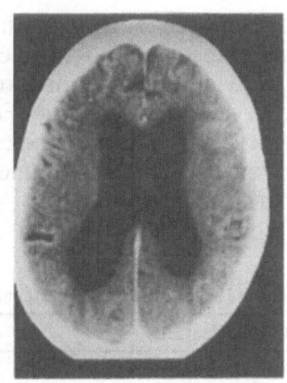

a   b, c

Fig. 18.1. CT scans: **a** a normal patient; **b** in cerebral atrophy, showing ventricular dilation and prominent sulci and sylvian fissures; **c** in normal pressure hydrocephalus, ventricles only are dilated. (By permission of Dr. M. Hourihan, University Hospital of Wales, Cardiff.)

with generalised cerebral atrophy (Fig. 18.1) and loss of nerve cells. The degree of pathological change correlates with the mental status of the patient and with a reduction in the level of the cortical enzymes, choline acetyl transferase (CAT) and acetylcholine esterase (AChE). This cholinergic deficit is widespread and severe in younger patients dying in their seventh or eighth decade and is accompanied by other abnormalities of noradrenaline, gamma-aminobutyric acid (GABA) and somatostatin. In the very elderly, dying in their ninth and tenth decades, there is a relatively pure cholinergic deficit confined to the temporal lobe and hippocampus. Thus there would seem to be two distinct age-related forms of Alzheimer's disease, and this is supported by evidence suggesting that younger patients (Type 2) tend to follow a more malignant clinical course than the very old (Type 1). The involvement of the cholinergic system appears to be an early feature of both forms of the disease and has led to considerable optimism concerning the discovery of an effective treatment.

Vascular Dementia

In contrast to Alzheimer's disease, vascular dementia is most often seen in patients in their sixties and seventies and is more common in men. There is generally evidence of other atheromatous disease, particularly hypertension and focal cerebral infarction, but vasculitis, clotting disorders, endocarditis and other causes of cardiac emboli should also be considered. Most cases of vascular dementia are caused by repeated small strokes resulting in multiple areas of cerebral infarction. Once the volume of infarcted brain is over 50 ml, the patient begins to exhibit symptoms of dementia.

Although multi-infarct dementia can only strictly be diagnosed by CT scan or autopsy, the clinical features are characteristic and have been incorporated into Hachinski's "Ischaemia Score" (Table 18.3) in which a total of 7 or over in a demented patient suggests a vascular aetiology. The onset of symptoms is usually sudden, with a subsequent "step-wise" progression of symptoms, with episodic worsening followed by a plateau or partial recovery, before further worsening as one infarct follows another. Personality, judgement and insight are relatively well-preserved but mood changes, particularly depression, are common and emotional lability, with inappropriate laughter and crying in response to minor provocation, is characteristic. Focal neurological symptoms and signs may range from aphasia, hemiplegia and convulsions to more subtle complaints of headache and dizziness and signs of unequal tendon reflexes, extensor plantar responses and parkinsonism.

Table 18.3. Hachinski's "Ischaemia score"

Clinical feature	Score
Abrupt onset	2
Stepwise deterioration	1
Fluctuating course	2
Nocturnal confusion	1
Relative preservation of personality	1
Depression	1
Somatic complaints	1
Emotional incontinence	1
History of hypertension	1
History of stroke	2
Evidence of associated atherosclerosis	1
Focal neurological signs	2
Focal neurological symptoms	2

A total score of 7 or more favours multi-infarct dementia.

An uncommon variant of vascular dementia is Binswanger's disease, or subcortical arteriosclerotic encephalopathy. A slowly developing dementia occurs and there is usually a history of hypertension, strokes and prominent bilateral but asymmetrical motor signs. Severe small vessel disease is associated with atrophy of multiple areas of subcortical white and grey matter, with relative preservation of the cerebral cortex. The CT scan appearances of white matter, low attenuation and mild atrophy help to distinguish the condition from multi-infarct dementia, in which multiple lesions compatible with infarcts or lacunae are usual. Although, like Alzheimer's disease, there is at present no specific treatment for the cognitive abnormalities of vascular dementia, the nature of the condition suggests that it should be possible to prevent progress of symptoms by appropriate management of vascular risk factors such as hypertension, smoking and diabetes.

Other Causes

The uncommon causes of dementia in general become even less common with increasing age but are important nevertheless because many are potentially treatable.

Normal pressure hydrocephalus most frequently occurs in the late middle-aged or the young elderly and there is often a previous history of subarachnoid haemorrhage, meningitis or head injury. Dementia tends to be mild, with memory most prominently affected, an associated progressive gait disturbance (gait dyspraxia) and urinary incontinence. A CT scan will show severely dilated ventricles in the absence of sulcal widening (Fig. 18.1) and appearances on isotope cisternography are diagnostic. About 50% of patients, particularly those with some known aetiological factor, are dramatically improved by the introduction of a ventriculo-atrial or peritoneal shunt.

Space-occupying lesions may initially present with progressive confusion in the absence of focal neurological signs or evidence of raised intracranial pressure. Slow-growing mid-line tumours and those involving the frontal lobes are most easily overlooked. Chronic subdural haematoma may not cause symptoms until months after head injury, which sometimes cannot be recalled. Confusion is usually associated with headaches and clouding of consciousness, symptoms tending to fluctuate from day to day. Outcome, even after surgical intervention, may be poor. Extracranial malignant disease, particularly carcinomas of the bronchus, stomach and ovary, may rarely be the cause of a dementia syndrome in the absence of secondary deposits, though acute confusion is more common. Patients with long-standing epilepsy may also develop cognitive impairment in later years, usually preceded by personality change and often associated with cessation of fits.

Neurosyphilis is now rare, but most commonly presents with simple dementia or depression and with the characteristic pupillary changes and positive serological tests. In hypothyroidism, cognitive loss occurs early and the typical physical symptoms of myxoedema may not at first be apparent. If the correct diagnosis is delayed replacement treatment with thyroxine may not result in complete recovery.

Parathyroid disease may also give rise to dementia and, even if advanced, the response to surgery is good. Deficiency of vitamin B_{12} may also cause a fluctuating dementia in about a quarter of patients, and this may occur without anaemia or other neurological changes. The serum B_{12} level is always low, though even the bone marrow may be normal. Folic acid deficiency has also been claimed to cause reversible dementia. Thiamine deficiency, usually secondary to alcoholism, gives rise to Wernicke–Korsakoff syndrome, characterised by a severe memory deficit and associated with ataxia, diplopia and disorders of gaze. Early treatment with parenteral vitamin B complex may prevent the development of permanent deficit. Chronic alcoholism may also not uncommonly cause a progressive dementia, possibly as frequently as vascular disease. Abstinence is the only beneficial treatment. Pseudo-dementia may result from long-term use of a wide range of drugs, most notably sedatives, certain anti-convulsants, anti-hypertensives, digoxin and corticosteroids. The confusion often associated with Parkinson's disease is as frequently related to drug treatment as to the underlying condition. Diabetics taking insulin or oral hypoglycaemics are at risk of confusion secondary to hypoglycaemia, sometimes developing unobtrusively and causing sustained cognitive impairment. Reducing drug dosage or changing to safer alternative management usually results in significant recovery.

Management

Much can be done to help patients with chronic confusion and, equally importantly, to help their relatives who generally carry the burden of care. The first principle must be to exclude reversible causes of confusion, to critically review the indications for all medication and to treat other concurrent medical conditions. Hearing and eyesight problems in particular should not be overlooked so that an optimum sensory input is ensured. Treatment of depressive symptoms may help the patient think more clearly and make best use of his or her remaining mental abilities. In the early stages of dementia, advice can be given on the use of simple memory aids, such as checklists of things to do, keeping a diary and having accurate clocks and calendars on view. Establishing routines, ensuring a safe and familiar environment and avoiding situations which will inevitably lead to a failure to cope, all help to avoid unnecessary domestic crises. Simple positive instruction and dealing with issues one at a time minimises confusion.

Continued objective assessment of the patient by a multi-disciplinary team is desirable and enables the family and health and social services to adapt to the changing situation. Attendance at a local day centre or day hospital can be arranged, relieving the family for a regular number of hours each week. Social services such as home-help and Meals-on-Wheels may help to maintain the patient's independence in the community and defer the need for institutional care. Community nursing services can help with emotional and behavioural problems, as well as offering practical care, such as bathing, if this is needed. Advice on management of incontinence, provision of commodes and special clothing and pads and, in some areas, a laundry service to provide and wash bed-linen may be invaluable in later stages of the condition. Voluntary organisations, such as the Alzheimer's Disease Society, can offer considerable support to relatives through regular meetings and by the provision of sitting or minding services. Most publish helpful literature for carers on dementia and on looking after people at home. Information concerning financial benefits, such as the Attendance Allowance, and on legal matters such as the Enduring Power of Attorney and Court of Protection should be forthcoming (see Chap. 27). Short-term admission to residential or hospital care gives carers a break and is a useful opportunity to review overall management. Permanent institutionalisation is generally required for social rather than clinical reasons and is often precipitated by illness or death of a spouse. Admission to "sheltered accommodation" is rarely successful.

Drug treatment in dementia may be to treat either the symptoms or the cause. Sleep disturbance is common and can rapidly exhaust carers. A short-acting hypnotic, such as temazepam or chlormethiazole, may allow a full night's sleep for all concerned. Daytime agitation, distressing hallucinations, wandering or "violent" behaviour may necessitate a sedative drug, such as haloperidol, thioridazine or chlormethiazole, though their use very often results in side effects. Doses should initially be small and increased very gradually until the minimum effective dose is established; whereupon it should be kept under constant review.

Drugs to treat the cause of dementia remain elusive and none currently available are proven to be of consistent value. Co-dergocrine mesylate in a daily dose of 4.5 mg or more is claimed to improve symptoms in Alzheimer's disease and there is some evidence to support the use of cyclandelate (1600 mg daily) in cases of vascular dementia. The absence of adequate controlled clinical trials makes assessment of their role difficult to determine. More recent understanding of the biochemical deficiencies in Alzheimer's disease has led to interest in the use of cholinergic drugs. Studies with the pre-synaptic agents choline and lecithin have been disappointing but the cholinesterase inhibitors physostigmine and most notably tetrahydroaminoacridine (THA) have resulted in improvements in both specific cognitive areas and overall functioning in many of the patients tested.

They are currently the most promising therapeutic approach to the disease and the subject of enormous research interest.

It must, however, always be remembered that drugs are not a substitute for diagnosis, practical advice or the organising of support services and some may indeed make symptoms worse. Early and more effective identification of confusional states should be the cornerstone of management. This enables the development of a clear plan for care; a basis for sustained contact between patient, family and services can be negotiated and the inevitable strain on both patients and carers can be kept to a minimum.

Further Reading

Arie T (ed) (1985) Recent advances in psychogeriatrics, 1. Churchill Livingstone, Edinburgh

Jolley D (1981) Acute confusional states in the elderly. In: Coakley D (ed) Acute geriatric medicine. Croom Helm, London, pp 175–189

Lipowski ZJ (1983) Transient cognitive disorders (delirium, acute confusional states) in the elderly. Am J Psychiatr 140:1426–1436

Mace NL, Rabins PV, Castleton B, Cloke C, McEwan E (1985) The 36 hour day. Hodder and Stoughton, Sevenoaks

Murphy E (1986) Dementia and mental illness in the old. Macmillan, London

Pitt B (ed) (1987) Dementia. Churchill Livingstone, Edinburgh

Report of the Royal College of Physicians (1981) Organic mental impairment in the elderly. J R Coll Phys Lond 15:141–167

Roth M, Iversen LL (eds) (1986) Alzheimer's disease and related disorders. Br Med Bull 42:1

Depression

Delyth Alldrick

Introduction

Traditionally, the psychiatry of old age has been associated with the management of dementia. It is often forgotten that elderly people suffer from a wide range of psychiatric disorders, not least among them being depression. With people of all ages, differences in terminology and the use of various rating scales result in disagreement regarding the diagnosis and hence the prevalence of the problem.

The peak prevalence of depression requiring hospital admission occurs in late middle age and subsequently declines. As there is a close association between physical illness and depression, many elderly depressives are probably admitted to non-psychiatric wards where their problem is not always recognised. Alternatively they may remain undiagnosed at home, their low mood seeming appropriate to their circumstances. A Swedish study has found that 18% of men and 27% of women admitted to feeling "depressed frequently or for long periods" during the previous year. At any given time, some 2%–3% of old people are suffering from a primary depressive illness while a further 11%–12% have "senile dysphoria".

While a continuum exists in the spectrum of depressive illness, distinct patterns are recognised which are of clinical relevance because their management differs. It should be borne in mind that the pattern of illness can change and what, for example, starts off as a neurotic depression can develop into a more serious type of disorder.

Affective illness refers to a severe disorder of mood. A patient with a unipolar affective illness suffers from depression only, whereas with a bipolar illness, mania or hypomania are additional features. Its prevalence among old people exceeds 1%. A psychotic form exists when there are delusional or hallucinatory symptoms with associated loss of insight.

Endogenous depression is a term used to differentiate a severe depressive illness, for which no external stress can be found, from less severe depression.

Neurotic or reactive depression occurs when the illness is precipitated by acute or chronic stress (e.g. physical illness, other psychiatric disorders, alcoholism, organic mental states, personality disorder, drug therapy, etc). The degree of mood disturbance is less in neurotic than in endogenous depression and it may be intermittent, with occasional lightening of mood occurring in response to a pleasant experience. Removal of the underlying cause does not always effect a cure and additional forms of treatment may be required. Its prevalence has been estimated at almost 10% of the elderly population.

Senile dysphoria describes a type of depression in old people which is not so severe as to qualify for the diagnosis of a major depressive disorder but which nevertheless is easily recognised as "depression". Long-standing personality problems, physical illness and disability all appear to be associated with this often intractable condition.

Suicide

Successful suicide is associated with depressive illness, increasing age, social isolation, bereavement, alcoholism, physical illness and the male sex. The peak age for suicide in women is about 60 years and about 80 years for men. The ratio of successful suicide to parasuicide (deliberate self-harm) and attempted suicide (an unsuccessful serious attempt) rises with age; the elderly choosing more immediately lethal methods such as hanging, shooting and drowning rather than drug overdose. Nevertheless, they communicate their intention no less commonly than younger people and may have consulted their general practitioners in the previous week. It is nearly always a mistake to dismiss suicidal gestures in the elderly as "manipulative".

Aetiology (Table 19.1)

Table 19.1.   Aetiology of depression in old age

Genetic factors
Life events: bereavement, retirement, change of residence, acute illness
Chronic stress: physical illness, disability, poor housing, poverty
Abnormal pre-morbid personality
Ageing brain: lowered brain density, larger ventricles, increased MAO activity

Genetic Factors

It is generally held that genetic factors are not so important in the aetiology of severe depressive illness in older patients as they are in illness developing at an earlier age. In one study however, 44% of patients with severe depression requiring hospitalisation and who had psychotic symptoms had first degree relatives who were affected. Other hospitalised patients without psychotic symptoms had affected relatives in 31% of cases.

Life Events

The elderly experience life events, especially of a "loss" kind, much more frequently than younger people. Acute illness, retirement, death of a spouse, moving to live with relatives or into institutional care are all major changes which occur either more frequently or entirely in old age and which can precipitate depression. Surprisingly, life events do not precede neurotic depression more often than they precede endogenous depression. One study has found that only in 15% of depressive patients could an independent and severe precipitant not be found. Such patients had experienced more severe life events, more social difficulties and poorer physical health during the preceding year than had a control group of old people.

Bereavement, one of the most common and most severe losses suffered by the elderly, has been extensively studied. Approximately half of widowed people still described themselves as depressed five months after the death of their spouse, while 25% of women still appeared depressed almost two years after being widowed. Widowed people commit suicide at an increased rate during the first four years and especially the first year following bereavement. The most significant loss for most people is that of the spouse, though loss of another relative, friend, neighbour or even a pet may be important.

Chronic Illness and Disability

Physical illness is a frequent accompaniment of old age and several studies have shown that depression is more common among the elderly who have recently been ill or who have chronic disability (Table 19.2).

Table 19.2. Physical conditions associated with depression

Neurological: Alzheimer's disease, Parkinson's disease, cerebral infarction, sub-dural haematoma, brain tumour, normal pressure hydrocephalus

Cardiac: heart failure, myocardial infarction

Infective: viral diseases, tuberculosis, tertiary syphilis

Metabolic: hyponatraemia and hypokalaemia

Endrocrine: thyroid and parathyroid dysfunction

Renal: chronic renal failure

Neoplastic: especially carcinoma of lung and pancreas

Drugs: reserpine, methyldopa, corticosteroids, digoxin, alcohol

Although it is probably commoner in medical practice to fail to diagnose depression altogether, there are times when depression is wrongly diagnosed instead, because the patient just complains of vague feelings of being "run down" or "tired". An occult malignancy may present with depressive symptoms as may other less serious illnesses. Tuberculosis, bacterial endocarditis and osteomyelitis may all present with vague non-specific complaints and be missed if the index of suspicion is low.

Depression after stroke is thought to be especially common, though this is not universally accepted. Several workers have studied depression after stroke and its relationship with the site of damage. While there is no conclusive proof that damage in any specific site is particularly likely to lead to depression, it is said to be more common in aphasic patients and in those with left hemisphere damage who are right hemisphere dominant. Depression after stroke may, however, largely be determined by social factors.

Giant cell arteritis can present predominantly with depressive symptoms, usually in combination with anaemia, a high ESR and systemic disturbance. Treatment with steroids usually relieves the depressive symptoms along with the other clinical features.

It is often difficult to know how far to go in investigating elderly subjects who present with depressive symptoms. All patients with depression of sufficient severity to be admitted to hospital generally undergo a battery of investigations, usually comprising full blood count, ESR, serum urea and electrolytes, liver function tests, blood sugar, urine analysis, thyroid function and chest X-ray. In general practice, if milder depression does not respond to first line treatments then it is usual to investigate these patients while at the same time enquiring further into the home and family circumstances, relationship problems, etc.

Drugs

Certain drugs are well-known for causing depression in old people (Table 19.2). Fortunately, most can be replaced by others less likely to cause the same problem.

Pre-morbid Personality

Severely affected late life depressives have been found to have rather more stable pre-morbid personalities than younger patients, whereas senile dysphorics are often people who enter old age with poor socialisation and coping abilities. They lack a "confidante", a problem found to be relevant in younger-age depression also, not just because of the general losses of old age but due to lifelong personality defects.

Chronic Stress

In both men and women, "depression" is commoner in those with poorer education and financial status living in poorer accommodation as well as those who are widowed, separated or divorced. Dysphorics tend to complain of a multitude of physical complaints often of a trivial nature (rather than more serious ones) and are more likely to be housebound.

The Ageing Brain

The ageing brain has been postulated as having an increased tendency to depression. Cohort studies have shown that in the 7th and 8th decades of life, mood remained steady or improved in 46.6% of subjects while it dropped slightly in 53.4%. Lowered mood levels were thought to be caused by many interacting factors including age changes in the hypothalamic–pituitary–thyroid axis, gonadal and other functions together with monoamine oxidase activity, always higher in females, which rises with age.

It was at one time thought that depression in old age might be a portent of dementia to come, but this has not been found to occur more frequently than by chance, both being common conditions. However, greater age, later onset of depression and the presence of minor organic signs do seem to be associated with a less favourable outcome. It has been shown that during the illness many elderly depressives have deficits on certain cognitive and neurophysiological tests which nevertheless do not amount to pseudo-dementia. These and other findings, such as the correlation of ventricular enlargement, decreased brain densities and poor outcome, together with the increased monoamine oxidase activity with age, point to the likelihood of the ageing central nervous system and endocrine system having an important role in the aetiology of depression in late life.

Clinical Evaluation

Many authors have remarked on the difficulty in diagnosing some depressive illnesses in elderly people. The classic picture of "involutional melancholia", with severe agitation, nihilistic delusional symptoms and loss of insight is now far from typical of the presentation of depressive illness in late life; but there are a variety of other presentations which may give rise to a missed or a mistaken diagnosis.

All too often the symptoms and signs of depression are attributed by the medical profession, by the patient's family and not least by the patient himself, to being part of growing old. They often expect to be slower in thought and movement, to suffer from insomnia (as opposed to requiring less sleep), to go off their food (as opposed to requiring less to eat) and to lose some interest in life. A careful history with direct questioning about mood, pleasure taken in life and hopes and fears for the future will usually reveal the diagnosis. Speed of onset of the symptoms will usually distinguish depression from senile dementia, a rapid decline into bewildered self-neglect is much more likely to be due to depressive illness.

Some elderly people are reluctant to complain about "depression" seeing this as an admission of weakness; instead they may complain about various "respectable" physical symptoms and even deny being depressed on direct questioning. Typical complaints include constipation, headache, "rheumatic" pains, blurred vision, shakiness, weakness, etc., which can easily mislead the doctor. This tendency to hypochondriasis is the only symptom which has clearly been shown to differentiate depression in old age from that in younger people.

Minor aches and pains which normally would not bother an elderly person of normal mood may become severe and handicapping when that person becomes depressed. The pain is then blamed for the insomnia, the inactivity, the enforced dependence on others and often for suicidal thoughts and/or behaviour. The history often reveals other evidence of depression such as a bereavement or other adverse life event, the effect of which has been minimised by the patient. Successful treatment may not eradicate the pain completely (a common example being post-herpetic neuralgia), but it is seen in perspective once again and does not grossly interfere with daily living.

Depressive Pseudo-dementia

This syndrome has attracted a great deal of attention from researchers over the years, although in practice the diagnosis may be difficult to establish except with hindsight. The differentiating factors between dementia and depressive pseudo-dementia can be summarised in Table 19.3. The main point is that any depressive pathology, whether accompanied by cognitive failure or not, should be vigorously treated.

Table 19.3.   Comparison of dementia and pseudo-dementia

	Dementia	Pseudo-dementia
History	Long history of steady or step-wise decline	Short history with a relatively acute onset
Memory/orientation	Little insight into memory loss and disorientation	Complains of memory loss and disorientation
Constancy	Answers to questions consistently inaccurate	Fluctuating. Answers sometimes appropriate
Answers	Tries hard or confabulates	"I don't know answers" common
Other features	Consistent with global dementia	Other depressive symptoms usually found

Hospitalised Depressives

Of the elderly who are sufficiently depressed to be admitted to hospital, just over a third have severe and psychotic depressive illness. They tend to be very ill in terms of agitation or retardation and are easily recognised as of low mood or sometimes frightened and perplexed. Delusions are common and are often of the nihilistic type (e.g. of having no bowels or blocked bowels, rotten bones, decaying brain, etc.). They may be convinced they are dying of cancer. Typically they feel dirty, guilty of past misdeeds and plead poverty. Quite often they feel they deserve to be mistreated, to suffer misfortune or to be shunned by others. Some have auditory hallucinations, usually in the form of voices calling them obscene or deprecatory names. In those who are extremely retarded, verging on stupor, it is impossible to guess at thought content except from their very distressed or depressed expression. The majority of this group will have sleep disturbance: typically early morning wakening, and often additional trouble getting to sleep, waking repeatedly or even complete insomnia. They have usually lost their appetites and have lost weight and become constipated as a result; this latter symptom may fuel their nihilistic delusions. They may show diurnal variation of mood, being worse in the morning, but in the severest cases mood remains equally low all day. The main manifestations of depression are outlined in Table 19.4.

Around a quarter of hospitalised depressives seem less seriously ill and do not cause so much concern over their behaviour on the ward. They usually continue to eat and drink, are less restless and may not even appear to be particularly depressed. They still tend to have delusional ideas as described above but may present them with a more "paranoid flavour"; with ideas of persecution arising from guilt or other delusions. The fact that their paranoid ideas arise out of their

Table 19.4.   Symptoms and signs of depression (adapted from the Hamilton rating scale)

Mood: sad, pessimistic, tendency to cry or "can't cry"

Anxiety: "tension", irritability, trivial worries

Suicide: death wishes, suicidal ideas or attempts

Hypochondriasis: bodily preoccupation, preoccupation with health

Interest: poor concentration, no interest in work or hobbies, difficulty in making decisions, decreased social activity

Guilt: self-reproach, ideas of guilt/punishment, delusions of guilt

Paranoid symptoms: suspicion, persecutory delusions/hallucinations

Somatic symptoms: anorexia, weight loss, constipation, poor energy

Insomnia: problems falling asleep , waking at night or early morning

Agitation: restlessness, pacing up and down, "wringing of hands"

Retardation: slowness of thought, speech or action, apathy, stupor

Diurnal variation: Symptoms worse in the morning or evening

Insight: full, partial or nil

depressive mood distinguishes these patients from those with paranoid psychosis who have no self-blame and feel unjustly persecuted.

The remainder of hospitalised depressives are usually diagnosed as suffering from neurotic depression. They tend to be preoccupied with somatic complaints, often bowel disturbances such as constipation. In contrast to those with endogenous or psychotic depression they often blame others for their predicament while also showing some self-reproach and low self-esteem. Quite often, these patients have been admitted at the behest of family, neighbours or other carers who are often at their wits end trying to deal with what seems to them to be a person who is doing his or her best to be a nuisance.

Management

Some of the first considerations for a clinician who diagnoses depressive illness in an elderly person are: How serious is it? Is there a significant risk of suicide? Is there a likelihood of self-neglect? The answers or "best guesses" to these questions determine not only the method of treatment employed but also whether the patient requires admission to hospital or not. In general, a patient who presents voluntarily complaining of depressed mood, often with diminished appetite, some insomnia, lack of interest and concentration while retaining insight but without any psychotic symptoms (such as persecutory or hypochondriacal delusions) and who denies any suicidal intention, can usually be satisfactorily treated by his or her general practitioner. A careful eye must be kept on progress or the lack of it; signs of deterioration despite treatment include failure to attend for follow-up, further weight loss, signs of self-neglect and increasing concern from family members or neighbours.

Even when psychotic features are elicited this is not necessarily an indication for immediate admission to hospital, especially if there are carers available to look after the patient and to supervise medication. As soon as delusions begin to "take over" however, with, for example, "blocked bowels" leading to a refusal to eat or take medication, or derogatory auditory hallucinations leading to aggressive behaviour, then there is little doubt that skilled psychiatric nursing is required. If insight is completely lost and the patient refuses hospitalisation, or cannot understand the reason for recommending it, then steps may be taken under the appropriate sections of the Mental Health Act 1983 (see Chap. 27).

An alternative to in-patient admission is regular psychiatric day hospital attendance where progress and medication can be monitored by experienced staff. This option avoids the inevitable disruption that inpatient admission entails and may make working with the patient's family easier. Even electroconvulsive therapy can be administered successfully to a day patient.

Occasionally the decision to admit does not just depend on the patient's condition but also on the despair expressed by the patient's carers, especially where histrionic or attention-seeking behaviour is exhibited. In these cases it is usually wise to admit earlier rather than later, when the carer may have become so desperate as to cut off all ties with the patient and subsequently refuse to consider having him home following treatment.

Perhaps more so in this age group than in any other, close cooperation with the family is essential, not only during an acute episode but also in order to prevent, or at least delay, relapse. Close attention may have to be paid to family dynamics, living conditions and physical disability as well as the treatment for the depressive illness itself.

Treatment for the acute attack usually consists of one or more of the following:

Antidepressant medication (see Table 19.5)

Electroconvulsive therapy (ECT)

Psychotherapy

Table 19.5. Properties and side effects of antidepressant drugs

Drug	Properties	Side effects/precautions
Tricyclics		
Amitryptyline	Sedative	
Dothiepin	Sedative	Anticholinergic and cardiac effects can be troublesome in
Imipramine	Neutral	old people
Clomipramine	Neutral	
Lofepramine	Neutral	
Fluvoxamine	Neutral	Fewer anticholinergic and cardiac side effects
Newer drugs		
Mianserin	Sedative	Few anticholinergic effects. Safe in overdose. Risk of blood dyscrasias
Trazodone	Sedative	Few anticholinergic/cardiac effects
MAOIs		
Phenelzine	Useful for "atypical" depression	Need for dietary precautions (avoid tyramine-containing foodstuffs)
Trytophan	Useful adjunct	Few or no side effects. Has a therapeutic window

Antidepressants

For patients dealt with in general practice the usual choice is antidepressant medication together with general support from the primary care team. Compliance with medication is often a problem in old people and must be considered together with efficacy, safety and side effects when prescribing.

There have recently been several studies examining the special problems in prescribing antidepressants for old people. The tried and tested drugs are tricyclic antidepressants. These used to be considered cardiotoxic for elderly patients even in therapeutic doses, though recent research has refuted this. However, tricyclics are still best avoided in patients with intraventricular conduction defects since they prolong the P–R interval and broaden QRS complexes. Imipramine has been found to have a quinidine-like anti-arrhythmic property suggesting that tricyclics may be beneficial in certain cardiac conditions. Tricyclics have been demonstrated not to have any significant effect on ventricular function in arteriosclerotic or hypertensive cardiac disease. Orthostatic hypotension has been found to be associated with imipramine therapy; this is not dose related and is found predominantly in patients with pre-treatment orthostatic hypotension. The new tricyclic agents, lofepramine and fluvoxamine have both been particularly recommended for the elderly because of their lower incidence of side effects, especially anti-cholinergic and cardiac, while maintaining efficacy similar to that of imipramine. Although tricyclics have been marketed with a label of "sedative" or "alerting", in practice the success of a particular drug in particular types of depression has not been convincing.

Newer antidepressants are usually compared in trials to the traditional tricyclics and most have been found to be of equal efficacy with the advantage of fewer side effects. Mianserin has been found to be of equal efficacy to amitriptyline whilst producing less deterioration in cognitive function; it also has the added advantage of being anxiolytic and safer in overdosage. However, recent studies have indicated that mianserin may provoke blood dyscrasias in the elderly. Blood tests are recommended every 4 weeks during the first 3 months of treatment. If the patient develops fever, sore throat or other signs of infection, treatment should be stopped and a full blood count obtained (Committee on Safety of Medicines, 1989). Trazodone has been compared with imipramine and found to be equally effective, although no more rapid in action or any better for agitation.

Monoamine oxidase inhibitors (MAOIs), although rarely used in the elderly as a first-line drug, may have a role in resistant or refractory depression or where anxiety or phobic symptoms are prominent. Side effects most often reported are dizziness, orthostatic hypotension and weight gain.

Tryptophan is an amino acid which is a precursor of 5-hydroxytryptamine. Although known for some time to potentiate certain other antidepressants (MAOIs, clomipramine and amitriptyline), it is now known to be an antidepressant in its own right. Having few or no side effects it is a very useful adjunct in resistant depression or in those who cannot tolerate sufficiently high doses of other antidepressants.

Lithium can be successfully used in the elderly both for the acute episode and for prophylaxis as long as certain safeguards are borne in mind. Lithium added to antidepressants when the initial response is poor seems to accelerate improvement, although there have been no systematic evaluations of lithium therapy for unipolar depression in the elderly. For recurrent depression lithium is the best know preventative treatment and is effective in about two-thirds of patients. Therapeutic plasma levels are best kept to the lower end of the advised range for adults, i.e. 0.4–0.8 mmol/l, as renal failure, cardiac failure and diuretic therapy (all more prevalent in elderly patients) can all lead to accumulation of lithium salts and toxicity. In the long term thyroid function should be monitored as hypothyroidism can result.

Carbamazepine as a prophylactic compound has not been fully evaluated in the elderly but may be safer and better tolerated than lithium. Leucopenia has been known to occur so that monitoring of the white cell count is necessary.

Whichever drug is chosen it is imperative to start with relatively low doses in the elderly patient but to increase the dose incrementally to the level of tolerance. Tricyclics have long half-lives and can often be given once a day thus improving compliance and, if sedative, helping to reduce insomnia when administered at night. At least 2 weeks must be expected to elapse before any significant improvement occurs. This must be carefully explained to both patients and relatives to avoid disappointment and dissatisfaction with the treatment (and, therefore, the therapist). Side effects also require explanation, especially the commoner ones which can usually be expected to abate with continued usage. The commonest complaints in the elderly are due to the anti-cholinergic properties of some drugs and consist of constipation (often already present due to the depressive illness), urine retention, dry mouth, blurred vision and, rarely, exacerbation of glaucoma. Increased confusion, especially in those with pre-existing dementia, and occasionally visual hallucinations can occur, both of which are an indication to discontinue the offending drug.

Antidepressants need to be continued in full dosage for several months following recovery, with a gradual reduction after this to a maintenance level of perhaps half the therapeutic dose. The elderly are probably best advised to continue on this regimen indefinitely rather than risk relapse by stopping the drug. However, this strategy should not be confused with the pointless exercise of prescribing antidepressants continuously despite the absence of any worthwhile response. Careful follow-up is essential for the maintenance of compliance and to spot early signs of relapse.

Electroconvulsive Therapy

Electroconvulsive therapy (ECT) can be a life-saving procedure in severe depressive illness and may be a safer alternative in the elderly who cannot tolerate antidepressants. The indications for ECT include the failure of antidepressant medication in alleviating depression even when they have been given in adequate dosage for sufficient time (i.e. at least 6 weeks with proven compliance). In the elderly "adequate dosage" may fail to be achieved due to troublesome side effects.

When psychotic symptoms are present then ECT is probably the treatment of choice, although success may also be achieved by combining an antidepressant with an antipsychotic agent such as a phenothiazine. It must be remembered that the side effects of the additional drug can cause further difficulties.

In depressive stupor or distressing agitated depression, ECT can be literally life-saving. In such circumstances one treatment can be given without the patient's consent as long as steps are then taken to place the patient on a treatment section of the Mental Health Act 1983 followed by a second opinion from another psychiatrist so that the course of ECT can be completed.

When explaining the ECT procedure to an elderly patient or their relatives it must be recognised that some will remember when ECT was given without anaesthetic or muscle-relaxants and may be frightened of the prospect. Nowadays they can be reassured that as long as they are considered fit for a short-acting anaesthetic then ECT is an extremely safe procedure.

It has been advocated that ECT should be administered unilaterally to the non-dominant hemisphere in the elderly as this leads to a shorter duration of memory loss surrounding the event. However, this may prolong the duration of treatment required. Perhaps the best course is to give unilateral ECT initially and if the response appears to be slow then to change to bilateral ECT. The frequency of treatment is usually twice per week, most patients beginning to show some improvement after the second or third treatment, with improvement being transient initially. The improvement lasts longer with successive treatments until eventually there is no relapse between treatments. The average number of treatments required is about seven or eight, there being little advantage in carrying on if there is no response after ten or twelve treatments.

General Supportive Measures

The patient requires careful observation in the early stages of improvement, whether this is a result of drugs and/or ECT, as it is often at this stage that suicidal thoughts are acted upon, the patient having been too ill previously to carry out his intention. As the patient improves the distressing symptoms of agitation, anxiety, hypochondriasis, delusions and feelings of guilt gradually fade away. The progress is often patchy and it is worth warning the patient about the occurrence of occasional "bad days" in the early stages. These should become less frequent with time.

One of the problems associated with recovery is a continuing lack of confidence in skills which were lost when the depression was at its worst. Conversation, decision making, shopping, paying bills and so on are functions which may well have been taken over by relatives. If so, patients will need to be gradually reintroduced to these skills and "reclaimed" from well-meaning carers. This is the point at which some form of formal psychotherapy is most useful. No systematic evaluation of psychotherapy for the treatment of depression in old age has so far been attempted but it has been suggested that the use of cognitive psychotherapy, where the negative thought processes of depression are challenged and replaced by positive ones, may be adapted to the special needs of the elderly and aid recovery.

Groups of recovering patients can often help each other in the process of "re-entering" life once more. Home assessments and shopping trips in the company of occupational therapists can help to overcome initial resistance to relinquishing the sick role. Family dynamics can be just as easily disrupted by a member becoming well again as when they became ill in the first place and this is the time when the whole family may need to become involved in order to effect full recovery.

Prognosis

Treatment of the acute attack of depressive illness in the elderly is usually successful and rewarding although some 15% will be resistant to the treatments described above. Often this is due to co-existing physical disease which may be undiagnosed, or sometimes to slowly progressive dementia. Poor environmental conditions, continuing interpersonal conflicts and long-standing personality difficulties are also associated with a poor prognosis.

For those with a "pure" depressive illness which fails to respond to conventional treatments, various cocktails of therapeutic measures have been devised which are beyond the scope of this chapter. Even in the elderly, when all else fails, psychosurgery may need to be considered.

Elderly patients are prone to frequent relapse even when the treatment of the initial attack is successful. In a recent study 22% of elderly hospitalised patients made a lasting recovery from a depressive episode over a follow-up period of between four and nine years, 38% had further episodes but recovered completely in between and 32% continued to suffer from "depressive invalidism" while only 8% were continuously ill throughout. The presence or absence of health problems were associated with a very poor and very good outcome respectively and men were more likely to have a poor outcome. Other variables such as a past history of depression, a long duration of illness, the presence or absence of precipitating life events and whether suicide had been attempted did not seem to predict outcome.

There seems no doubt that as the numbers of the elderly increase the demands on primary care and psychiatric services by the victims of depression will continue to mount. Research continually throws up newer and supposedly better drugs and therapeutic regimens but as with all other conditions, prevention is better than cure. Further research would seem to be indicated into the social and physical forerunners of depressive illness and senile dysphoria.

Further Reading

Baldwin RC, Jolley DJ (1987) The prognosis of depression in old age. B J Psychiatr 149:574–583
Blazer D, Williams CD (1980) Epidemiology of dysphoria and depression in an elderly population. Am J Psychiatr 137:439–444
House A (1986) Depression after stroke. Br Med J 294:76–78
Kay WK, Bergmann K (1980) Epidemiology of mental disorders among the aged in the community. In: Birren IE, Slone RB (eds) Handbook of mental health and ageing. Prentice-Hall, Englewood Cliffs, pp 34–56
Murphy E (1982) Functional disorders. In Levy R, Post F (eds) The psychiatry of late life. Blackwell Scientific Publications, Oxford, pp 176–221
Post F, Shulman K (1985) New views on old age affective disorders. In: Arie T (ed) Recent advances in psychogeriatrics. Churchill Livingstone, Edinburgh, pp 119–140
Shaw DM (1986) Handbook of affective disorders. The Boots Pure Drug Company PLC, Nottingham

Chapter 20

Anaemia

R. D. Hutton

Introduction

Modern blood cell analysers have radically altered both the diagnosis and the concept of anaemia. It is no longer enough to recognise anaemia as a condition in which the haemoglobin concentration is abnormally low. Instead attention must now be given to the concepts of relative anaemia and pre-anaemia. These conceptual changes are particularly relevant if the maximum benefit is to be obtained from the full blood count when used as a screening test. Whereas anaemia, as traditionally defined, is common in the elderly, relative anaemia and pre-anaemia are very common. Throughout this chapter the use of the word anaemia should be understood to include both relative anaemia and pre-anaemia.

Anaemia

Traditionally anaemia has been recognised when the haemoglobin concentration falls below pre-set reference values. For younger adults this level is usually accepted as 115 g/l (11.5 g/dl) for females and 130 g/l (13.0 g/dl) for males. In elderly people the lower reference value tends to be decreased. This applies particularly to males, where decreased testosterone production reduces the sex difference in haemoglobin concentrations. As a general guide, the haemoglobin level in old people should be above 110 g/l (11.0 g/dl).

Relative Anaemia

Even if the haemoglobin concentration is within the normal reference range, its level may have dropped or may be inappropriately low for the individual. The presence of relative anaemia may be deduced from historic data, when a significantly higher haemoglobin concentration was recorded in the past. Alternatively, the haemoglobin concentration may be lower than expected in a given set of circumstances. Thus, a "normal" concentration may be inappropriately low for a person who is chronically hypoxic.

Pre-anaemia

Pre-anaemia refers to a change in an individual's red cell indices, which may herald the development of anaemia. The mean cell volume (MCV) and the mean cell haemoglobin (MCH) are very stable in health throughout adult life. The MCH is the more robust indicator across time, as the MCV may vary according to the methods used to measure it. The normal range for the MCV should therefore be determined locally, while the reference range for the MCH is 27.5–32.5 pg. As with the haemoglobin concentration, it is far better to know an individual's "normal" value than the overall "normal range". Such data may be available from the person's medical records.

A patient with an overtly abnormal MCV or MCH should be investigated, regardless of the haemoglobin concentration. Similarly, a progressive increase or decrease in either the MCH or MCV should prompt appropriate investigation. This will allow a diagnosis to be made before the patient becomes symptomatic. Therapeutic intervention may be easier at an early stage and severe clinical anaemia will be avoided. There is no sense in waiting for values to fall outside the reference range or for the haemoglobin concentration to drop before taking action.

The mortality rate from anaemia itself is very low; death in anaemic patients being usually related to the underlying disease. Occasionally however, patients present with severe anaemia and die despite intervention. In such cases, a review of previous blood counts sometimes reveals abnormalities which, had they been investigated, would have led to an earlier diagnosis of treatable disease.

Incidence

Most types of anaemia are more prevalent in older people than in the general population, the trend increasing with advancing years. The exceptions are the inherited anaemias that reduce longevity (e.g. thalassaemia major) and iron deficiency. The latter is most common during periods of rapid growth and in females during their reproductive years. However, inherited anaemias such as hereditary spherocytosis and thalassaemia trait are often not diagnosed until the later years of life. As with other types of anaemia, they may be discovered as an incidental finding when the patient presents with other conditions.

Anaemias are classified as microcytic hypochromic, macrocytic hyperchromic or normocytic normochromic according to cellular morphology. The principle causes of each type are listed in Table 20.1. Table 20.2 indicates the effect of these underlying conditions on the red cell indices, their relative frequency and associated clinical features.

As with other problems in the elderly patient, anaemia may be due to more than one cause. This must be borne in mind when making a diagnosis and when assessing the response to treatment.

Table 20.1. The underlying causes of different types of anaemia

1. *Microcytic hypochromic (MCH<27.5 pg)*
   or
   Falling MCV/MCH
   or
   Subpopulation of microcytes

   Iron deficiency
   Haemoglobinopathy
   Secondary anaemia
   Lead poisoning
   Aluminium toxicity
   Sideroblastic anaemia
   Some myeloproliferative states

2. *Macrocytic hyperchromic (MCH>32.5 pg)*
   or
   Increasing MCV/MCH
   or
   Subpopulation of macrocytes

   B_{12}/folate deficiency
   Ethanol
   Myelodysplastic, leukaemic and hypoplastic conditions
   Liver disease
   Hypoxia
   Reticulocytosis
   Cytotoxic drugs
   Myxoedema

3. *Normochromic normocytic (MCH 27.5–32.5 pg)*
   or
   Falling haemoglobin concentration

   Acute blood loss
   Secondary anaemia
   Renal failure
   Combination of conditions in 1 and 2
   Developing condition in 1 and 2
   Hypopituitarism

Common Forms of Anaemia

Iron Deficiency

Iron deficiency leads to a hypochromic microcytic anaemia though it is important to appreciate that in the early stages the anaemia is normochromic and normocytic. It is usually caused by increased iron loss but may also reflect a decreased dietary intake, impaired absorption or a combination of these factors. Absorption is decreased when gastric acid is deficient and this may be secondary to gastric surgery, atrophic gastritis or the effects of medicines given specifically to decrease acid production. Malabsorption may occur if there is disease of the duodenum and upper jejunum. Pathological loss of iron usually occurs through gastrointestinal bleeding but may be due to chronic blood loss from other organ systems. Rarely, it is due to the occult loss of intracellular iron from the urinary tract, skin or lungs.

Table 20.2.   Common causes and features of anaemia

	Usual effect on MCV/MCH	Relative frequency	Associated features
Decreased production			
Iron deficiency	↓	+++	Angular stomatitis, dysphagia, atrophic glossitis, blood loss, koilonychia, gastric surgery
B_{12} and/or folate deficiency	↑	+++	Anorexia, nausea, bowel disturbance, weight loss, glossitis, fever, jaundice
B_{12} deficiency	↑	++	Peripheral neuropathy, dementia, subacute combined degeneration of spinal cord
Hypoplasia/aplasia	↑	–	Petechia, infection, fever, exposure to marrow toxins
Dysplasia	↕	+	Often symptomless. May be marrow failure, splenomegaly
Erythropoietin deficiency	N or ↓	+	Features of renal impairment
Secondary to other disease	↓	+++	Features of other diseases (e.g. chronic inflammation)
Marrow replacement	↑	+	Features of malignancy, splenomegaly, lymphadenopathy
Heterozygous haemoglobinopathy	↓	V	Usually none. Family history important
Increased turnover			
Acute blood loss	N or ↑	+	Visible bleeding, hypovolaemia
Haemolysis	↑	–	Jaundice, discoloured urine, splenomegaly
Homozygous haemoglobinopathy	↓ or N	V	Skeletal deformities, jaundice, iron overload

N: normal; V: varies with population groups; ↓: decreased; ↑: increased; ↕: may be increased or decreased.

Iron deficiency always indicates an underlying disorder which should be identified and treated. Investigation will always require exclusion of a source of gastrointestinal blood loss by appropriate means.

Folic Acid and B_{12} Deficiency

Folic acid and B_{12} deficiency may both lead to macrocytic hyperchromic anaemia, though a hypochromic or normochromic anaemia may result where there is a complicating factor which would otherwise cause hypochromia. Deficiencies may be caused by a dietary lack, malabsorption or increased requirements of folic acid and/or B_{12}.

Folic Acid Deficiency

Folic acid deficiency is very common in old people and frequently is related to poor diet and/or ethanol abuse. In addition, many conditions lead to increased requirements and if the diet is inadequate to provide them, deficiency will result. Increased requirements are seen in many haematological conditions (e.g. myeloproliferative, myelodysplastic and haemolytic processes) together with all forms of malignancy and infective/inflammatory disorders. Drugs which impair folate utilisation include trimethoprim, triamterene, methotrexate (all dihydrofolate reductase inhibitors), anticonvulsants and ethanol. Wherever possible, the cause of the folate deficiency should be identified and remedied. Specific supplemental therapy is discussed later in the chapter.

B_{12} Deficiency

B_{12} deficiency is rarely due to dietary deficiency, although this may be seen in vegans. For absorption B_{12} needs to be bound to intrinsic factor, which is produced in the stomach. It is a lack of intrinsic factor which most commonly results in deficiency, secondary to either gastric surgery or pernicious anaemia. The B_{12}/intrinsic factor complex is absorbed in the terminal ileum and hence disease affecting this part of the intestine can also result in malabsorption.

Secondary Anaemias

Secondary anaemias may be normochromic or hypochromic in nature. They are extremely common in elderly people and may result from chronic infection, inflammation, malignancy or renal failure. In some cases the aetiology remains unclear. When possible, the underlying condition should be remedied but often this is not possible. It is essential to exclude reversible elements of the anaemia such as haematinic deficiencies as these are frequently associated and easily treated. Few cases are severe enough to warrant blood transfusion. When transfusion is necessary, the haemoglobin concentration will rapidly fall again unless the underlying problem is resolved. Therapeutic trials are currently being undertaken of erythropoietin in patients with severe anaemia secondary to renal failure and such therapy may become more widely applicable.

Refractory Anaemias

Refractory anaemias may be secondary to myelodysplastic syndromes, hypoplastic states or myeloproliferative diseases. Again it is essential to exclude any reversible elements of the anaemia, such as haematinic deficiencies or hypersplenism. In part, the diagnosis of myelodysplastic syndromes relies upon the failure to respond to a trial of appropriate vitamins. Folate deficiency is particularly common in these conditions as there is often increased haemopoiesis and prophylactic supplements may be justified. In some cases, particularly where there are associated bleeding problems, it is also important to exclude iron deficiency. Patients with myeloproliferative diseases complicated by anaemia sometimes show an improvement in their haemoglobin concentration if their myeloproliferation is controlled with appropriate therapy.

If such patients become symptomatically anaemic despite the therapeutic options considered above, the only additional measure is to commence a regular programme of repeated blood transfusions. Problems with infection and bleeding should be anticipated as far as possible and treated as they occur. At present there is considerable research interest in myelodysplasia and although specific therapy cannot yet be recommended, the situation may well change.

Haemolytic Anaemias

Haemolytic anaemias are caused by several mechanisms including inherited red cell defects, affecting either the membrane or the metabolism of the red cell, and acquired defects resulting from immune damage, mechanical trauma or chemical damage to the red cell membrane. Classically haemolysis results in jaundice and decreased plasma haem-binding proteins such as haptoglobins. Reticulocytosis is usual and this may result in macrocytosis, but a reticulocyte response may be absent if the bone marrow is suppressed for any reason (e.g. infection or other physiological stress). The combination of haemolysis and failed marrow response may rapidly lead to life-threatening anaemia and will usually require transfusion support until the marrow recovers.

The peripheral blood film may well suggest the cause of a haemolytic anaemia and suggest further appropriate investigations. The presence of immune-mediated haemolysis should be excluded by performing a Coomb's test to look for antibody or complement coating the red cells. Problems with providing compatible blood in cases of immune-mediated haemolysis should be anticipated early.

Intravascular haemolysis may lead to large amounts of iron being lost in the urine as frank haemoglobinuria or as occult haemosiderinuria. Iron deficiency may result and alter the laboratory profile of the anaemia. Where haemolysis is due to red cell trauma (e.g. from a heart valve or other vascular prosthesis), then iron deficiency can increase the rate of haemolysis substantially whereupon replacement therapy should be given.

The management of haemolytic anaemia depends on the underlying cause which must be identified and modified where possible. Co-existing iron deficiency and infection should be corrected when found. All patients with haemolysis have high requirements for folic acid and supplements should be given routinely. Transfusion should be avoided if possible but can sometimes be life saving.

In cases where the haemolysis is mediated by exposure to cold the patient should be kept as warm as possible. If intravenous therapy (including transfusion) is required the products should be prewarmed, but only in a purpose built warmer. Blood products should be complement free. Steroid therapy and splenectomy are not usually appropriate therapy as the haemolysis is usually intravascular.

In warm autoimmune haemolytic anaemia, steroids should be given in high doses (e.g. prednisolone: 0.5–1 mg/kg/day) initially and tailed off very slowly once the haemolysis is controlled. Patients must be monitored carefully and the dose of steroids immediately increased if there is evidence of increasing haemolysis. If the patient cannot be maintained without steroids, splenectomy is indicated. Where this is not practicable, the use of other immunosuppressive agents should be considered.

Clinical Evaluation

The clinical features found in the elderly are very variable and may differ substantially from those seen in younger patients. The speed of onset of the anaemia and the patient's level of activity greatly modify the severity of symptoms. Anaemia of rapid onset in an active patient is likely to be noticed early. Conversely, immobility can delay diagnosis as exercise-related symptoms will be minimal or absent. The ability of the haemoglobin to release oxygen to the tissues is also very important. This is increased in acidosis and with low affinity haemoglobins (e.g. sickle cell haemoglobin (HbS)) and decreased in alkalosis and with high affinity haemoglobins (including carboxyhaemoglobin). Co-existing pathology such as cardiorespiratory disease or hyperviscosity states will also exacerbate symptoms of anaemia.

A careful history and examination will often provide a working diagnosis and guide further investigation. The associated features listed in Table 20.2 should be sought. Frequently, history taking will need to be extended to relatives, attendants and other carers due to communication difficulties with the patient. This is essential where there is any doubt about the reliability of information, particularly concerning such factors as diet, enthanol intake and drug history. A phone call to the general practitioner will often save much valuable time and may also provide the results of past investigations.

It should be appreciated that while anaemia may be diagnosed on clinical grounds, in most cases investigation follows the finding of an abnormality on a "routine" blood count.

Further Investigation

Patients should be investigated if the haemoglobin concentration is less than 110 g/l (11.0 g/dl), or is falling, or if there is a significant change in their MCV or MCH. Good clinical information is vital if the appropriate tests are to be performed; "blunderbuss" investigation wastes time and resources and is not to be commended. Unexpected results should always be confirmed by repeat blood sampling before undertaking unnecessary, unpleasant and expensive tests. A schema for investigation of microcytic hypochromic anaemia is summarised in Fig. 20.1 and one for macrocytic anaemia in Fig. 20.2. Consultation with the hospital haematology service will often lead to a quicker and cheaper diagnosis.

Many modern blood cell counters produce histograms showing the distribution of various red cell indices. These may indicate early problems. A "mean value" may be well within reference ranges but hide subpopulations of abnormal cells which could facilitate early diagnosis. A full profile from such an instrument and examples of such abnormalities are shown in Figs. 20.3 and 20.4. Interpretation of such complex data is not demanded of most clinicians. Nevertheless, they should appreciate the changing technology and be familiar with the techniques used in laboratories which they utilise.

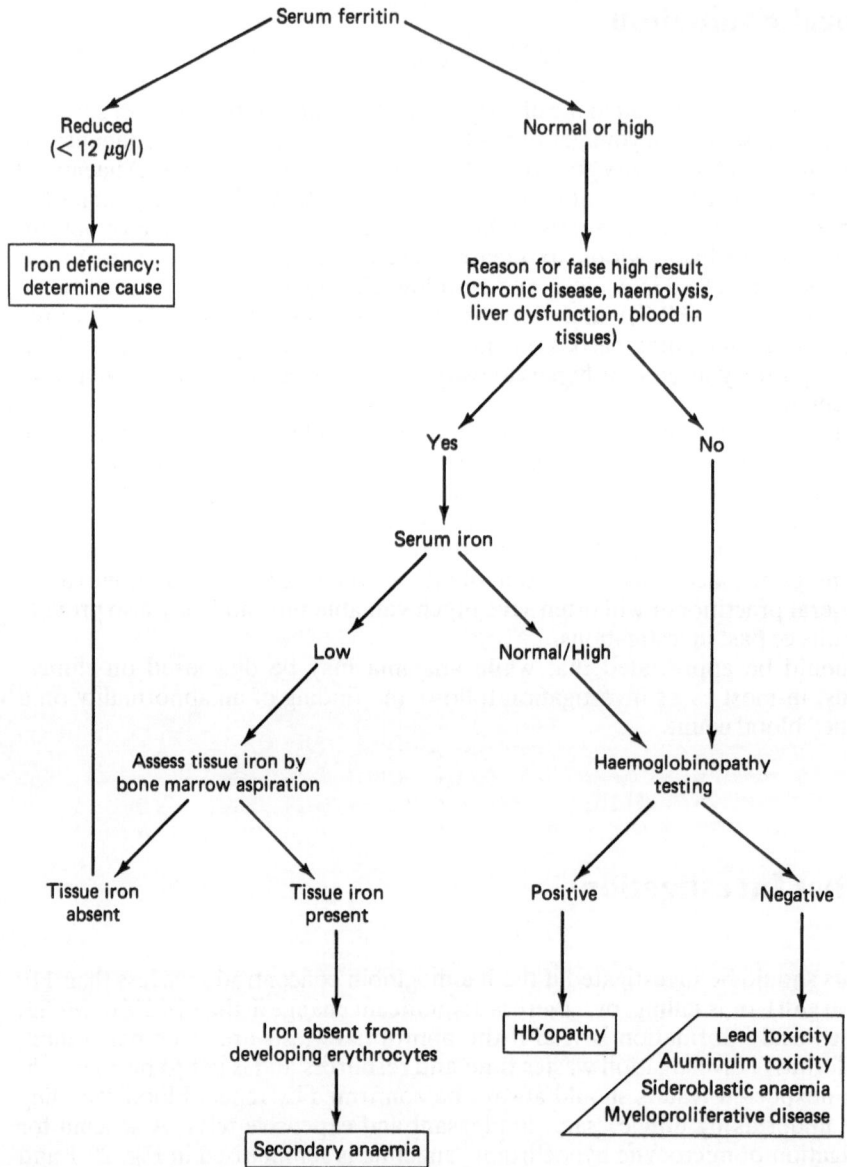

Fig. 20.1. Investigation of microcytic hypochromic anaemia.

Blood film examinations are now rarely routine, being only performed if the clinical information indicates such a need, or the laboratory staff think such an examination is likely to be productive. Further diagnostic investigation will depend on the clinical history, examination, laboratory data and diagnostic imaging results.

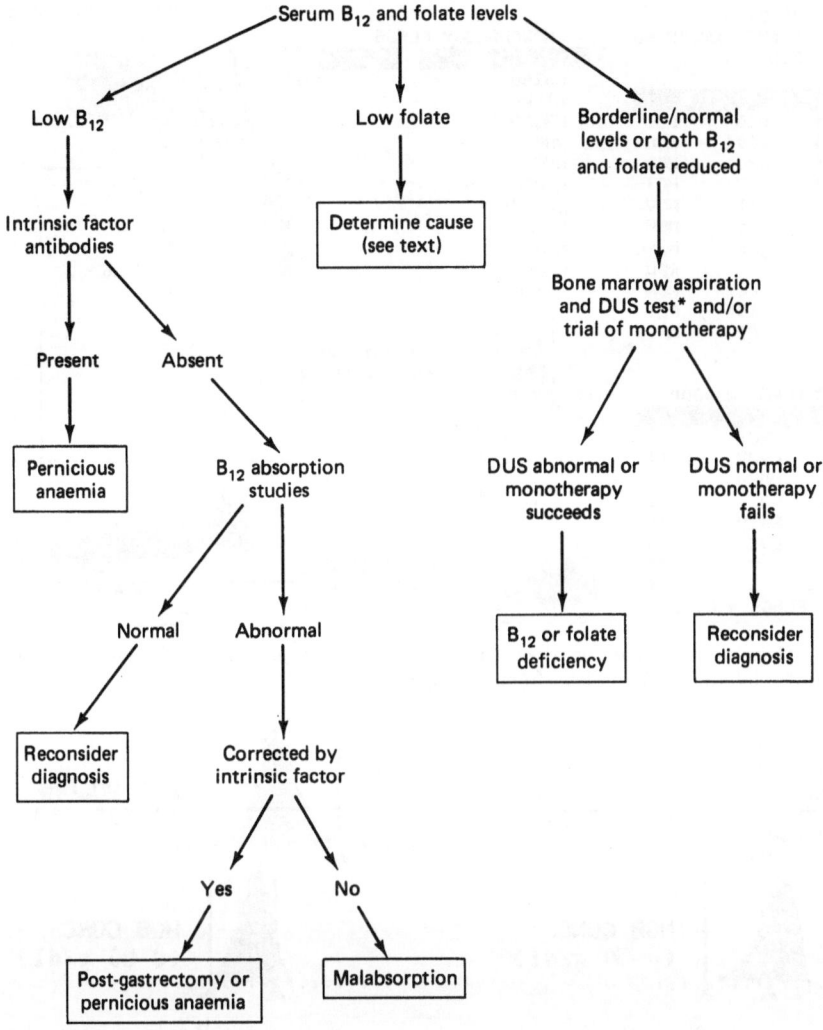

*DUS = deoxyuridine suppression test. This test is increasingly used to
provide a rapid biochemical diagnosis of B_{12} and folate deficiencies.

Fig. 20.2.   Investigation of macrocytic hyperchromic anaemia.

Management

Management will depend upon the underlying cause and it is therefore essential
to make a precise diagnosis whenever possible. Should it be necessary to begin
therapy before a diagnosis is reached, sufficient blood should first be taken to
allow haematinic assays and other appropriate tests to be performed. This will

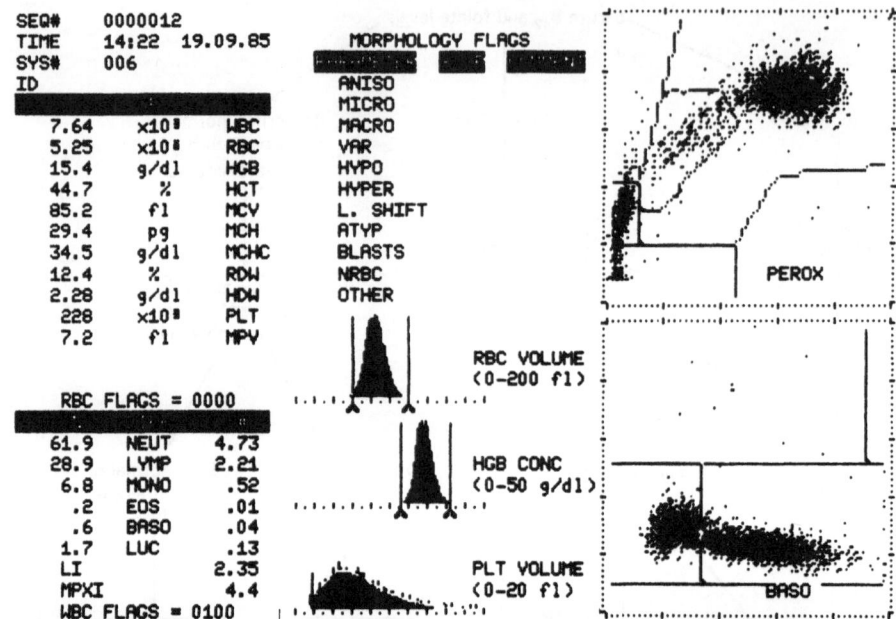

Fig. 20.3. Haematological data on a normal patient available from a Technicon HI blood cell counter. Further information is available from the inbuilt computer.

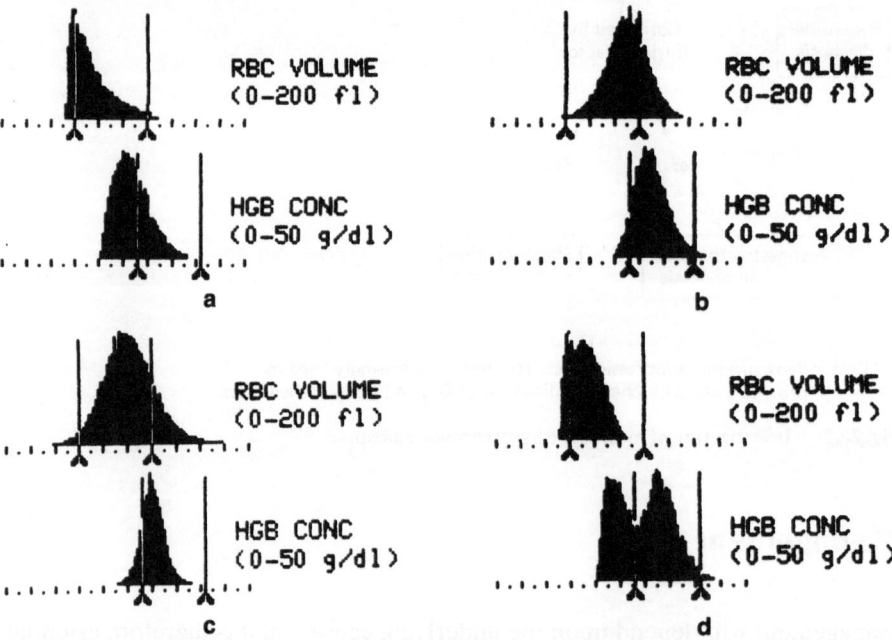

Fig. 20.4a–d. Red cell histograms from patients with: **a** iron deficiency; **b** B$_{12}$ deficiency; **c** myelodysplasia; **d** iron deficiency following blood transfusion. The upright bars enclose the normal reference values.

usually include a further blood count sample which will allow a blood film to be examined and additional tests, such as a reticulocyte count and direct Coomb's test to be performed where indicated. If appropriate a bone marrow sample should also be obtained before treatment is commenced.

Patients with symptomatic anaemia should rest until improved by treatment and then gradually encouraged to return to full mobility. Heart failure should be managed along established lines (see Chap. 7) and drug therapy gradually withdrawn as the haemoglobin concentration returns towards normal.

With severe anaemia there should be a rapid response to appropriate therapy. However with pre-anaemia or when the anaemia is mild, there will not be a reticulocyte response to specific therapy and the red cell indices may take up to 3 months in returning to normal. For this reason it is important that therapeutic trials in such patients are extended before deciding whether or not they are successful. Red cell histograms produced by modern blood cell counters (Fig. 20.3) are extremely useful in monitoring response and often make reticulocyte counts unnecessary.

Transfusion

Blood transfusion should be reserved for those patients with symptomatic refractory anaemia or for those whose anaemia is so severe that waiting for a response to conventional therapy could be dangerous. In the latter case the amount of blood transfused should be limited to that required for symptomatic relief or to allow urgent medical or surgical intervention. It should not prevent the immediate institution of specific therapy and should never be used as a substitute for such therapy. Transfusion must be preceded by obtaining the samples necessary to enable a specific diagnosis to be made.

If transfusion is required, packed red cells should be given slowly with diuretic cover as necessary. In life-threatening situations, exchange transfusion of volumes of blood between 50–100 ml should be considered.

For the management of refractory anaemia it is best to give small (2–3 units), frequent transfusions. This can be done on an out-patient basis. The haemoglobin concentration should always be kept above the level at which the patient is symptomatic. There is no sense in allowing patients to develop symptoms and then to admit them for a hazardous large volume transfusion. Before embarking on a long-term transfusion programme the blood bank should be informed so that the patient's extended blood groups can be determined. This will minimise the possibility of subsequent cross-matching difficulties.

Unless given to replace blood loss, repeated blood transfusion will produce iron overload. Each unit adds approximately 200 mg of iron to the body stores. Few old people requiring repeated transfusion are likely to live long enough to develop problems with iron overload so that routine use of expensive chelation therapy is seldom warranted. However there may be cases where chelation therapy should be considered. A decision regarding its use will be influenced by the presence of pre-existing iron overload, pathology that would be made worse by iron overload, the frequency of transfusion and the anticipated lifespan of the patient. Should a low cost, non-toxic oral chelating agent become available, its extended use might be justified.

Iron Supplementation

Iron deficiency is usually treated with an oral ferrous salt. About 100 mg of elemental iron should be given daily, as ferrous sulphate 200 mg twice daily or ferrous gluconate 300 mg three times daily. Slow release preparations should not be used as they have no therapeutic advantages and may be ineffective if the iron is released past the site of optimum absorption. Tetracycline should not be administered with oral iron as the absorption of both will be markedly impaired. Absorption of iron is also reduced by antacids, H_2 antagonists, zinc salts and trientine. Where appropriate these drugs should be administered at different times.

With treatment the haemoglobin concentration usually increases by about 10 g/l (1 g/dl) per week, the rate of response being proportional to the severity of the anaemia. It should be expected that the haemoglobin concentration will have returned to normal within 6 weeks; if it has not, a reason for failure of response should be sought. Assuming that the original diagnosis was correct, such reasons include non-compliance with treatment, the inappropriate use of slow-release formulations or co-administration of iron-binding preparations. Alternatively, there may be malabsorption, continuing severe blood loss or co-existing disease suppressing marrow response.

The red cell indices will take several months to return to normal. The duration of therapy should be determined by clinical considerations. If the cause of the deficiency is certain and has been remedied, then therapy should continue for a further 3 months in order to replenish the iron stores. In many cases, however, it is appropriate only to continue the course of treatment until the haemoglobin concentration has returned to normal, as a subsequent early fall in the haemoglobin concentration or red cell indices will then draw attention to a continuing unresolved problem. In a few patients continued iron therapy may be necessary but only at the minimum dose necessary to maintain the haemoglobin concentration.

Side effects are dose-related and can be reduced by taking tablets with food or by reducing the dose. Non-compliance with treatment often stems from a patient being given too high a dose. Patients and carers should be advised that stools will become black and that iron tablets represent a potentially lethal hazard to inquisitive children.

Parenteral iron therapy can cause severe allergic reactions, including anaphylaxis. This is more likely to occur if the iron-binding proteins in the blood are saturated, so it must only be given after the diagnosis of iron deficiency has been confirmed either by finding a low serum ferritin or a raised iron-binding capacity. One of the following criteria must also exist:

genuine intolerance to oral iron therapy (usually related to gastrointestinal disease);

intractable non-compliance with oral iron;

continued blood loss exceeding the therapeutic response obtainable from oral iron.

Before administration it is essential to ensure the absence of serious infection and to enquire about a history of allergy. Iron dextran is the preferred therapy – each millilitre contains 50 mg of elemental iron.

The intramuscular route is safest but not always practicable. Intravenous therapy should be used only if there is insufficient muscle bulk for intramuscular injection, if frequent repeated therapy is likely or if patient compliance is not achievable by the intramuscular route. Therapy must be preceded by a test dose and full resuscitation facilities must be available when the intravenous route is used. Whichever route is used it is essential that the manufacturer's guidelines are strictly adhered to.

Vitamin B$_{12}$ and Folic Acid Supplementation

These forms of treatment should only be given after blood has been taken for appropriate assays and when appropriate, after a bone marrow examination has been performed. In most patients it is possible and sensible to await the results of specific assays, but therapy should not be delayed in patients who are very sick, have severe neurological complications or who are likely to have their marrow reserves stressed (e.g. by surgery).

Folic Acid Supplementation

In extremely sick patients, particularly those who have received a dihydrofolate reductase antagonist (e.g. trimethoprim), initial therapy should be with parenteral folinic acid. In other cases, oral folic acid (5 mg daily) is sufficient treatment. In most cases the cause of the deficiency can be reversed so that long-term therapy is unnecessary. When the underlying cause of the deficiency cannot be modified or where there is chronic increased cell turnover (e.g. haemolytic anaemia, myelofibrosis), long-term prophylactic therapy with 5 mg of folic acid daily is necessary. Caution should be used in starting folate therapy in patients with epilepsy or uncontrolled malignancy and in megaloblastic patients in whom B$_{12}$ deficiency has not been totally excluded. It should be noted however that in some cases of malignancy, specific therapy can only be started when cytopenias secondary to folate deficiency have been remedied.

Patients on long-term folate therapy should have annual checks of their vitamin B$_{12}$ status. Checks should be more regular if there is evidence of neuropathy or dementia.

Vitamin B$_{12}$ Supplementation

As initial therapy a single 1 mg dose of hydroxocobalamin is sufficient for a full haematological and neurological recovery. Daily therapy is not required but a further dose may be given after one week when a check blood count should be taken to assess response.

Whenever practicable, long-term therapy should only be instituted when the diagnosis has been confirmed. The finding of a low serum B$_{12}$ is not sufficient justification for starting life-long therapy. However, therapy should be started immediately following either total gastrectomy or total ileal resection. The treatment regime of choice is hydroxocobalamin 1 mg intramuscularly at 3 monthly intervals. Once a diagnosis is established treatment is life-long and it is important that both the patient and their attendants appreciate this.

Where the diagnosis is in doubt, a therapeutic trial with 2 μg of B$_{12}$ should be given parenterally daily and the response assessed after 7 days. It is important to note that close scrutiny of a patient may lead to an improved dietary intake or decreased ethanol consumption. Patients with folate deficiency may therefore improve and this improvement may be erroneously attributed to B_{12}. On the other hand, there may be no observable response in a B_{12}-deficient patient if their initial haemoglobin concentration is relatively high, or if their bone marrow response is suppressed by other factors such as acute illness or renal failure.

Further Reading

Hoffbrand AV, Lewis SM (eds) (1981) Postgraduate haematology, 2nd edn. Heinemann, London

Chapter 21

Vomiting and Haematemesis

Jane Bradshaw

Vomiting is a reflex autonomic response to a wide range of stimuli. It may be provoked by irritation, inflammation, distension or compression of the gastrointestinal tract or of other abdominal viscera (Table 21.1) or be attributable to a variety of non-gastrointestinal disorders (Table 21.2). The vomiting centre in the medulla receives these stimuli and co-ordinates the response.

Forceful contraction of the abdominal and respiratory muscles causes a rise in the intra-abdominal pressure which, with relaxation of the stomach and oesophagus, closure of the larynx and elevation of the soft palate, leads to the forceful expulsion of the gastric and sometimes duodenal contents. Vomiting may be preceded by sweating, palpitation, excessive salivation and faintness, although the extent of the generalised autonomic upset varies.

Table 21.1. Gastrointestinal causes of vomiting

Pharyngeal pouch

Oesophageal lesions (diverticulum, oesophagitis, hiatus hernia, stricture, achalasia, tumour)

Gastric lesions (hiatus hernia, gastritis, pyloric stenosis, gastric ulcer, gastric carcinoma, acute gastric dilatation)

Duodenal lesions (duodenal ulcer, scarring and stenosis)

Bowel disease (appendicitis, small or large bowel obstruction, Crohn's disease, paralytic ileus, sigmoid volvulus)

Miscellaneous lesions (pancreatitis, cholecystitis, hepatitis, biliary obstruction, pyelonephritis)

Table 21.2. Non-gastrointestinal causes of vomiting

Metabolic disorders (uraemia, diabetic precoma)

Drug induced (digoxin, alcohol, poisoning, chemotherapeutic agents)

Neurological disorders (psychogenic, migraine, motion sickness, Ménière's disorder, raised intracranial pressure)

Infection (urinary tract infection, septicaemia, meningitis, etc.)

Miscellaneous causes (myocardial infarction, radiation sickness)

Gastrointestinal Causes of Vomiting

Oesophagitis

Reflux of gastric contents into the lower oesophagus after meals is a common occurrence, though only a proportion of patients with demonstrable reflux experience symptoms. Reflux is more likely to occur in the obese, in smokers and after alcohol consumption. The presence of a hiatus hernia predisposes to reflux, but reflux may occur in the absence of a hiatus hernia if the lower oesophageal sphincter is incompetent. Obesity and tight corsets increase the likelihood of reflux by raising the intra-abdominal pressure, whilst cigarette smoking and alcohol lower the resting tone of the lower oesophageal sphincter. Previous gastric surgery, especially if there is delayed gastric emptying or a small gastric remnant may also predispose to reflux.

The presence of food within the oesophagus usually induces secondary oesophageal contractions which rapidly "clear" refluxed material, thus preventing mucosal damage. Unlike the gastric mucosa, the oesophageal mucosa has no protective mucus barrier and is not designed to withstand injury by gastric acid. Any prolonged exposure will lead to inflammation, sometimes with ulceration, bleeding and ultimately stricture formation. Acid is not always the cause of oesophageal injury however, and bile, when present in gastric contents, is also an irritant. This is particularly likely to be present following gastric surgery. Other irritants, such as tablets containing potassium salts may cause injury if they lodge in the oesophagus as a result of impaired oesophageal motility. Elderly patients are particularly susceptible to oesophageal injury from tablets, not only because of the number of tablets consumed but also because oesophageal motility declines with age, a condition sometimes described by the term "presby-oesophagus".

The most common symptom is of "burning" retrosternal chest pain. The pain may occur when food and especially hot drinks are being swallowed or when reflux is provoked by bending, straining or lying flat. Occasionally oesophageal spasm occurs which may be of sufficient severity as to suggest myocardial ischaemia; as both conditions are relieved by nitrates an erroneous diagnosis of angina, or even myocardial infarction, may be made. Patients with severe oesophagitis may also experience dysphagia. This is usually due to marked inflammation and oedema of the mucosa, sometimes with associated oesophageal spasm. Long-standing oesophagitis may lead to the development of a benign oesophageal stricture (see below). Iron-deficiency anaemia or even frank haematemesis may occur in patients with bleeding oesophagitis or oesophageal erosions.

Endoscopy is the investigation of choice for the diagnosis of oesophagitis as it enables the inflamed mucosa to be visualised and biopsied if necessary. There is a poor correlation between the endoscopic appearance of the oesophageal mucosa and the severity of symptoms. Barium studies may be helpful in demonstrating gastro-oesophageal reflux, but oesophagitis can occur in the absence of demonstrable reflux and reflux is common in people without oesophagitis. Barium swallow may demonstrate oesophageal spasm which is not always detectable endoscopically. Hiatus hernias are commonly found in the elderly and are of importance only if associated with symptomatic reflux oesophagitis.

Reflux oesophagitis should be treated initially with simple anti-reflux measures. These consist of elevating the head of the bed at night, removing tight corsets and stopping cigarette smoking and alcohol consumption. Large meals late at night should also be avoided. Obese patients should be encouraged to lose weight. Medication includes alginates which react with gastric acid to form a floating barrier on the surface of the gastric contents, metoclopramide to increase the tone of the lower oesophageal sphincter and H_2 receptor antagonists which lower gastric acid secretion and volume. Antacids give symptomatic relief but will disrupt the alginate "raft" and the two should not be given together. Surgery may be considered in younger patients with troublesome symptoms or with an oesophageal stricture. Surgery is rarely indicated for hiatus hernia and most elderly patients are not suitable for traditional fundoplication procedures. The recent development of a silicone prosthesis to prevent reflux (Angelchik prosthesis) may prove to be an advance in the management of hiatus hernia with troublesome reflux.

Benign Oesophageal Stricture and Oesophageal Tumour

Benign oesophageal stricture and oesophageal tumour present in a similar fashion with dysphagia, initially for solid foods, but progressing until the patient can manage only a liquid diet. Weight loss (see Chap. 10) is usually marked. Both benign and malignant stricture may be accompanied by iron-deficiency anaemia or present as a haematemesis. A gastric carcinoma arising at the gastro-oesophageal junction may mimic an oesophageal neoplasm by presenting with dysphagia.

Benign oesophageal stricture is generally due to chronic oesophageal damage from acid reflux. It may be difficult to distinguish between a benign and malignant stricture on barium examination so that endoscopy and biopsy of the lesion is essential. Benign oesophageal stricture may respond to the same treatment as that described for oesophagitis. Most patients however require initial endoscopic dilatation followed by anti-reflux measures. Dilatation may need repeating from time to time according to the patients symptoms and nutritional status.

A rapid onset of dysphagia suggests malignancy, occurring most often in the lower third of the oesophagus. Most patients with an oesophageal neoplasm are unfit for a major operation but dysphagia can be relieved by the endoscopic insertion of a palliative feeding tube. Such a tube will however allow free reflux of gastric contents and may also be blocked by a large food bolus. Patients should be advised to masticate their food well or to eat semi-solid foods. Minor blockages of the feeding tube may be relieved by fizzy drinks while major obstructions can be relieved endoscopically.

Peptic Ulceration

Peptic ulceration in the elderly is a common and potentially serious disorder. While the prevalence of peptic ulcer disease has declined in younger age groups, it has remained unchanged in older individuals. Indeed, the prevalence of gastric ulceration in elderly women has probably increased, which may be related to the increased consumption of non-steroidal anti-inflammatory drugs. Mortality rates for the elderly patient with a peptic ulcer are 200–300 times higher than in the younger age groups.

Peptic ulceration may occur in the oesophagus, stomach or duodenum. Oesophageal ulcers occur primarily in patients with long-standing reflux and above a Barrett's epithelium, then described as a "Barrett's ulcer". Certain drugs, notably Slow K and emepronium bromide, may cause oesophageal ulceration. For this reason great care should be taken to ensure that evening medication is given with sufficient fluid and with the patient erect as tablets might otherwise remain in the oesophagus overnight. Gastric ulcers may be sited within a hiatus hernia, not infrequently at the level of the diaphragm itself, or within the body or antrum of the stomach. They may be acute or chronic, superficial, punched out or deeply penetrating, single, multiple or co-existing with duodenal ulceration. A deeply penetrating gastric ulcer may adhere to surrounding structures or erode into an artery leading to a potentially fatal haematemesis. Duodenal ulcers which penetrate deeply may also involve the pancreas or biliary system, leading to pancreatitis or obstructive jaundice.

Symptoms of anorexia, weight loss and occasional vomiting are non-specific. Dyspepsia is not a prominent symptom in old people, which makes the diagnosis difficult, though vomiting may occur with an acute exacerbation. The first indication of a peptic ulcer in an elderly patient may be an iron-deficiency anaemia or frank haematemesis.

Diagnosis is made by endoscopy, barium meal examination or both. A deeply penetrating gastric ulcer may mimic a gastric carcinoma radiologically. Endoscopy allows such ulcers to be biopsied and examined histologically.

Patients with peptic ulceration usually respond to H_2 receptor antagonists within a few days, although ulcer healing takes 8–12 weeks. Side effects include mental confusion which is more likely to occur if the H_2 receptor antagonist is given intravenously. Ranitidine is less likely to produce confusion than is cimetidine and the extent of the problem with the newer H_2 receptor antagonists, famotidine and nizatidine has yet to be determined. Colloidal bismuth (De-Nol) is also useful in ulcer healing and has a lower relapse rate than the H_2 receptor antagonists. Colloidal bismuth may also be of benefit in gastritis, particularly when *Campylobacter* organisms are demonstrated in the gastric mucosal biopsies. Recent evidence suggests that in smokers with duodenal ulceration, mucosally acting agents such as colloidal bismuth, sucralfate and the prostaglandin analogues are more effective than the H_2 receptor antagonists in promoting healing and prolonging the length of remission.

Gastric Outlet Obstruction

Gastric outlet obstruction is suggested by the regular, copious vomiting of foul-smelling vomitus, often with recognisable food eaten the previous day. There is generally an associated rapid weight loss. Gastric outlet obstruction may be due to *pyloric stenosis*, secondary to peptic ulceration and scarring or to an antral *gastric carcinoma*. A previous history of peptic ulceration suggests benign pyloric stenosis, as does a more gradual onset and progression of symptoms. Gastric carcinoma tends to present at a late stage, unless it arises close to the cardia or pylorus and causes early obstruction. The history is usually of a general decline, with weight loss, anorexia and anaemia. Vomiting is usually a late symptom and frank haematemesis is uncommon. The prognosis is generally poor as the tumour has already spread widely before the patient presents. Early lesions in the distal stomach, without evidence of metastatic spread may be managed by sub-total gastrectomy and this may occasionally effect a cure. Palliative treatment for lesions occluding the cardia is similar to oesophageal tumours with the passage of a feeding tube. If gastric obstruction is complete, a palliative by-pass procedure may be considered, otherwise a liquid diet and metoclopramide (to increase the rate of gastric emptying) may help. H_2 receptor antagonists may be used to relieve pain and to reduce the volume of gastric secretions.

Surgical Emergencies

A variety of acute surgical conditions can present with vomiting. They include acute appendicitis, bowel obstruction, sigmoid volvulus, biliary obstruction and acute mesenteric ischaemia. Their detailed description is outside the scope of this chapter.

Such emergencies in old people are notoriously difficult to detect, because the typical symptoms and signs seen in younger age groups are masked. The patient is often acutely confused and the history may be vague. Even in the presence of pancreatitis, cholecystitis or appendicitis, abdominal pain may not be a prominent feature and abdominal examination may not reveal noticeable guarding or rigidity. An acute abdominal surgical condition should always be considered in a shocked, profoundly ill or rapidly deteriorating elderly patient.

Non-gastrointestinal Causes of Vomiting

Vomiting can be a presenting symptom of a wide variety of disorders from myocardial infarction to uncontrolled diabetes mellitus. A brief list of possible causes is given in Table 21.2. Drug toxicity is a frequent cause and digoxin is probably the commonest offending agent.

Clinical Evaluation

When history taking it is important to clarify that the patient is truly vomiting, i.e. forcefully expelling gastric contents. Effortless regurgitation of undigested food is suggestive of a pharyngeal pouch or a lesion within the oesophagus such as an oesophageal diverticulum, stricture or tumour leading to a hold-up of food within the oesophagus. Vomiting with little effort occurs when the lower oesophageal sphincter is incompetent or when a hiatus hernia is present.

The duration and frequency of vomiting should be noted, together with the volume and character of the vomitus. Does it contain blood, bile or undigested food eaten many hours previously? Are there associated symptoms of dyspepsia, dysphagia or weight loss? These may give diagnostic pointers. Weight loss, for example, is uncommon with simple oesophagitis, but an expected symptom of oesophageal malignancy. Factors which exacerbate or relieve symptoms should be sought. Mundane causes, such as travel sickness, should not be overlooked in patients attending out-patient clinics or Day Hospital. Are there symptoms of bowel dysfunction? The importance of a drug history cannot be over-emphasised.

On examination, the general appearance of the patient, degree of hydration, together with the presence of anaemia, jaundice, toxaemia, acute confusion and lymphadenopathy should be noted. On abdominal examination, distension, visible peristalsis, tenderness, a mass, a succussion splash or abnormal bowel sounds should be noted. Examination of the hernial orifices and a rectal examination must never be omitted.

Further Investigation

It is often useful to tabulate the frequency and timing of vomiting and an examination of the vomit itself may be helpful in recognising undigested food, altered blood like "coffee grounds", food consumed a day ago and so on. Vomitus may be tested for acid (negative in the case of an oesophageal diverticulum) or occult blood.

Examination of the urine may reveal the presence of bile, sugar, protein or blood and indicate an underlying systemic disorder such as renal failure or diabetes mellitus. Urine microscopy and culture will identify lesions within the urinary tract. Blood cultures should be taken in acutely ill patients in whom a gram-negative septicaemia is suspected secondary to intra-abdominal pathology. Laboratory investigations will confirm any suspected metabolic cause of vomiting or conditions such as hepatitis, pancreatitis or cholecystitis.

Plain radiography of the abdomen may be of use in identifying gallstones, renal stones or pancreatic calcification. Supine and decubitus films should be requested if a perforation is suspected, although the absence of demonstrable free gas does not exclude a perforation. Ultrasound scanning of the abdomen is extremely useful in the investigation of the elderly patient. Lesions within, or abnormalities of, the stomach, pancreas, liver, gallbladder, biliary tree and kidneys may be identified with little distress to the patient. Abnormalities and masses within the lower abdomen and pelvis can also be demonstrated.

Barium studies of the upper gastrointestinal tract may be necessary where there is no easy access to upper gastrointestinal endoscopy, but is generally recognised to be less informative than endoscopy. Upper gastrointestinal endoscopy is safe and well-tolerated by old people and is better able to detect mucosal lesions, such as oesophagitis, gastritis and gastric erosions. It also allows lesions to be biopsied where carcinoma is suspected. Barium studies may, however, be better at detecting early benign oesophageal strictures or achalasia of the cardia. Gastric washouts may be required in the presence of gastric outlet obstruction before adequate views of the stomach are obtained, by either barium meal or endoscopy.

Management

The general management of the vomiting patient depends on his or her general condition and on the underlying cause. Patients who are shocked or dehydrated require intravenous replacement of fluids and correction of any electrolyte imbalance. Nasogastric suction will be necessary in those with intestinal obstruction, pancreatitis and sometimes in those with cholecystitis. Antibiotic cover should be given to those with pancreatitis or cholecystitis after blood cultures have been taken.

Patients who are distressed by nausea and vomiting may benefit from a short course of an anti-emetic agent. The phenothiazine derivatives (e.g. chlorpromazine, prochlorperazine) are effective. These act centrally and may cause sedation (which is occasionally desirable). They are dopamine antagonists and can rarely cause severe extra-pyramidal side effects. Metoclopramide closely resembles the phenothiazine derivatives but has an additional action on the gut which is an advantage in vomiting due to gastrointestinal disease. Domperidone acts peripherally on the chemoreceptors and does not readily cross the blood–brain barrier. It is a preferable drug if sedation needs to be avoided and in patients with Parkinson's disease, in whom dopamine antagonists should be avoided. Domperidone is also useful in managing the nausea following radiotherapy or chemotherapy as it can be given in large doses without causing side effects.

Remember that drugs may be a cause of rather than a solution to vomiting and any drugs which could be incriminated should be discontinued.

Haematemesis

Old people represent an increasing proportion of all hospital admissions for haematemesis. It is a serious problem in the elderly patient because it carries a high mortality despite being usually due to a "benign" condition. In one study, 58% of all cases were 60 years of age or more and 37% were 70 years or over. Only 4% of those under 60 years died as a result of their haematemesis compared to 20% of those in the 70 years and over age group.

About half the patients have peptic ulceration, with the remainder having bleeding oesophagitis, a Mallory–Weiss tear, gastritis, gastric erosions or duodenitis. Non-steroidal anti-inflammatory agents are frequently implicated. Bleeding varices are rarely seen in old people whilst patients with gastric carcinoma are more likely to present with symptoms of weight loss, vomiting and iron-deficiency anaemia than with haematemesis. Haematemesis is occasionally attributable to angiodysplasia, particularly if there is a history of recurrent obscure bleeding. It can also be due to a primary bleeding diathesis or to poorly controlled anticoagulation.

Clinical Evaluation

Clinical evaluation of patients with haematemesis may be difficult. It is important not to underestimate the potentially serious nature of a gastrointestinal bleed.

Firstly confirm the source of bleeding. Some patients may themselves be uncertain as to whether the blood was produced by coughing or vomiting. Occasionally patients with a profuse nose bleed vomit altered blood which has been swallowed, having trickled down the posterior pharynx from the nose.

Many elderly patients with peptic ulceration have no previous history of peptic ulcer disease and no symptoms of indigestion or abdominal pain. Indeed, the first indication of their peptic ulcer may be when they present with a life-threatening haematemesis. Patients with bleeding oesophagitis may give a history of burning retrosternal chest pain, acid reflux or a previously diagnosed hiatus hernia. A drug history is of great relevance as over 50% of old people with peptic ulceration, bleeding oesophagitis, gastritis or gastric erosions will be taking non-steroidal anti-inflammatory agents. It is obviously of paramount importance to know if a patient is taking anticoagulant drugs.

The general condition of the patient is a better guide to the size of the bleed than any estimate of the amount of blood vomited. Confusion, hypotension, tachycardia or shock indicate a major bleed, requiring prompt resuscitation and immediate transfusion. The initial haemoglobin may be of little help in determining the extent of blood loss, if taken before haemodilution has had time to occur and may be misleadingly reassuring.

Further Investigation

Endoscopy should be performed in every patient with a haematemesis. An emergency endoscopy is only required in those patients for whom surgery is contemplated. For most an elective procedure will suffice so long as the person's condition is stable. Better visualisation is obtained once the bleeding has stopped, allowing a more accurate assessment. At endoscopy the presence and location of fresh or altered blood is noted. Peptic ulcers may show the stigmata of recent bleeding – small red or black dots on the ulcer surface – or there may be a visible vessel protruding from the ulcer base. Blood present several days after the initial bleed indicates continuing bleeding or a re-bleed.

Where the source of bleeding remains obscure, angiography or radionucleotide scanning may help in locating the site, providing the patient is bleeding at the time of the procedure. These techniques are especially useful in the detection of bleeding angiodysplastic patches.

Management

Haematemesis should always be regarded as serious in the elderly patient. As a small initial bleed may be followed by a larger bleed, all patients with haematemesis should have their blood group checked and have donor blood cross-matched. If the patient is not shocked leave an intravenous cannula in situ, but avoid overloading the patient with fluid.

Patients with a haemoglobin of 10 g/dl or less should be transfused, initially with whole blood, unless there is concomitant heart failure. If several units are to be transfused, some may be given as packed cells. Avoid giving saline before or during the transfusion as this may precipitate heart failure and further complicate management. If blood is not available use plasma to restore the circulating volume. It may be necessary to use a pump or a number of intravenous lines to keep pace with transfusion requirements in a patient who is bleeding profusely. A blood warmer should also be used in such circumstances. A prompt surgical opinion should be requested in all patients who require transfusion. In some departments the surgical team is notified whenever a patient with haematemesis is admitted. Patients who have had a large bleed require an urgent endoscopy which, if necessary, can be performed in theatre immediately prior to operation.

Patients with minor haematemesis should be closely monitored for evidence of re-bleeding, with a careful watch kept on pulse rate and blood pressure. Endoscopy should be arranged within the following few days as superficial lesions such as erosions or a Mallory–Weiss tear may heal rapidly.

The adverse prognostic features of haematemesis are given in Table 21.3, together with those features which predict a poor outcome following surgery. It must always be remembered that elderly patients are a high risk group. They are more likely to have prolonged bleeding and to re-bleed. If transfused large amounts of blood they tend to fare badly – becoming confused and lapsing into heart failure – unless closely monitored. Strict fluid balance charts should be maintained and care taken to maintain an adequate urinary output. Central venous pressure should be monitored in patients being transfused with several units of blood. Surgical intervention should be considered early as the elderly patient's general condition tends to deteriorate the longer the bleeding and transfusion continues.

Table 21.3. Prognostic indicators in patients with haematemesis

Adverse prognostic features in the outcome of haematemesis	Adverse prognostic features in the outcome of surgery
Increasing age of patient	Age over 60 years
Shock	Concurrent disease
Transfusion requirement >10 units	Tranfusion requirement >10 units
Prolonged bleed (>24 hours)	Re-bleeding
Re-bleeding	Delayed surgery
Visible vessel on endoscopy	

H_2 receptor antagonists are often given to patients with haematemesis, although there is no evidence that these influence bleeding. Intravenous administration in particular may precipitate confusion and it is reasonable to commence oral H_2 receptor antagonists once the patient has begun to take oral fluids. Providing surgery is not contemplated a light diet can be introduced once the patient has settled and the bleeding stopped; food is an excellent antacid.

Other techniques are undergoing evaluation in the treatment of haematemesis, but are not yet generally available except in specialised units. These include electrocoagulation or laser coagulation of the bleeding point by endoscopic procedures and embolisation of the bleeding vessel by selective angiography.

Further Reading

Cooper BT, Neumann CS (1986) Upper gastrointestinal endoscopy in patients aged 80 years or more. Age Ageing 15:343–349
Dronfield MW (1979) Medical or surgical treatment for haematemesis and melaena. J R Coll Phys 13:84–86

Chapter 22

Accidental Hypothermia

R. T. M. Edwards

Accidental hypothermia refers to environmentally induced hypothermia and exists when the core body temperature reaches 35°C or less. This is in contrast to hypothermia which is artificially induced, as in some surgical procedures, for example. Exposure to cold is a prerequisite for accidental hypothermia, though the cold need not be profound. The severity of hypothermia is classified according to the core body temperature and is divided into three classes as shown in Figure 22.1.

It is only in the last two decades that studies have been undertaken to elucidate the incidence of accidental hypothermia in old people. In 1966 a British study estimated that 0.28% of all people aged over 65 years being admitted to hospital had hypothermia. A 1975 study found that 3.6% of elderly people were hypothermic on admission to two London hospitals. It is likely that there are many more old people in the community who are either acutely or chronically hypothermic but are not admitted to hospital. A community survey found that 10% of elderly people, living normally at home, excreted early morning urine the temperature of which indicated hypothermia.

Reported mortality rates among hospitalised patients range from 20%–80% and a study by McLean and Emslie-Smith showed a mortality rate of 50% during the first month after admission to hospital, with most dying from an underlying disorder rather than the hypothermia. The principal factors adversely affecting the prognosis are the severity and duration of the hypothermia, the presence of underlying predisposing conditions, the development of complications and the

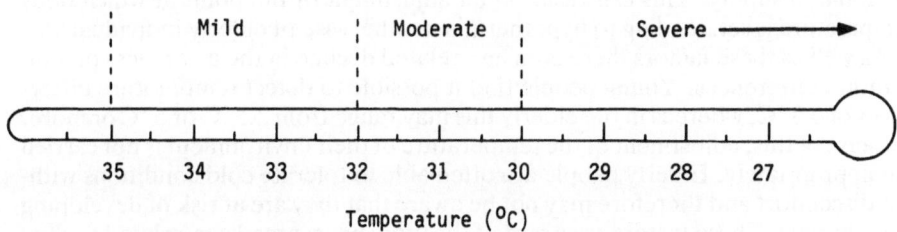

Fig. 22.1.   Degrees of hypothermia.

age of the patient. The prognosis is worst in those who have several of these factors and especially if there is a severe irreversible underlying disorder. There is an increased risk of recurring hypothermia in those successfully treated.

Factors Predisposing to Hypothermia

A lowered body temperature results from a combination of physiological, environmental and pathological factors, each of which are more prevalent in elderly people. As with so many disorders in old age, the cause is usually multi-factorial (Table 22.1).

Table 22.1.   Factors predisposing to hypothermia in old age

Neurological disorders:	depression, dementia, brain tumour, Wernicke's encephalopathy, Parkinson's disease, cerebrovascular disease
Endocrine disorders:	hypothyroidism, hypoglycaemia, hypoadrenalism, diabetes mellitus
Cardiovascular disorders:	myocardial infarction, peripheral vascular disease, congestive heart failure, pulmonary embolism
Infections:	septicaemia, bronchopneumonia
Musculo-skeletal disorders:	immobility, arthritis, Paget's disease
Drugs:	phenothiazines, hypnotics and sedatives
Miscellaneous:	erythematous skin rashes, renal failure, severe gastrointestinal bleeding

Physiological Changes

Physiological changes with ageing result in impaired thermoregulation. Cutaneous vaso-constriction is a powerful mechanism by which heat loss through the skin is conserved. Normally, there is a core/shell temperature difference of 4.5°C which is maintained and regulated by vaso-constriction and vaso-dilatation. In old people there is a diminished capacity for such a mechanism, many having low peripheral blood flow, so that a fall in the deep-body temperature results. Shivering is a method whereby heat can be generated, but this diminishes with age because of a reduction in lean body mass and muscle mass, impairment of the reflex arc and a decrease in sweat gland activity. Centrally there is a decrease in neuron cell activity in the thermoregulating centre of the hypothalamus with a reduction in its blood supply. This can result in an adjustment of the point at which body temperature is set, leading to hypothermia in otherwise fit elderly individuals.

As well as these factors there is an age-related decline in the awareness of temperature differences. Young people find it possible to detect temperature differences of 0.8 °C, whereas in the elderly this may range from 2.5 °C or 5 °C or more. Because of this, adjustment of the temperature of their environment is not carried out appropriately. Elderly people are often able to tolerate cold conditions without discomfort and therefore may not be aware that they are at risk of developing hypothermia. These factors are a part of the more widespread age-related decline in function of the autonomic nervous system.

Environmental Factors

Environmental factors causing a low ambient temperature predispose to hypothermia, the incidence of which increases as the temperature drops, especially below freezing point. A national survey in Britain in 1973 estimated that 75% of people aged over 65 years, and living at home, had their living-room temperature below the recommended cold weather minimum of 18.3 °C set by the Parker Morris Committee. In 10% of cases the living-room temperature was below 12 °C and in some below 3 °C. In addition, the temperatures in bedrooms were considerably lower as 30% had no heating and the majority had unheated halls and toilets.

A large percentage of the elderly did not use more heating because of the expense, even though they did not feel warm enough in the cold weather. Many were unaware of the financial help available from the Department of Social Security (DSS) towards heating costs. Characteristically the elderly who develop hypothermia are more likely to be living alone and have poor housing conditions, have a tendency to fall and are socially isolated.

Pathological Conditions

Pathological conditions predisposing to hypothermia are listed in Table 22.1. They lower body temperatures by either decreasing heat production, increasing heat loss or by deranging thermoregulation.

An example of decreased heat production is myxoedema in which the basal metabolic rate is reduced to such a level that it is not possible to maintain normal body temperature. The concomitant diagnosis of hypothermia and hypothyroidism can be difficult.

Increased heat loss occurs, for example, in alcohol intoxication and is due to vasodilatation. With Paget's disease, the increased peripheral blood supply causes heat loss for which the body is unable to compensate, thus reducing the body core temperature.

Derangement of thermoregulation occurs especially in neurological diseases, often because hypothalamic function is disturbed. Following a cerebrovascular accident, immobility may exacerbate this tendency in an elderly hemiplegic patient. Drugs such as phenothiazines may act upon the hypothalamus and interfere with normal temperature control. Patients with acute confusion or dementia may have deranged hypothalamic function. They may also be unaware of their surroundings or react inappropriately to them as, for example, when clothes are removed as body temperature falls.

Clinical Evaluation

Symptoms and signs are often vague and develop insidiously over a period of time. Unfortunately, the symptom of feeling cold seems to diminish once the core body temperature has fallen below 35 °C. Once within the hypothermic range the symptoms are varied and depend upon the core body temperature and any under-lying condition. Initially patients are less alert than normal and may have slurred speech. Muscular movements are often uncoordinated and clumsy. As the condition worsens, they become more drowsy, confused and can eventually become comatose.

The diagnosis is made by the observation that the core body temperature is below 35 °C. If the diagnosis is considered, a low-reading thermometer should be used preferably using a rectal temperature probe as oesophageal temperature probes can lead to ventricular fibrillation in hypothermic patients.

In addition to the general appearance of a pale skin, peripheral cyanosis and a puffy facial appearance, hypothermia affects each of the organ systems.

Cardiovascular System

Initially, homeostatic mechanisms cause the cooling body to shiver, in an attempt to raise its temperature. This increases the heart rate, blood pressure and oxygen consumption. When the temperature falls below 35 °C the heart rate and blood pressure start to fall progressively, this being most marked below 30 °C. The main signs of cardiac involvement are arrhythmias and hypotension with sinus bradycardia or atrial fibrillation occurring commonly as the temperature falls into the moderate range of hypothermia. As the temperature reaches 29 °C then there is an increased risk of more serious arrhythmias and especially ventricular fibrillation.

The electrocardiogram usually shows a degree of heart block with increasing P–R interval, a widening of the QRS complex and T waves are occasionally inverted. There is often a fine oscillation of the base-line indicating a minimal shivering response. The J wave which is a deflection at the junction of the QRS complex and ST segment is said to be a characteristic finding (Fig. 22.2) but even in severe cases it may be absent. It is not related to the severity of the hypothermia and does not seem to have any prognostic value.

Respiratory System

The respiratory rate and minute volume decrease so that patients present with a very slow and shallow respiratory pattern. The cough reflex diminishes as does mucociliary function and these, together with altered consciousness, predispose

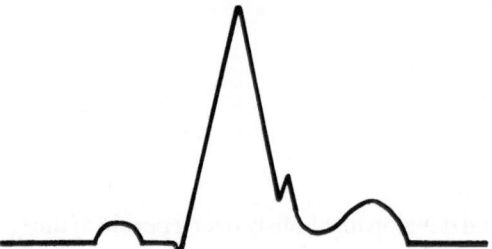

Fig. 22.2.   The ECG in hypothermia showing a J wave.

to pulmonary infection and aspiration. Pulmonary oedema not associated with cardiac failure is a common finding, especially if the hypothermia is relatively long-standing and the oedema can be exacerbated by rewarming especially when intravenous fluid is given. Hypoventilation is reflected in a high PCO_2. The PO_2 falls and because of changes in the oxyhaemoglobin dissociation curve there is an increase in tissue hypoxia.

Renal System

Hypovolaemia is a common finding in hypothermia and is multifactorial in origin. A diuresis is common due to a compensatory reduction in anti-diuretic hormone secretion, this despite a reduction in the glomerular filtration rate. Acute tubular necrosis is not infrequently found, especially if severe dehydration occurs.

Central Nervous System

There is a progressive decline in mental function as the temperature drops, with coma appearing commonly at 29 °C and below. Multiple other neurological abnormalities occur, with the posture resembling that of rigor mortis because of hypertonicity of the musculature. Reflexes, including the pupillary arc reflex, are lost at 26–27 °C and the pupils appear to be fixed, dilated and unresponsive to light.

Gastrointestinal Tract

Pancreatitis is common and is usually mild, though acute haemorrhagic pancreatitis can occur. There is gastric dilatation with slowing of bowel motility which can lead to aspiration of gastric contents. Acute gastric ulcers can cause bleeding.

Laboratory Abnormalities

The haematocrit will rise secondary to haemoconcentration and there is often a leucocytosis secondary to infection. Thrombocytopenia due to sequestration of platelets in the hepatic and splenic circulation is a common finding, but may reflect other disorders such as disseminated intravascular coagulation. Bone marrow failure can occur.

The blood glucose is often raised but severe hypoglycaemia can occur. Insulin is not active below 31 °C and diabetic patients requiring insulin should be warmed to above 30 °C before it is given. The sodium concentration falls as sodium passes into the cells and potassium rises simultaneously. Raised levels of creatine phosphokinase, aspartate aminotransferase and hydroxobutyrate dehydrogenase are often found. Low levels of thyroid hormone and raised cortisol levels are also commonly found.

Management

All hypothermic patients should be referred to hospital, though treatment should begin immediately the diagnosis is suspected. The following first aid measures should be undertaken:

Temperature Stabilisation

The patient must be protected from the wind, wet clothing should be removed and blankets or other insulating material applied. Warmed oxygen relieves anoxia and reduces heat loss from the respiratory system.

Circulatory Support

External cardiac massage should only be undertaken when there is unequivocal evidence of ventricular fibrillation or asystole. The mechanical stimulation of resuscitation can induce ventricular fibrillation in a hypothermic patient in sinus rhythm. Respiration may also need to be assisted.

Transportation

Transportation to hospital should be carried out as swiftly as possible. Caution should be exercised when moving the patient to reduce the risk of ventricular fibrillation which can be induced by movement.

Rewarming

Once in hospital the priority is to rewarm the patient, either actively or passively. Active rewarming can be accomplished by an external or internal route. The rate and method of rewarming hypothermic patients has been a matter of controversy for years.

Active external rewarming with hot water bottles, electric blankets, hot baths etc. is rapid and theoretically should prevent some of the complications of continuing hypothermia. However, it is hazardous, especially for elderly patients, as it is associated with cardiovascular collapse and after-drop. The reflex vaso-dilation caused by externally applied heat causes relatively warm central core blood to flow to the periphery where it is cooled and returns to the core. Thus there is a paradoxical drop in the central core temperature on warming – the so-called "after-drop". Cardiac arrhythmias can occur due to electrolyte imbalance and lactic acidosis. For these reasons active external rewarming is not recommended for old people.

Active internal rewarming is achieved by peritoneal dialysis, heated humidified oxygen and colonic or bladder lavage. It is of use in life-threatening hypothermia and has the advantages of limited after-drop due to delayed mobilisation of peripheral blood. It is expensive, may be difficult to undertake and is associated with a high morbidity and mortality.

Passive external rewarming involves placing the patient in an environment of between 25 °C and 30 °C and adjusting the ambient temperature to maintain an increase in the core body (rectal) temperature of 0.5 °C/h. More time is available to solve any metabolic, cardiac or biochemical problems that may appear, making this the treatment of choice for elderly patients.

Supportive Measures

Supportive measures may be required in those patients who develop complications. Those most commonly encountered include cardiac arrhythmias, hypovolaemia, electrolyte disturbances and hypoxia.

Most atrial arrhythmias will revert spontaneously on rewarming and need no specific treatment. Ventricular arrhythmias, especially ventricular fibrillation, are common with low temperatures and can be triggered by rough handling or by an invasive procedure (e.g. insertion of a naso-gastric tube or central venous pressure line). They are often resistant to treatment and electrical defibrillation is ineffective below 30 °C. Bretylium can be effective in this situation and can be given prophylactically if the risk of ventricular fibrillation is great. For bradycardia, atropine or isoprenaline are usually effective and asystolic cardiac arrest can be tolerated for a considerable time.

A reduced cardiac output can occur on rewarming due to peripheral vasodilation and decreased venous return to the heart. Intravenous fluids may be required, the volume to be given depending on the central venous pressure, whose measurement is critical in minimising the risk of pulmonary oedema. All intravenous fluids should be warmed prior to being given. Non-diabetic patients should be given a mixture of dextrose and saline at a rate of 100–200 ml/h. Hyperkalaemia can be a problem and should be treated aggressively as the risk of associated arrhythmia is high.

Adequate oxygenation of the patient must be ensured and some may need mechanical ventilation using intermittent positive pressure ventilation (IPPV). It is important that the oxygen given is warmed and humidified as this will also help the rewarming of the body core. Measurement of arterial blood gases taken from a hypothermic patient will be slightly inaccurate at room temperature, giving a falsely high PO_2 and PCO_2 and a low pH. This can be overcome by either measuring the gases at the hypothermic temperature or by the use of conversion tables.

Laboratory Investigation

Laboratory investigation should routinely consist of a blood count and measurement of electrolytes, glucose and arterial blood gases. Blood culture and a chest X-ray should be obtained in a search for a septic focus. An ECG must always be obtained and serum amylase measured for evidence of pancreatitis.

As hypothermia is often secondary to underlying conditions (Table 22.1), appropriate investigation may be required to elucidate them. Thyroid function tests, drug toxicological analysis, cardiac enzymes and skull X-ray are the investigations most likely to be of use.

Prevention

There are several measures which the elderly themselves can undertake so as to minimise the risk of developing hypothermia.

Diet

Diet should be adequate and provide sufficient calories, especially during the cold months. The local Meals-on-Wheels Service or luncheon club can supply a warm mid-day meal to a disabled person unable to provide one for himself. The grocery cupboard should be kept well-stocked, especially during the winter if an elderly person has difficulty in getting to the shops. It is important to have hot drinks, particularly between meals and a vacuum flask at the bedside will allow ready access to hot drinks during the night.

Conservation of Body Heat

Exercise will help to keep the body warm, thus activity should be encouraged and sitting down for long periods of time avoided. Adequate clothing should be worn; several thin layers of clothing are more effective than a few heavy layers. One can lose a large amount of body heat through the head, thus wearing a woollen cap will reduce this. At night, bedding should be arranged so as to prevent heat loss.

Insulation

Insulation of the home will reduce both heat loss and heating bills. Up to 25% of heat loss can be through an uninsulated loft, grants for the insulation of which can be obtained from the local authority in Britain. Draught-proofing of windows, doors and floors should be undertaken. Windows can be double-glazed cheaply using plastic sheets attached to the window frames as double-glazing proper is expensive. Draught excluders should be fitted to doors and old newspapers placed under the carpets to prevent draughts from under the floorboards. The hot water tank should be insulated as this will reduce heating costs. There are many local schemes whereby, for the cost of the materials, draught-proofing can be carried out; details can be obtained from the local Citizens Advice Bureau.

Money Matters

Many elderly people do not adequately heat their homes through fear of accumulating electricity and gas bills which they will be unable to pay. In Britain, a code of practice has been drawn up by the Electricity and Gas Boards in which they have agreed not to cut off the supply to any pensioner during the winter months. For those on income support, part of the benefit can be paid directly from the DSS to either the Gas or Electricity Boards who should be contacted for information on various schemes. A pensioner on income support is entitled to a weekly heating allowance and in very cold weather, to an "exceptionally severe weather" payment. One is also entitled to grants and payments to help with draught-proofing and provision of a new hot water-tank jacket.

Notwithstanding what pensioners can do for themselves, people who are particularly vulnerable should be visited frequently by relatives and neighbours during spells of cold weather. Advertising campaigns have been organised to encourage this. The family doctor should seek to identify patients at risk, attempt to minimise predisposing factors and thereby lower the number of people who continue to die each year from hypothermia, a testament to an uncaring society.

Further Reading

McLean D, Emslie-Smith D (1977) Accidental hypothermia. Blackwell Scientific Publications, Oxford
Paton BC (1983) Accidental hypothermia. Pharmacol Ther 22:331–377
Royal College of Physicians of London (1966) Report of the Committee on Accidental Hypothermia

Chapter 23

Pruritus

G. V. Boswell

Pruritus or itching can be defined as a cutaneous sensation leading to the desire to scratch. Scratching in response to itch is a spinal reflex which can be modulated by the brain. Free nerve endings in the skin act as itch receptors. Following their activation, slowly conducting C nerve fibres (which also transmit pain sensation) transmit the itch sensation to the spinal cord and via the lateral spinothalamic tract to the thalamus. Additional impulses may be carried by rapidly conducting delta fibres and by the activation of adjacent neurones within the sensory relay areas of the cord. Pharmacological mediators (e.g. opioid peptides) in the periphery or within the central nervous system influence the perceived quality of itch.

Degenerative changes in the skin lead to a variety of lesions which predispose to itching so that its prevalence increases with age. While hereditary factors are mainly responsible for the rate of ageing of the skin, environmental factors (e.g. excessive exposure to sun and wind, long-term steroid therapy) may also play a part. The skin in elderly Caucasians often appears yellow, dry, wrinkled, inelastic and thin. Dryness is due to dehydration of the surface layers of epithelium follow-

Table 23.1. Causes of pruritus

Skin disease
Xerosis
Lichen simplex chronicus
Anogenital pruritus
Dermatitis (allergic contact, seborrhoeic, gravitational)
Dermatitis herpetiformis
Urticaria
Infestations (scabies, lice, fleas, bedbugs)
Neoplasia (mycosis fungoides)

Systemic disease
Hepatobiliary disease
Renal disease
Haematological disorders (polycythaemia, anaemia, paraproteinaemia)
Endocrine disorders (thyroid dysfunction, carcinoid syndrome)
Malignant disease (lymphoma, leukaemia, carcinoma)
Drugs (opiates, aspirin, quinidine)
Psychogenic illness (stress, delusional states, psychogenic pruritus)

ing its atrophy and subsequently diminished oiliness. Pruritus may often accompany these age-related changes, dry skin in particular tending to itch.

While pruritus may be due to physiological rather than pathological causes, it must always be taken seriously as a symptom. The severity of the itch and the patient's response to it is variable. While some find it a minor nuisance which is promptly relieved by scratching, others may be severely distressed by it and continue scratching even to the point of drawing blood. Persistence of the symptom can lead to the interruption of daily life, loss of sleep, depression and even suicide. It must also be remembered that pruritus may be the first symptom of serious systemic disease. Various reports have estimated the prevalence of such underlying disorders at between 10% and 50%.

Pruritus is caused by either dermatological or systemic disorders, as listed in Table 23.1.

Dermatological Disorders

Most of the primary skin diseases listed in Table 23.1 have a typical appearance and present few problems with diagnosis. However, persistent scratching of the skin will lead to its secondary lichenification. This may make the original condition unrecognisable so that skin biopsy is required for diagnosis. Primary skin disorders can be either localised or generalised.

Xerosis

Xerosis (senile pruritus) refers to chapping of the hands as a result of drying of the horny layer of the skin. It can affect between 40% and 80% of old people in areas where atmospheric humidity is low. It is often worse in winter when itch receptors are stimulated by frequent changes in skin temperature. It is exacerbated by excessive bathing, frequent washing with soap and water and diuretic therapy. Irritants such as residues of soap, detergents and "biological" washing powders left in clothes also predispose to it as does the low humidity of centrally heated and air-conditioned rooms.

The skin is rough and looks flaky. Management consists of educating the patient to avoid exacerbating factors. An emollient ointment will help to relieve the itch.

Lichen Simplex Chronicus

Lichen simplex chronicus is an extremely itchy localised skin disorder found particularly in old people. Raised red patches are typically found in sites such as the occipital area of the scalp, the dorsum of the foot, the wrists and knees. Thickening of the skin results from its continually being scratched. There is often an associated psychological disorder and unless this is treated, the condition is usually resistant to all forms of treatment.

Anogenital Pruritus

Anogenital pruritus refers to an irritation in the areas of moist skin surrounding the anus, perineum and external genitalia. The condition tends to be either acute with an obvious local cause or longstanding with no obvious cause. The skin is irritated by endogenous or exogenous factors.

Endogenous irritant factors include urine and faecal matter. The latter is a problem in those patients with haemorrhoids, an anal fissure, diarrhoea or faecal incontinence. Symptoms may be made worse by the use of poorly absorbent underwear and tight-fitting outer garments which lead to prolonged skin contact with the irritant. A chronic vaginal discharge may complicate malignancy of the cervix, vagina or vulva or complicate infection with trichomonas or candida and lead to pruritus. Such factors are exacerbated by poor anogenital hygiene. Other causes include infestation of the anogenital area, enterobiasis, candidiasis and a bacterial skin infection. Intrinsic skin diseases such as intertrigo, psoriasis and seborrhoeic dermatitis can also underlie it.

Exogenous irritant factors include chemicals (e.g. antiseptic solutions) which are added to bath water and topical drugs (e.g. anti-histamines and antibiotics) which sensitise the skin. Harsh toilet paper and frequent enemas may lead to trauma around the anal margin.

Dermatitis

Dermatitis (eczema) has a variety of forms all of which are itchy. *Allergic contact dermatitis* results when the skin becomes sensitised to a variety of metals, chemicals (including locally applied drugs), adhesives, dyes or plants. The area of skin in contact with the allergen becomes involved initially, though the inflammation can spread to involve other areas. If the skin is removed from contact with the allergen, the inflammation will gradually subside, though emollient and steroid creams will speed up the process and give symptomatic relief. *Seborrhoeic dermatitis* predominantly affects the scalp and the face. In the early stages it looks like severe dandruff, while later it may spread to involve the face and possibly the limbs and trunk. Again emollient and topical steroid preparations may be required to keep the problem in check. *Gravitational* (stasis) *dermatitis* is often found in the presence of chronic venous insufficiency in the lower limbs (see Chap. 9). There is often associated gravitational skin ulceration, pigmentation and lipodermatosclerosis. Attempts to scratch the skin surrounding an ulcer may make the ulcer bigger. The management of chronic venous insufficiency is discussed in Chap. 9. The itch can be helped with an emollient cream and, if the inflammation is severe, with a weak topical corticosteroid.

Dermatitis Herpetiformis

Dermatitis herpetiformis occasionally presents for the first time in old age. The association with coeliac disease (see Chap. 10) is seen in old people as in all age groups. A gluten-free diet causes the rash to improve. Dapsone usually causes a dramatic improvement in symptoms. One should begin with a small dose (100 mg) and increase this gradually until symptoms improve or side effects occur.

Urticaria

Urticaria can cause severe, though usually transient pruritus. It is primarily due to the release of histamine from mast cells as a manifestation of a type 1 hypersensitivity reaction. The stimuli triggering histamine release are mainly extrinsic and include a variety of chemical and physical agents. Drugs are causative in up to a third of severe urticarial reactions, antibiotics, aspirin and opiate drugs being most often implicated. Occasionally, urticaria is found in associated with vasculitis, Henoch–Schonlein purpura and systemic lupus erythematosus. Other atopic manifestations such as bronchospasm and even anaphylactic shock are found in severe cases. Anti-histamine preparations will give good subjective relief.

Infestation

Infestations are not uncommon and can spread rapidly in institutions for the elderly. Scabies and lice are the commonest problems found in Britain. *Scabies* which is caused by the mite *Sarcoptes scabiei*, produces an often intense and generalised itch. The mites are most often found in burrows in the interdigital areas and palms of the hands, wrists, axillae, genitalia and buttocks though secondary skin changes from scratching may cover their tracks. Treatment is with either benzyl benzoate or gamma benzene hexachloride. Other members of the family and close contacts must also be treated even if they are asymptomatic and show no clinical features.

The body louse *Pediculosis corporis* is found mainly on elderly neglected people where it causes itch and often leads to secondary impetigination. Specific treatment is with malathion or carbaryl as lice are now resistant to DDT. However, they usually disappear once infested clothing is removed. Clothing should be "deloused" by boiling.

Fleas and other mites from pets need to be considered and these as well as household furniture may need to be treated.

Cutaneous Neoplasms

Cutaneous neoplasms such as mycosis fungoides can cause a rash which is very itchy. This T-cell lymphoma is most commonly found in late middle aged and elderly patients. In the early stages it responds to phototherapy and emollients; topical corticosteroids are useful in controlling the pruritus. Radiotherapy to the skin and systemic chemotherapy may be required in advanced disease. Mastocytosis is a proliferative disorder of mast cells which is occasionally seen in old age.

Systemic Disorders

Hepatobiliary Disease

In 80% of jaundiced patients, the cause is bile duct obstruction. Some 16% have hepatocellular disease while 4% have haemolysis. Of those with obstructive jaundice, over half will have a malignant obstruction while over one third will have a calculous obstruction. Infection leads to ascending cholangitis, often secondary to gallstones or previous biliary surgery. This, together with drug-induced cholestasis and primary biliary cirrhosis are other important causes of biliary obstruction. While primary biliary cirrhosis is most common in middle-aged women, it can present in old age.

Jaundice due to obstruction is usually associated with pruritus, which may be the initial complaint. In one study 50% of patients with carcinoma of the head of the pancreas had pruritus as their first symptom. Pruritus is not a feature of haemolytic jaundice.

Raised levels of bile salts are primarily responsible for the pruritus though other factors such as metabolites of cholesterol have also been implicated. Treatment is aimed at lowering the bile salt pool with cholestyramine, which binds to bile salts in the gut, preventing their reabsorption.

Renal Disease

The incidence of itching in uraemic patients has been reported at between 10% and 40%. Its cause is unknown and there is no direct relationship with disease severity. Symptoms sometimes respond to either non-specific treatment with emollients and anti-histamines or more specific measures, including cholestyramine, low-protein diets, ultraviolet phototherapy, oral charcoal and parathyroidectomy.

Haematological Disorders

Pruritus is associated with iron deficiency, even in the absence of anaemia and it resolves when the deficiency is corrected. Pruritus following a hot bath or shower occurs in 10% to 30% of people with polycythaemia rubra vera. This symptom is non-specific and also occurs in myeloid metaplasia and Hodgkin's lymphoma. It must be differentiated from benign aquagenic pruritus in which a change in skin temperature leads to vasoactive changes in the skin and enhancement of itching.

Endocrine Disorders

Both hyperthyroidism (by increasing the skin temperature) and hypothyroidism (by causing excessive dryness of the skin) can result in pruritus. When it involves the anogenital area, the itching is usually due to fungal infection. Carcinoid syndrome causes itching by the alteration of skin temperature and by the effect of serotonin on itch receptors. There is no evidence to support the widely held view that generalised pruritus is a manifestation of diabetes mellitus, although diabetes does predispose to localised skin infections that can be itchy.

Malignant Disease

Haematological and lymphoproliferative disorders are often associated with pruritus. Up to 30% of patients with Hodgkin's disease are affected and it may be the initial symptom. The itching may be localised or generalised and associated with secondary changes leading to misdiagnoses of papular urticaria, infestation or neurotic excoriation. Carcinoma of any organ may produce symptoms of pruritus whether the liver is secondarily involved or not. Treatment may lead to disappearance of pruritus with recurrence of the symptom should the disease relapse.

Drugs

As discussed in Chapter 24 reactions to drugs are common in old people and pruritus is a common feature. Urticaria is often an associated finding. Symptoms usually resolve within 2 weeks of discontinuing the offending drug.

Psychogenic Illness

Psychogenic illnesses can be characterised by pruritus, though as a rule other causes must be excluded before this diagnosis is made. Features of anxiety are generally present. Delusional parasitosis is one of the most common complaints and delusions of ill health in relation to other systems are often found.

Clinical Evaluation

All too often, pruritus in old people is seen by doctors as a non-specific problem requiring non-specific treatment aimed at symptom relief. Unless the underlying cause is self-limiting, such an approach is unsatisfactory. Rather, a cause of the pruritus must be sought and if possible removed. Identifying the cause of pruritus is sometimes difficult despite appropriate assessment and investigation. Should unexplained pruritus continue as a symptom, regular review of the patient will be necessary as the cause will eventually come to light. Establishing the cause of pruritus requires a sensible approach so as to save a patient from a battery of unnecessary tests and undue worry.

As always, a good history is important. One should enquire as to whether the itch is localised or generalised though with some underlying conditions it can be either. Its mode of onset and course should be elucidated. A knowledge of provoking and relieving factors is important (e.g. bathing can exacerbate the itching associated with polycythaemia rubra vera) as is its character (e.g. a burning sensation is usually experienced with dermatitis herpetiformis). The severity of the symptom and the time when it is worst are important (e.g. itching is usually worst at night, especially when due to infestations).

A knowledge of treatments already tried, together with the results of such treatments may be useful. Remember that "remedies" can themselves cause itching. An assessment of the patient's personality and mental state, a social history and information on hobbies and on household pets may give valuable diagnostic clues.

On examination, the skin must be inspected for evidence of a primary dermatological disorder, but remember that the appearance may be camouflaged by secondary skin changes. These include excoriations, eczematisation, purpura and hyper-pigmentation. Unreachable areas, especially over the back, will be spared and the nails may be burnished from excessive rubbing. Following this a search for systemic illness should be made with initial screening tests followed by more intensive investigation if such is clinically indicated.

Management

Where possible any underlying disorder should be identified and treated. If this is not feasible, symptomatic treatment should be undertaken as outlined below.

Reduction of Exacerbating Factors and Patient Education

Dryness of the skin should be minimised by avoiding excessive bathing, by using mild soaps and using emollients afterwards. Oils added to the bath, although helpful to the skin, cause people to slip. It is therefore essential to use an adequate non-slip bath mat as a safety precaution. Dryness of the air is particularly common in centrally heated atmospheres in winter and can be corrected with a humidifier. The wearing of too much clothing and irritating fabrics should be avoided as should hot spicy foods which cause vasodilatation.

Physical Methods

Local application of a cool cloth or taking a cold bath may help stop scratching and break the scratch cycle. Gently rubbing a large area of surrounding skin may help, while transcutaneous nerve stimulation and acupuncture are also sometimes beneficial.

Symptomatic Topical Treatment

Simple emollients such as *Unguentun Merck*, white soft paraffin or emulsifying ointment, perhaps with the addition of bath oils, will moisten a dry itchy skin.

Aqueous preparations such as calamine lotion promote further drying of the skin and may thus exacerbate pruritus. Some other medicines and creams which are available without prescription may well exacerbate symptoms and should be avoided, especially if lasting relief is not promptly obtained.

Systemic Drug Treatment

Specific treatments are available for pruritus which is secondary to underlying disease as outlined above (e.g. cholestyramine in obstructive jaundice). In the symptomatic treatment of pruritus it is often difficult to separate a true therapeutic benefit from a placebo effect. There is no evidence that anti-histamines are of benefit except in those conditions characterised by histamine release (e.g. urticaria). As they cause drowsiness they should be used with caution in old people. A large number of preparations are available with little to choose between them.

Further Reading

Hanna MJD, MacMillan AL (1978) Ageing and the skin. In: Brocklehurst JC (ed) Textbook of geriatric medicine and gerontology, 2nd edn. Churchill Livingstone, Edinburgh
Marks R (1985) Skin disorders. In: Pathy MSP (ed) Principles and practice of geriatric medicine. John Wiley, Chichester, pp 873–897
Marks R (1987) Skin diseases in old age. Martin Dunitz, London
Savin J (1980) Itching. In: Rook A, Savin J (eds) Recent advances in dermatology 5. Churchill Livingstone, Edinburgh, pp 221–235
Waisman M (1979) A clinical look at the ageing skin. Postgrad Med 66:87–96

Aspects of Medical Care in the Elderly

Chapter 24

Drug Therapy

C. G. Swift

There is ample evidence that the likelihood of receiving drug therapy increases for any individual as he or she grows older. The proportion of total drug expenditure by the National Health Service in Britain accounted for by elderly people is about two and a half times greater than the proportion of the total population that this age group comprises. Several studies have shown a stepwise increase in the prescription rate for certain drug groups with advancing age. This occurs particularly with psychotropic drugs, analgesics (including NSAIDs) and drugs acting on the cardiovascular system, in particularly diuretics. In addition to prescribed medication, older people purchase substantial amounts of "over-the-counter" medication.

The success of drug therapy depends on achieving a satisfactory therapeutic outcome while avoiding unwanted or adverse effects. Given such a high level of prescribing, it is clearly important to try and monitor the success rate for individual older patients and the elderly population as a whole.

Unfortunately there is evidence that the risk-to-benefit ratio for prescribed drugs is increased amongst older recipients. Drug surveillance studies of hospital populations have shown that the likelihood of suffering an adverse drug reaction is several times greater for patients in their 70s and 80s than for those in their 20s. Such findings, backed up by the clinical experience of geriatricians, have led some clinicians to question deeply the value of drug treatment for the elderly, almost to the point of "therapeutic nihilism".

What in fact is needed, as with most aspects of the medicine of old age, is a more cautious, thorough and careful approach to each patient, based on a better knowledge of the interacting factors which influence both the characteristics of illness and the response to medication in the elderly.

It has been argued that the high incidence of adverse reactions amongst elderly patients is solely the result of the high levels of prescribing. Such a direct relationship has been shown in the case of the "yellow card" side effect reporting system operated by the UK Committee on Safety of Medicines. The proportion of total unwanted drug effects amongst the elderly detected in this way is, however, likely to be quite small since many are simply the outcome of apparently excessive dosage (therefore not "reportable"); it is also likely that many go undetected, except when special drug surveillance initiatives are undertaken.

Some studies have clearly shown that the age-related increase in adverse reactions can be reduced or abolished by giving smaller doses (e.g. the benzodiazepine hypnotics), while the importance of dose reduction for some drugs (e.g. digoxin) has been well known to clinicians for years. These observations emphasise the importance of changes with age in the biological mechanisms which affect the handling of drugs (pharmacokinetics) and the characteristics of drug response (pharmacodynamics).

A key objective of the science of clinical pharmacology is to try to make the outcome of drug therapy more predictable. This entails trying to define and measure factors which contribute to inter-individual variability in drug handling and response. Since the margins of therapeutic benefit and safety are narrowed in the elderly, it is particularly important to achieve this objective. The body of knowledge implicating age as an important variable has been steadily growing and information of this kind is now required by drug regulatory authorities for all new compounds. More importantly, guidelines can be drawn up for the practising clinician.

Indications for Prescribing

Success and safety in the use of drugs presupposes a correct diagnosis and that the chosen medication is of proven benefit for the patient population concerned. Much drug-induced morbidity amongst old people has arisen from the problems of diagnosis they present and from the assumption that the results of successful drug trials in the young can be automatically extrapolated to the old. Some of the more important diagnostic pitfalls are covered elsewhere in this volume and will not be reviewed here. Neurological and psychiatric disorders are often singled out as presenting special difficulty. Examples include the differentiation of parkinsonism from other causes of tremor, of anxiety states from phobic disorders and of dementia from depressive illness. Diagnostic errors of this kind readily result in inappropriate prescribing and drug-induced morbidity.

The demonstration of benefit from drug therapy in conditions affecting younger adults may not be instantly applicable to the old. The natural history of a disease process may be different in the elderly, whether the disease is of late onset or at an advanced stage. The existence of concurrent disease processes often requires careful consideration before embarking on a course of treatment for what would otherwise be a "standard" indication. Weighing up the likely benefit under such circumstances requires good clinical judgement.

Examples include the coexistence of dementia with parkinsonism, the reversibility or otherwise of advanced chronic airflow obstruction and the likely therapeutic benefit of controlling high blood pressure in very advanced age. In respect of the latter, the findings of the European Working Party on Hypertension in the Elderly have helped to clarify the advantages of anti-hypertensive therapy in the 7th and 8th decades, but generalisation becomes progressively more difficult in older subgroups of the aged. Equally, the possible advantages of some forms of medication may be relatively under-exploited, for example, the treatment of depression presenting with pseudo-dementia and perhaps the limited place of the cardiac glycosides in patients with resistant heart failure in sinus rhythm.

Perhaps the most important lesson is that there is no place for casual or cavalier use of loosely indicated drug treatment. It is essential to arrive at a firm and clear rationale for therapy, based on an awareness of diagnostic pitfalls and difficulties in the elderly, a knowledge of the available evidence from controlled studies of drug treatment in this age group and carefully individualised clinical judgement.

It is important also to consider alternatives to drug therapy, especially in the treatment of comparatively trivial disorders such as sleep disturbance. The latter may be a symptom of an underlying disease state (e.g. depression, prostatism or pulmonary oedema), which should itself be the target of intervention rather than the presenting insomnia. Even where there is no causal diagnosis, the correct approach should entail counselling, minor adjustments to life-style or correction of an adverse environmental problem.

Practicalities of Drug Administration

In order for the writing of a prescription to be meaningful, a mutual agreement or contract is assumed to have taken place between prescriber and patient. The role of the pharmacist as the supplier of medication is also crucial, assuming that the prescription will be presented to the pharmacist for dispensing. The drug supply must be presented to the patient in a way which is comprehensible, accessible and manageable. Acquisition of supplies may depend on relatives or neighbours or on professionals such as district nurses, home helps and pharmacists who are prepared to interpret their job descriptions flexibly to the extent that patients are assured of receiving their medication. Actual administration of the drug therapy in accordance with prescribed instructions will then depend on both adequate understanding of the regime by the patient and a disciplined willingness on his or her part to carry out the instructions given.

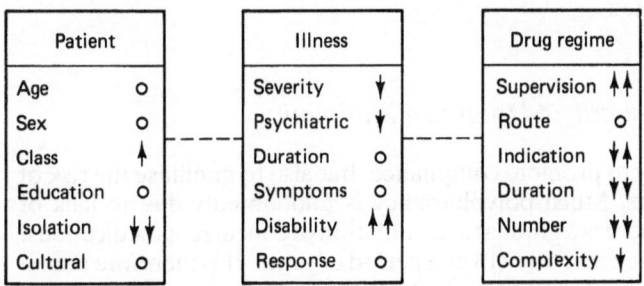

Patient		Illness		Drug regime	
Age	o	Severity	↓	Supervision	↑↑
Sex	o	Psychiatric	↓	Route	o
Class	↑	Duration	o	Indication	↓↑
Education	o	Symptoms	o	Duration	↓↓
Isolation	↓↓	Disability	↑↑	Number	↓↓
Cultural	o	Response	o	Complexity	↓

↑ Improves compliance
↓ Impairs compliance
o No effect on compliance

Fig. 24.1. Factors influencing drug compliance in old age.

With all these possible pitfalls, it is perhaps surprising that advanced age in and of itself has not been shown to be a major factor in non-adherence to prescribed drug regimes (non-compliance). Figure 24.1 gives an outline of the results of a range of studies carried out to try to determine the most important factors. From this evidence it is possible to put together a profile of the patient most likely to exhibit problems of adherence to prescribed regimes. Such an individual will be socially isolated, suffering from severe, protracted illness (particularly psychiatric illness) and will be required to take a large number of drugs at various times of the day over a long period of time. Such a patient profile in varying degrees should register strong warning signs to the prescriber that special measures will need to be taken if the act of prescribing is not to be rendered a total nonsense.

The following measures may be regarded as generally applicable.

Achieve Concordance Between Prescriber and Patient in the Range of Drugs Being Taken

Several studies have shown marked discrepancy between a prescriber's perception of what his or her patient is receiving and the information obtained from patients themselves. The best way to minimise this problem is to insist that all patients (irrespective of age) physically bring with them their complete supplies of medication to every consultation whether in surgery or in out-patient clinic. In some cases, to start with, a wheelbarrow might be necessary, but that is a measure of the scale of the problem rather than the unrealism of the solution!

Ensure the Removal of Stockpiles of Old Drugs

The retention of such domestic supplies, often "for a rainy day", undoubtedly contributes to confusion about drug therapy (let alone the risk of interactions). While removal of these stockpiles cannot be enforced, since they are strictly the patient's personal property, the author's experience is that there are few patients who cannot be persuaded to dispose of their old medications, once the reasons have been clearly explained.

Keep the Number of Prescribed Drugs to a Minimum

This is necessary not only to promote compliance, but also to minimise the risk of adverse drug interactions. Much polypharmacy is undoubtedly due to lack of proper review. Hence, there is a gradual accumulation of concurrent medications, often on repeat prescription and often over a period of years. It is therefore necessary for each prescriber to ensure that he or she has a built-in system for stopping or reviewing medication, which is just as important as the mechanics of prescribing. For the hospital clinician this may best be achieved through the presence and advice of a staff pharmacist at the regular ward meeting. For the general practitioner, appropriate programming of computer software dealing with prescriptions to ensure review after a given period of time, may be the method of choice.

Where a patient is required to take four or more different preparations, the likelihood of errors is high and rises exponentially above that number. Under such circumstances, scrupulous rationalisation of therapy is clearly essential.

Prescribe the Simplest Possible Regime

Once or twice daily regimes of therapy are desirable wherever possible. This objective may have to be a factor influencing the choice of drug for some elderly patients (for example beta-blocking agents or oral hypoglycaemic drugs). The further development of sustained release preparations may prove helpful in this respect (for example levodopa preparations in Parkinson's disease), but the benefits in terms of compliance require to be measured against the loss of flexibility in dose adjustment. Reduction in the rates of elimination of some drugs with age (see below) may reduce the necessity for divided dose regimes of some standard preparations.

Ensure that Drug Presentation is Satisfactory

The use of clear rather than tinted containers facilitates tablet identification. Container labelling should be clearly typed or printed and state clearly the name of the drug, the dose and the number and frequency of tablets, capsules, 5 ml teaspoons or other forms of administration. Access to the container should not cause the patient difficulty (as is unfortunately the case with some childproof containers). The drug vehicle should be acceptable to the patient (e.g. fluid or soluble formulation or alternative route where swallowing tablets or capsules is a problem).

Ensure that Supervision or Practical Help is Available when Necessary

Memory impairment and some other disabilities may render a patient unable to manage their own medication or obtain their own supplies. It is clearly pointless to prescribe under such circumstances until a reliable provider of help and supervision has been identified and instructed.

Ensure that Adequate Patient Instruction is Given

Although measurement of drug compliance presents difficulties and the results of interventions are difficult to measure, at least one controlled study has shown significant and sustained benefits from patient counselling, with a proper explanation of drug therapy. Another study in general practice showed marked differences in levels of drug compliance between the patients of different partners. These findings point strongly to the importance of good communication in forestalling compliance problems. There may be an important health education role for professionals other than doctors (e.g. pharmacists or district nurses) in achieving this objective.

Consider the Use of Compliance Aids

The effectiveness, or otherwise, of diaries and mechanical devices remains controversial. However, for certain patients, devices such as the "Dosette" may provide an answer and should be considered where difficulties are being encountered.

Determination of Dose and Dose Regime

As already indicated, adjustments in dosage with some drugs have been found to be necessary to insure against the occurrence of adverse reactions due to excessive drug effect in elderly patients. Reasons for this have been found in the pharmacokinetic and pharmacodynamic changes in some drugs which accompany increasing age. Such changes do not occur in all drugs, even those within the same pharmacological category. It has been found necessary to examine each drug individually, although a number of broad age-related trends in drug handling mechanisms have emerged. These are mostly (though not entirely) explained by a number of age-related changes in physiology, as listed in Table 24.1. The most important of these changes are as follows:

Table 24.1. Age-related changes which influence drug handling

Gastric pH increased
Gastric emptying impaired
Splanchnic blood flow reduced
Gastrointestinal motility reduced
Gastrointestinal absorptive surface reduced and thinned
Total body size reduced (in advanced age)
Total body fat relatively increased (until advanced age)
Metabolically active tissue decreased
Total body water decreased
Plasma albumin concentration reduced
Alpha-1 acid glycoprotein increased (slight and variable)
Liver mass reduced
Hepatic microsomal enzyme activity reduced
Regional blood flow from liver and kidney redistributed
Glomerular filtration rate reduced
Renal tubular function impaired

Absorption and Bio-availability

The age changes in the upper gastrointestinal tract shown in Table 24.1 might, in general, be expected to reduce the efficiency of drug absorption in old age. In reality, drug absorption, which is substantially a process of passive diffusion, has been found with few exceptions to be unaltered in elderly subjects. In the case of digoxin a very slight decrease in the rate (but not the extent) of absorption, too small to be of clinical significance, occurs. There may also be some reduction in the absorption of prazosin in the elderly.

In practice, it is more useful to consider the *bio-availability* of a drug (that is the amount reaching the systemic circulation after administration by any route). This is usually given as a percentage compared with intravenous administration (which is 100% by definition).

A factor which may influence bio-availability after oral administration of a drug is the amount of liver metabolism which takes place as the drug passes through the portal circulation. Comparatively few drugs undergo this so-called "first pass" effect, but for those compounds where this is extensive, only a small fraction of the administered drug reaches the systemic circulation. Examples include chlormethiazole, propanolol, metoprolol, labetalol, verapamil and some tricyclic and related antidepressants. The bio-availability of these compounds after a single, oral dose is increased in the elderly because the extent of first-pass metabolism by the liver is reduced. As a result of this, one would expect to see an accentuated effect of the drug after a single dose. This may be the case with chlormethiazole, but with the beta-blockers the effect may be offset by changes in pharmacodynamics (see below), and the immediate effects of verapamil and antidepressants are rather difficult to measure.

Distribution

Once present in the systemic circulation, a drug distributes into the extravascular tissues and fluid compartments of the body and, to a greater or lesser extent, to drug-binding proteins (albumin and alpha-1 acid glycoprotein in particular) in the plasma. The extent and characteristics of such distribution depend very much on the physico-chemical properties of the drug concerned. The same applies to the anticipated changes with age, which can on the whole be predicted from the alterations in body composition and binding proteins listed in Tables 24.1 and 24.2.

Table 24.2. Effect of age on plasma protein binding of drugs

Fraction bound decreased	Fraction bound increased	Fraction bound unaffected
Acetazolamide	Chlorpromazine*	Amitriptyline
Carbenoxolone	Disopyramide*	Atropine
Ceftriaxone	Lignocaine*	Atenolol
Clobazam	Propranolol*	Caffeine
Diazepam		Chlorthalidone
Lorazepam		Desmethyldiazepam
Naproxen		Frusemide
Phenytoin		Ibuprofen
Salicylic acid		Imipramine*
Tolbutamide		Maprotiline
Theophylline		Midazolam
Valproic acid		Oxazepam
Warfarin		Penicillin G
		Pethidine*
		Phenobarbitone
		Piroxicam
		Quinidine*
		Sulphadiazine
		Vancomycin

*Denotes substantial binding to alpha-1 acid glycoprotein.

Drug distribution is commonly expressed as the apparent volume of distribution (Vd) which indicates the proportion of drug in the body as a whole relative to that in the plasma. Drugs which are water soluble (e.g. digoxin, penicillin) distribute into body water and metabolically active tissue and, as a consequence, the distribution volume of these compounds tends to be reduced in the elderly. The relative amount of drug remaining in the plasma is therefore greater and the concentrations measurable in plasma after administration by any route are higher. This is of little clinical significance in the case of penicillin, a drug with low toxicity; the importance for digoxin, however, is in the size of the loading dose. While it is still appropriate in the elderly to use a loading dose where reasonably prompt digitalisation is required, the size of the loading dose should be smaller as a rule, particularly in the very elderly and those of small body size.

Conversely, lipid-soluble drugs distribute extensively into fatty tissue. The distribution volume of these drugs consequently increases with age due to the relative increases in total body fat. This has been shown to occur with the more lipid-soluble benzodiazepines, lignocaine, chlormethiazole, thiopentone, tolbutamide and amitriptyline. This increase in distribution volume actually slows down the rate of elimination (plasma half-life) of a single dose and so tends to prolong the duration of action of the compound.

Where drugs bind substantially to carrier proteins, only the free (unbound) fraction is pharmacologically active and available for presentation to the liver or kidney for elimination. A small reduction in binding may represent a substantial percentage increase in the free fraction. Studies of drug protein binding in the elderly, in most cases, have shown an increase in the free fraction, which is proportional to the small reduction in serum albumin (Table 24.2). With illness, this effect may be more pronounced. As a result of this change, the pharmacological effect of a single dose may be enhanced (higher plasma concentrations of free, pharmacologically active drug), and the rate of elimination may be increased (more free drug presenting to the liver or kidney for elimination). It has been suggested that episodes of hypoglycaemia in the elderly receiving initial doses of tolbutamide might be explained on this basis. Where the tissue distribution of drugs is extensive (e.g. diazepam) the net result is a further increase in distribution volume with few clinically significant pharmacological consequences.

The importance of alpha-1 acid glycoprotein as a drug-binding protein has only been recognised recently. Lipophilic drugs, which are basic rather than acidic, tend to bind to this protein rather than to albumin. Age is associated with a minimal increase in plasma concentrations of alpha-1 acid glycoprotein. However, the protein behaves reactively, with substantial increases occurring during acute illness, which far outweigh any effects of age. The free fraction of drugs bound in this way is minimally decreased or unchanged with age, but may decrease substantially (with the possibility of decreased pharmacological effect) in acute illness. This may perhaps be of some clinical significance for drugs such as propanolol.

The significance of possible changes with age in the extent of binding of drugs to other macromolecules, such as erythrocyte haemoglobin, lipoproteins and globulins, has been little studied and is uncertain.

Metabolic Biotransformation

Drugs which are lipid soluble and relatively non-polar require metabolic breakdown to more water-soluble (usually inactive) metabolites in order for renal or biliary excretion to take place. In some cases, active metabolites are produced and may be principally responsible for the desired pharmacological action, in which case the parent compound may function as a pro-drug, particularly if the initial metabolic step is rapid. The metabolism of many drugs takes place in the liver microsomes, via pathways of oxidation, reduction or hydrolysis, catalysed by enzyme systems dependent on cytochrome P450 and its subtypes (the so-called mixed function oxidase system). These processes are commonly referred to as Phase I reactions. Further reactions involve synthetic processes, such as conjugation with glucuronic acid, sulphate, glycine, and other groups, the so-called Phase II reactions. Some drugs undergo both phases of metabolism prior to excretion.

The possible effect of age on Phase I metabolic processes was initially studied using the marker drug, antipyrine, which undergoes slow hydroxylation in the liver. Comparisons of the rate of clearance of antipyrine between elderly and young subjects show reduced clearance rates in the former. An important point, however, is that variability between subjects in antipyrine clearance is high, presumably due to other factors such as genetic differences, environmental and dietary determinants of liver enzyme function and the possible involvement of different cytochromes. Gender has also been implicated by some investigators, the age-related reduction occurring to a much lesser extent in females. The clinical importance of this is that while, as a group, the elderly differ significantly from the young, the 95% confidence limits for the magnitude of reduction in any group of subjects are very wide.

Findings with other drugs undergoing Phase I oxidative metabolic processes have broadly corresponded to those with antipyrine. Examples include some of the more slowly eliminated benzodiazepines, tricyclic antidepressants, theophylline and a number of NSAIDs. Such a reduction in metabolic clearance in elderly recipients results in prolongation of the plasma half-life and the accumulation of higher, possibly toxic, steady-state plasma concentrations of the drug if given in regular, standard adult doses. Such accumulation has rightly been implicated in the occurrence of clinical toxicity with these drugs in elderly patients. It is therefore appropriate to use reduced initial doses where toxicity may be clinically relevant. Because of the marked variability, however, it is likely that a proportion of elderly patients may eventually require full dosage to achieve the required response. There is, at present, no practical alternative to titrating doses in this way.

There is some evidence that certain oxidative pathways of metabolism may be more impaired by age than others (e.g. demethylation more than hydroxylation). Further work is still needed to clarify the situation.

By contrast, most studies of Phase II drug metabolic processes have demonstrated only slight or negligible effects of age. Examples of drugs whose principal routes of metabolism are Phase II include paracetamol, isoniazide, ethanol, oxprenolol and the benzodiazepines, oxazepam, temazepam and lorazepam. While accumulation of some of these compounds still occurs on repeated dosage, this is generally not significantly greater in elderly than in young patients. There may, however, be other reasons to give reduced doses to the elderly (see below).

A further group of drugs undergoes such rapid metabolism in the liver that their metabolic clearance depends on liver blood flow. Since the latter falls gradually with age in proportion to the reduction in cardiac output, a reduced rate of metabolic clearance may be found (as is the case with propranolol, for example). Because of the rapidity of elimination, however, clinically important drug accumulation is not usually a consequence.

Renal Excretion

The well known, gradual decline in renal tubular and glomerular function with advancing age is due to the slowly progressive reduction in the numbers of intact nephrons. For drugs which are excreted by the kidney, without the necessity for prior metabolic biotransformation, the reduction in renal clearance is therefore fairly easy to predict, irrespective of whether the mechanism of excretion is glomerular filtration or tubular secretion. In practice there is usually a close correlation with the glomerular filtration rate as estimated by creatinine clearance. Direct measurement of the latter, involving 24 hour collections of urine, is rather cumbersome and serum creatinine alone is an unreliable index of renal function in the elderly, because it also depends on the amount of muscle mass (which itself declines with age). In practice, creatinine clearance can be successfully estimated using specially derived and readily available nomograms and formulae, such as those of Siersback-Nielsen et al. (1971) and Cockcroft and Gault (1976) respectively.

These methods have been developed primarily to assist in gauging the maintenance dosage of digoxin and it is surprising that they are not more consistently employed, even though the occurrence of digoxin toxicity has almost certainly declined with greater awareness of the need to reduce doses in many elderly patients.

Other cardiovascular drugs showing reduced renal clearance in the elderly include procainamide, practolol and atenolol. The same holds true for many of the commonly used antimicrobial compounds, including the penicillins, several sulphonamides, tetracycline, a number of cephalosporins and various aminoglycosides.

Where toxicity might have serious consequences therapeutic monitoring of plasma concentrations is essential, with reduced starting doses usually indicated for elderly subjects based on estimated creatinine clearance. This has been borne out by long clinical experience with, for example, the antimanic preparation, lithium.

Drug Sensitivity

The changes in drug-handling mechanisms outlined above go some way to explaining the occurrence of dose-related adverse drug reactions in the elderly and provide some broad guidelines for adjustments in dosage for some drugs. There is, however, additional evidence that differences in drug responsiveness may be found in older people which are independent of pharmacokinetic mechanisms. These pharmacodynamic differences may relate to changes in the processes taking place at or beyond the drug receptor site, within the target organ or within the broader homeostatic defence mechanisms which normally balance the pharmacological action of the drug. Such changes in "sensitivity" to drugs have been described in the elderly, although the precise mechanisms are ill understood as yet.

In the cardiovascular system, sensitivity to the effects of drugs acting on cardiac beta-receptors has been clearly shown to be reduced. The dose of isoprenaline required to increase the heart rate by 25 beats/minute increases linearly with advancing age, while the dose of propanolol required to reverse this process shows a similar age-related increase. This is likely to be due to change in post-receptor mechanisms (such as adenylate cyclase activity), but there may also be reduced density or affinity of cardiac beta-receptors. The reduction in sensitivity may, in practice, offset the increased propanolol concentrations which occur after administration of single oral doses to elderly patients (see above). Whether or not sensitivity to drug effects mediated via beta-receptors in blood vessels and in the bronchial tree is similarly changed, is not known.

The situation with alpha-adrenergic receptors is more complex, particularly as more receptor subtypes involved in vascular tone have been identified. Presynaptic and postsynaptic alpha-1 receptors seem to show no change in sensitivity with age, but several studies have shown a marked reduction in the responsiveness of alpha-II receptors.

In the central nervous system the most interesting finding has been an increase in the apparent sensitivity of the brain to the sedative effects of benzodiazepines. Indeed, dose and target organ sensitivity seem to be more important determinants of both the extent and duration of response to these compounds than the pharmacokinetic characteristics of the drugs concerned. The extent of use of these preparations is now rapidly declining, following greater awareness of the risks of benzodiazepine dependence. There is, however, still a place for their use in carefully selected circumstances and in anaesthetic premedication. In these circumstances, reduced dosage is usually appropriate for the elderly, at least initially.

Assessing the Outcome

Because of the increased susceptibility of elderly people to unwanted and exaggerated effects from drug treatment, the necessity for particular vigilance following the introduction of prescribed medication cannot be over-emphasised, particularly during the initial stages of treatment. The argument is strengthened by growing evidence that elderly people may show less subjective awareness of drug-induced symptoms and may therefore be unreliable in reporting back when problems occur. This seems to be a particular problem with the sedative effects produced by some psychoactive drugs, but a high index of suspicion of iatrogenic disease is, in any case, an important general principle of geriatric medicine.

It is important to make a point of enlisting the help of other independent observers, such as relatives, friends and neighbours, home helps, district nurses, wardens, officers of residential homes or hospital staff in detecting unwanted drug effects at an early stage. If in any doubt at all, the offending drug should be discontinued pending review.

In addition to the dose-related mechanisms above, drug response may be affected by a reduction in the efficiency of a number of homeostatic mechanisms. These are sufficient to maintain normal function under conditions of sound health, but there is a reduction in the effective reserve to such an extent that ill health or drugs may precipitate a situation of decompensation. Particular attention should be paid to the following:

Postural Stability

The frequency and amplitude of corrective movements involved in maintaining the upright posture increase gradually from early adult life into old age. Postural stability may, therefore, be compromised by illnesses and it is well known that falls are a common presenting symptom of disease (see Chap. 17). Similarly, drug side effects may present as impaired postural stability, especially in the case of psychoactive or sedative compounds.

Baroreceptor Function

Maintenance of blood pressure and the response of heart rate to standing from the supine position are both impaired in the elderly. Drugs which directly affect vascular tone, either via peripheral (e.g. vasodilating anti-hypertensive drugs, neuroleptics and antidepressants) or central (e.g. opiate analgesics) mechanisms, as well as drugs which cause intravascular volume depletion (i.e. diuretics) are particularly prone to cause symptomatic postural hypotension in the elderly. Measurement of both supine and standing blood pressure should be a routine part of the clinical assessment of any elderly patient and yet this procedure is still frequently omitted from routine clinical examination and the diagnosis remains commonly missed.

Thermoregulation

The role of drugs, particularly sedative agents and more specifically phenothiazine derivatives in the pathogenesis of accidental hypothermia is well recognised. It is still often overlooked however, particularly when the patient develops the condition in a normal, ambient temperature. The symptoms and signs may be non-specific (see Chap. 22). Failure to obtain an accurate rectal temperature recording using a low-reading thermometer will leave the problem undetected, when withdrawal of the offending drug could prove life-saving.

Maintenance of Orientation

Drugs which affect cholinergic transmission, centrally and peripherally, can particularly induce confusional states in older patients. The mental changes may be subtle and unless cognitive function is specifically tested (e.g. using the abbreviated mental test), an important drug-induced problem will be overlooked. In relation to drug therapy, maintenance of normal mental function is appropriately categorised as a homeostatic mechanism.

Pupillary Autonomic Responses

Paralysis of accommodation is a further well-recognised problem with anticholinergic compounds, though it is usually asymptomatic. The functional consequences of impaired vision are more likely to present, and unless thought of, these may not be specifically related to the offending drug.

Neurological Control of Bladder and Bowel Function

Marginal degrees of bladder instability are common in old people, so that problems of incontinence are readily induced by the rapid rise in intravesical pressure generated by loop diuretics. Conversely, compounds acting on the cholinergic system (e.g. tricyclic antidepressants) may precipitate urinary retention with overflow. Faecal impaction with spurious diarrhoea may also occur via the same mechanism.

Conclusions

In evaluating drug response it is vitally important to consider that the above "common problems of the elderly" may well be iatrogenic in origin.

In spite of the pitfalls of drug therapy, a gratifying response to treatment is characteristic of the medicine of old age. Given such a satisfactory therapeutic outcome a key question should then be "Can the drug treatment be stopped?" Historically, older people have often been left on drugs without review for an indefinite period. Sometimes this is right, but it should be the outcome of a positive decision on therapeutic management. Many studies have shown the drugs can often be withdrawn completely or the doses substantially reduced. Examples include the use of both digoxin and diuretics in acute heart failure and of NSAIDs in acute exacerbations of arthritis or non-articular rheumatism. These strategies should be taken seriously because of the heightened risk which such drug therapy carries.

It will be apparent that the answer to the particular problems of drug treatment presented by elderly patients lies essentially in the amount of care taken by clinicians in the individualisation of therapy. The broad guidelines given above should assist in defining the indications, tackling the practicalities, deciding on the best dose regime and assessing the outcome of treatment. It remains a fact, however, that success in the therapeutics of old age (as in diagnosis) requires greater thoroughness, skill, attention to detail and vigilance than may be the case for many younger patients. There is now an encouraging increase in the database available to prescribers, but further research is needed in the form of better clinical trials, a fuller understanding of pharmacological mechanisms and perhaps the development of specific strategies to individualise dose regimes.

Further Reading

Caird FI (1985) Towards rational drug therapy in old age (the F.E.Williams Memorial Lecture). J R Coll Phys 19:235–239
O'Malley K, Waddington JL (eds)(1985) Therapeutics in the elderly. Excerpta Medica, Amsterdam
Royal College of Physicians (1984) Medication for the elderly. J R Coll Phys 18:7–17
Swift CG (ed) (1987) Clinical pharmacology in the elderly. Marcel Dekker, New York
Vestal RE (ed) (1984) Drug treatment in the elderly. Adis Health Science Press, Sydney

Chapter 25

Rehabilitation

Gladys M. Tinker

> *It is possible for anyone, given a lot of guts and a bit of luck, to overcome gigantic misfortunes and terrible illness.*
>
> Roald Dahl

Rehabilitation describes the process whereby disabled people work towards attaining the maximum degree of physical and psychological independence possible. Healthy people convalesce rapidly from trivial illnesses. However, if the illness is severe or if the person's general health is poor (as is often the case with old people), spontaneous recovery may be delayed or incomplete. For such people, participation in a rehabilitation programme will often make the difference between leading a dependent rather than an independent life. It may allow them to continue to live in their normal environment rather than having to move into institutional care.

Rehabilitation will be of benefit to a wide range of people, suffering from an equally wide variety of disorders. Because certain disabilities are associated with unique problems and require specific management, it is often advantageous to treat people in special centres. Thus "stroke units", "orthopaedic rehabilitation units" and other units dealing with specific problems have come into being. However the general principles of rehabilitation are applicable to practically all patients irrespective of the nature of their illness. They can be implemented outside of special centres and even (perhaps especially) in the patient's own home.

The Rehabilitation Team

Successful rehabilitation requires a team approach as the skills of health workers from many disciplines are required. This multi-disciplinary team should include those who can contribute to the improvement of the patient and possible members

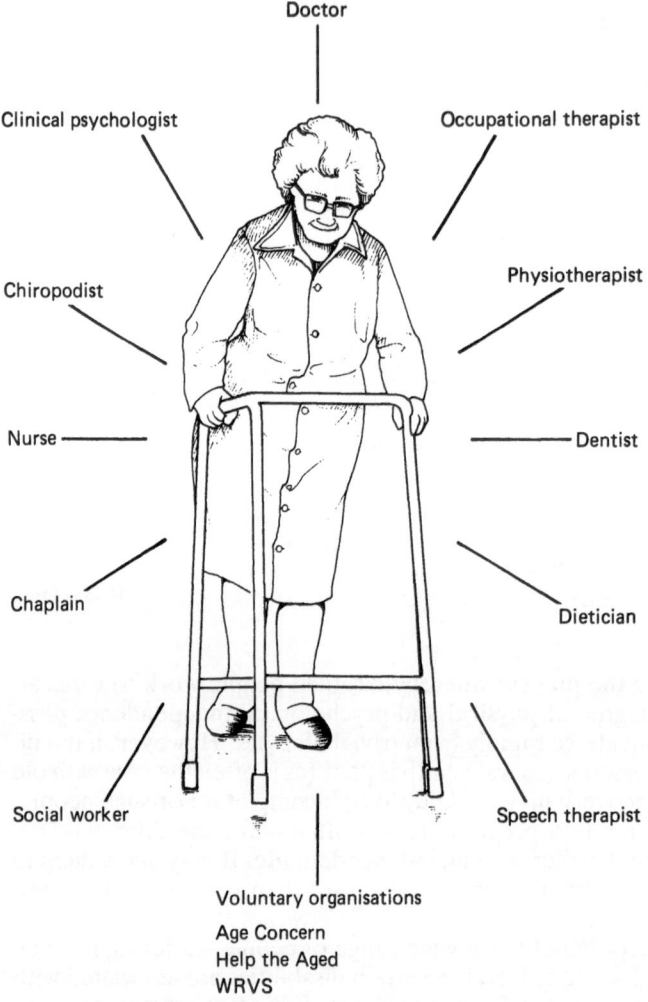

Doctor

Clinical psychologist

Occupational therapist

Chiropodist

Physiotherapist

Nurse

Dentist

Chaplain

Dietician

Social worker

Speech therapist

Voluntary organisations

Age Concern

Help the Aged

WRVS

Fig. 25.1.   Possible members of the multidisciplinary rehabilitation team.

are listed in Fig. 25.1. The composition of the team should be flexible. Not every patient will require the services of all members of the team. Sometimes help will be required from professionals who are not normally part of the team but who are seconded to it in order to deal with a specific problem in a specific patient.

In a rehabilitation unit there is normally frequent daily contact between the various members of the team. This affords continuous sharing of information and ideas. In addition, it is important that the team meet formally on a regular basis to discuss each and every patient being treated in the unit. In most units, weekly meetings are found to be ideal. Each member should inform the team of the patient's current functional state and whether this has changed from the previous meeting. An assessment of the potential for further improvement should be given and the plans towards achieving treatment goals should be proposed.

Team meetings also have an educational dimension, the exchange of information between the various experts ensuring this. Meetings should also be used as a discussion forum for new ideas and new techniques. When members of the team have learnt something new from their own reading, attending educational courses or seminars, etc., their knowledge should be shared with the group. This serves to consolidate the professional status of the team as well as allowing it to be updated on new advances.

The role of some key members of the team is outlined below. Roles often overlap, so job descriptions should not be adhered to rigidly. Thus, for example, the ward domestic staff should be encouraged to reposition hemiplegic limbs and all staff must know how to transfer disabled patients without causing injury to the patient or to themselves.

The Team Leader

The team leader is first and foremost the chairman at the team meeting. Here, he or she must sift through the innumerable facts brought into the meeting, collate them, form a joint assessment and then plan a coordinated programme of care for the long as well as short term.

At the team meeting all relevant shades of opinion on a given problem should be voiced and it is the leader's responsibility to ensure that this occurs. Members of the team who are reticent should be encouraged to contribute and no member of the team (not even the team leader) should be allowed to dictate. If the approach of the leader is truly democratic, all members of the team will realise that they have a voice which is listened to when formulating the care plan. This increases morale and motivation among the staff, which in turn makes successful rehabilitation of the patient more likely.

The leader must ensure that the team effort is coordinated. Should conflict arise within the team, its cause must be identified and dealt with rationally by all involved. Part of the art of leadership involves ensuring that this process works.

The rate of progress in many cases is frustratingly slow for both the patient and staff. If the long-term goals are still feasible, the leader is responsible for maintaining optimism and enthusiasm so that all concerned continue to give of their best. People may need reminding of the progress already made and to be made to understand that rehabilitation is often a long process.

The team leader is also the spokesman for the unit. There is often a political aspect to this when for example, further resources are required.

The Doctor

The doctor is involved in monitoring such ongoing medical conditions as may require further investigation and treatment. He must also be aware of those intercurrent problems which are likely to arise and if unable to prevent them, then to deal with them when they occur. His role differs to that traditionally taught in medical school; now the doctor is but one small part of a multi-disciplinary team. The programme of care differs to that found in acute medical wards; it can be indefinite in time and the emphasis is on functional recovery rather than curing disease.

Usually the doctor is also the team leader, though in some centres this is now changing. Being a good physician does not necessarily imply that one will have good leadership qualities and some doctors have an autocratic approach which militates against successful leadership.

Remedial Therapists

Remedial therapists such as physiotherapists, occupational therapists and speech therapists are the pivotal members of the rehabilitation team. It is with them that patients spend most of their working day. Their individual roles are outlined later.

Nursing Staff

Nursing staff are present on rehabilitation wards at all times whereas other members of the team are present for just a few hours each day. They have, therefore, a unique opportunity to influence the outcome of treatment. In the early stages an immobile patient may require frequent turning in bed and stroke patients will need careful positioning if spasticity and joint contractures are to be avoided. Following limb amputation wounds may need dressing for a long period. The skin over pressure areas must be frequently inspected and pressure sores prevented. Nursing staff have a critical role in ensuring an adequate fluid and dietary intake and in the care of the bowels and bladder.

Early mobilisation of the patient is as much the responsibility of the nursing staff as it is of remedial therapists. The patient should be encouraged to do as much as possible for himself at the earliest possible opportunity. It is often appropriate to encourage a disabled person to feed himself, tie his shoelaces, make his bed, etc., even if this involves a struggle, rather than do these tasks for him. In this way, the nursing staff complement the work of the occupational therapist.

The Patient

It seems a truism to state that the patient has an important role in his own rehabilitation. Yet patients are often not adequately involved in the therapeutic process. An informed patient is more likely to work hard and make rapid progress. Both the patient and the carer must be involved in setting goals, monitoring progress and deciding on future care. Many patients find it an awesome undertaking to take part in a formal multi-disciplinary meeting so that it is best if such discussions are informal.

The Rehabilitation Centre

During the period of rehabilitation, it is important that the surrounding environment be as stimulating as possible. When housed in multi-storey buildings, rehabilitation units should be on the ground floor giving easy access to the hospital grounds which can then be used in the rehabilitation programme. Thus a patient can be encouraged to walk there following a limb amputation, or to garden there following a stroke. Getting out of the ward, even if only in a wheelchair, breaks the monotony of institutional life. A breath of fresh air may not necessarily improve someone's PO_2 but it may improve temperament and morale.

The ward itself should be bright and pleasant and have a stimulating colour scheme. The presence of brightly coloured birds will add colour and life to a room. There are advantages in having a self-contained unit where the ward adjoins the gymnasium and other rooms used by remedial therapists. This facilitates regular contact between members of staff and minimises the time spent in travelling from one section to another. A "day area" should be available for recreational purposes and likewise a dining area. There should be a wide variety of furniture to try to meet the needs of all. Chairs are particularly important: they should be stable, have arms and firm seats and be of different heights and depths. Virtually no patient should need to be restrained in a so-called "Geriatric" chair.

Clothing should ideally be the patient's own; the use of clothes provided by the hospital reinforces the patient's sense of institutionalisation. If hospital clothing must be used this should be well-fitting and of adequate variety and abundance; there is no excuse for any patient being without proper underwear. Laundering can be carried out by the patients themselves or their carers on the ward, using ward facilities; otherwise a personalised district laundry service can be employed. In some units where both men and women have therapy simultaneously, the use of pretty track suits and training shoes for older women has been found to be very practical. Such clothing also has the psychological effect of motivating the patient to work hard at therapy.

Mirrors, hairdressing and barber facilities will all contribute to a more positive approach by staff and patients alike, the latter benefiting from a boost in dignity and self-esteem.

If rehabilitation is prolonged then access to social facilities, either within the hospital or preferably outside, will be necessary to maintain morale. Something as simple as the staff or relatives taking a patient to the local café or pub will demonstrate to that patient that he or she is making progress, will remind him of normal life outside the institution and encourage him to make further improvement. It is often useful for a patient who has an obvious disability, or who requires an aid, to appear in public for the first time with a staff member or friend for moral support. Practical efforts must be made to minimise the institutionalisation that accompanies a long period of rehabilitation. Ward routines should be flexible, with individual programmes of care and freedom of choice where possible.

The Rehabilitation Process

Assessment

The first step is to make a full assessment of the patient's current status. What is the nature and extent of functional impairment (*disability*) and what disadvantage (*handicap*) results from it? Psychological disability such as anxiety and depression can be as important as physical disability and must not be overlooked. Remedial therapists are best equipped to make an evaluation of physical disability, while the opinion of a clinical psychologist can be invaluable in assessing the mental state. Patient assessment is a dynamic process, requiring repeated review. One of the principal functions of the ward meeting is to facilitate this continuing re-evaluation.

It is essential to be aware of the patient's pre-morbid level of function and the circumstances in which he was living. How mobile was the patient and how did he cope with activities of daily living such as washing, dressing, toileting, cooking and shopping? What supports are available to him at home and to what extent had he been dependent on these? While this information is usually available from the patient, it sometimes needs to be verified by those in close contact with the patient such as a spouse, other relatives or carers, community nurses, Home Help, etc. Without this information, appropriate therapeutic goals cannot be set.

Remediation

With so many personnel involved, the day to day work of the therapists must be planned and coordinated. It must be ensured for example, that patients are not seen by several therapists on one day and by none on the next. In some units a weekly programme is drawn up, while in others a very brief meeting of the relevant team members occurs on a daily basis to discuss strategy.

Having identified the nature of the disability in a given patient, the *physiotherapist* must design a programme of exercise which will reverse it. For instance, in a patient with osteoarthritis and weakness of knee extension, exercises will be given to strengthen the quadriceps muscles. The process of recovery must often be allowed to take place in a stepwise fashion. Thus, in a hemiplegic patient, abnormal tone in the trunk muscles must be tackled before he can sit properly. The person must have good sitting balance before he can realistically be expected to stand, and he must be able to stand before walking is attempted. The philosophy of physiotherapy in hemiplegic patients has changed in recent years; whereas formerly early mobilisation was brought about by concentrating on the unaffected side, the more modern Bobath technique concentrates on the affected side and encourages bilateral patterns of movement. While progress tends to be slower with the latter approach, it results in better functional recovery (i.e. better rehabilitation).

Occupational therapists particularly concern themselves with the ability of people to cope with the activities of daily living. Where handicap exists, they devise ways of surmounting it. This can involve either retraining the patient or altering his environment. Thus the arthritic patient can be taught new dressing techniques, a raised toilet seat can be provided for the person with proximal myopathy and the provision of a new downstairs toilet can be recommended for the amputee. Particular skill is required in knowing when to provide a mechanical aid. If used inappropriately, aids can be counterproductive by preventing the return of function and encouraging dependence. However, for some patients, the provision of modified cutlery, a walking aid or a wheelchair may allow the person to feed himself, walk or go out of doors when without them this would not be possible.

The work of the *speech therapist* is primarily concerned with the treatment of communication disorders, though increasingly it includes the management of swallowing problems and other cranial nerve disorders.

Discharge

As the limit of the patient's potential is being approached consideration must be given to problems that may arise after discharge from hospital. For the vast majority of patients early return to their own home is the goal. Should residual disability be a problem, however, the patient may need support in order to continue living in the community. The support available to vulnerable old people in Britain is discussed in detail in Chapter 28. The likely needs of the patient must be assessed well in advance of discharge so that relevant community supports are in place when the person leaves hospital. Even a short delay in the provision of essential services can result in a crisis, loss of confidence, early re-admission to hospital and, perhaps, an avoidable move into institutional care.

Should the person be unable or unwilling to continue living in his own home, alternative arrangements must be made. Sheltered housing consisting of small, modified flats with a resident warden will allow many people to return to semi-independent life in the community. In Britain, unfortunately, the demand for such housing greatly exceeds the supply. Fostering schemes are becoming increasingly popular and are preferable to institutional care for many people. Some people, usually those with significant residual disability, will require institutional care in residential homes, nursing homes or long-stay hospital beds. These options are discussed in more detail in Chapter 28.

Inspection of the patient's home should always be considered prior to discharge. An initial visit can be carried out by the therapist alone, to see whether the patient can be realistically accommodated there. It is then valuable to make a repeat visit with the patient to see how he or she functions in that environment; this is often a revelation, as patients who function poorly in an unfamiliar hospital environment fare much better in their own surroundings. There are no set rules as to which members of the team take part in the home visit, the selection being entirely dependent on the individual patient's circumstances.

The transition between hospitalisation and returning to live at home is often best made in phases. The next step may be to leave the patient at home for a few hours, possibly being monitored by the therapist or a community Health Visitor. This can lead on to an overnight or week-end stay, gradually building up the patient's independence and the carers' confidence. After each visit home problems that have arisen should be reported to the team who can review the situation, and decide whether any changes or adaptations can be made to improve the patient's independence.

After-care

The rehabilitation process does not end once the patient returns home. As most people will have some degree of residual disability, they should be encouraged to continue with those exercise programmes taught to them while in the unit. Continued input from remedial therapists may be required; this can be provided in the home and many areas in Britain now have a domiciliary occupational therapy, speech therapy and physiotherapy service. Alternatively, continuing remedial therapy can be carried out in a day hospital.

All patients, after a long period of rehabilitation, require some form of follow-up assessment after discharge home. This can be undertaken by the domiciliary therapist and combined with further treatment. If no follow-up by therapist or hospital is required than an occasional visit from a specialist geriatric health visitor can be used to re-assess the situation, identify problems before they develop into a crisis and instigate active intervention at an early stage.

Rehabilitation at Home

The principles of rehabilitation can be readily applied outside the framework of a specialised rehabilitation centre. Thus a patient can be assessed and have remedial therapy at home. The home setting has natural advantages in that institutionalisation is avoided and the patient does not have to face the often difficult transition between hospital and home. Home care will require the enthusiasm of the carer as well as the patient if it is to be successful. The family doctor will often find himself in the position of leader of the multi-disciplinary team, even if on an informal basis.

The decision on whether or not to admit patients to hospital for rehabilitation should be based on the patient's circumstances. The most important factors influencing the decision will be the degree of disability and the amount of support available at home. In general, the elderly patient who requires more than one form of remedial therapy is best cared for in a rehabilitation centre, be it a day hospital or an in-patient unit, where there is input from the entire multi-disciplinary team, including the doctor and nurse.

Further Reading

Andrews K (1985) Rehabilitation in the elderly. In: Pathy MSJ (ed) Principles and practice of geriatric medicine. John Wiley, Chichester, pp 1213–1232
Caird FI, Kennedy RD, Williams BO (1983) Practical rehabilitation of the elderly, Pitman, London

Chapter 26

Terminal Care

Rhian E. Owen

> *"The field of terminal care presents an immediate problem. Where the dying are concerned there is no possibility of trying harder next time. The dead cannot complain and despite the resentments and grief, the bereaved do so with surprising rarity."*
>
> (Wilkes Report 1980)

Terminal care encompasses the care of an individual who is dying as a result of a progressive condition which cannot be reversed by treatment. It does not refer simply to the last hours of life, but may involve weeks or months prior to death and should entail not only the care of the patient but also his relatives.

Caring for the dying is an important and essential part of the geriatrician's work. Though one cannot always achieve a cure one must always strive to care for the patient. Professional staff should not view death as a failure. As far as the dying patient is concerned the only failure is not ensuring that the period before death is as comfortable as possible. The main aims of those providing terminal care should be to improve the quality of daily life by alleviating unpleasant symptoms and helping to prevent the patient from suffering fear and loneliness.

In recent years terminal care has become synonymous with the Hospice Movement for the Care of the Dying. The term hospice (L. hospis, way station or resting place) was derived by Dame Cecily Saunders in 1960 when she recognised and addressed the needs of her dying patients. While hospices specialise in the care of the terminally ill, the philosophy of terminal care can be applied in any unit and even in the patient's own home. As the needs of the dying patient are complex, with physical, psychological, social and spiritual aspects, no one person will have the expertise to deal with all of them. A multi-disciplinary team approach is required with input from a doctor, psychologist, social worker, physiotherapist, occupational therapist, dietician, chaplain and others. Success depends primarily on enlightened professional attitudes. Mutual respect and understanding of each other's roles is vital and there should be no rigid role barriers. The patient's confidence and trust are obviously essential and adequate communication is the corner-stone of good practice.

Clinical Assessment

Caring for the elderly dying patient emphasises the need for careful history taking. Multiple pathology is the rule and it is usually wrong to attribute all symptoms to the terminal disease. It is essential to listen to the patient and evaluate each problem without pre-conceived ideas. Pain may not necessarily be related to the malignant process so that a patient with carcinoma of the head of the pancreas may still experience angina or gout. While pain is the symptom most commonly associated with terminal disease, a plethora of symptoms may be experienced. Due to a reluctance to communicate all their problems, it is usually necessary to ask direct questions about those symptoms commonly experienced by people with terminal illness. The dying patient requires regular reassessment. Problems need to be evaluated daily so that changes in treatment can be instigated without delay.

Symptom Control

Pain

It is important to appreciate that not all patients with cancer experience pain and not all pain in a patient suffering with cancer is caused by the cancer. In many instances more than one pain may be experienced. In the care of the terminally ill it is important to appreciate that chronic pain serves no useful purpose. It cannot, for example, be compared with the pain of an acute appendicitis, which serves to point at the diagnosis and towards successful treatment. In achieving symptom control it is essential that documentation is precise and explicit. The site, frequency and type of pain should be recorded. A body chart may be useful. In the treatment of constant pain there is no place for "as required" medication; rather analgesia should be prescribed on a regular basis. Each pain needs separate assessment, treatment and subsequent review.

It is only when the nature of the pain is known that a management regime can be devised. The pain may not necessarily be connected with the underlying terminal disease and with elderly people particularly, the presentation may not be typical. Co-existing diseases such as ischaemic heart disease, urinary tract infections and pulmonary embolus may cause confusion. There is no rationale for multiple drug use and it has been shown that use of more than one analgesic reduces the efficacy of treatment. A stepped approach is advocated beginning with a non-narcotic agent, subsequently rising to a weak opioid and eventually reaching the strong opioids (Fig. 26.1). All medication is normally prescribed on a 4 hourly basis though occasionally it may be required 3 hourly. In the very elderly renal handling may be delayed and morphine in particular may accumulate. In such instances 5 hourly or even 6 hourly administration may be required.

When initially prescribing strong opioids the use of morphine sulphate or hydrochloride salt mixture allows flexibility of dosage until the pain is adequately controlled. To aid compliance and ease drug administration at home, the 24 hour total dose can subsequently be calculated and given as a long-acting preparation twice

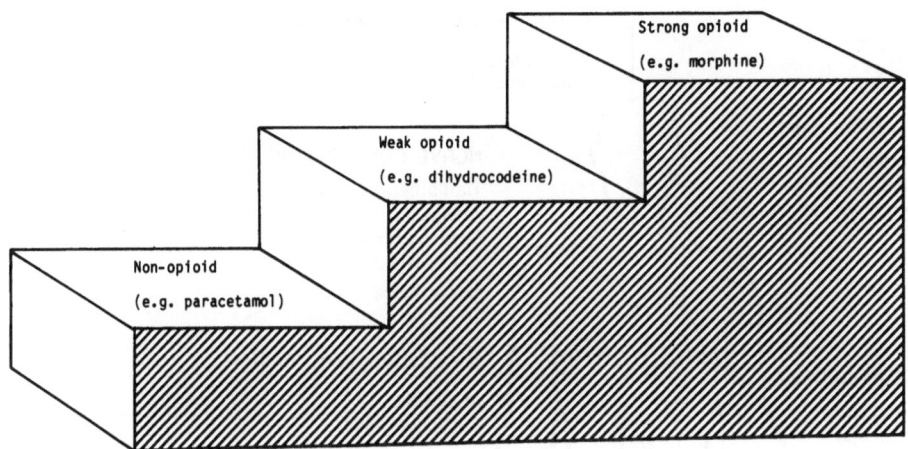

Fig. 26.1. The stepped approach with analgesic therapy in terminal care.

daily. If pain breaks through on this regime the dosage can be divided into an 8 hourly regime. Additional analgesic agents are usually unnecessary, though oxycodone suppositories 30 mg t.d.s. provide an alternative administration route. Phenazocine may be useful in narcotic-resistant individuals.

Patients unable to comply with oral medication may be considered for morphine by injection. Intra-muscular injections are painful and should therefore be avoided. The subcutaneous route is less painful and drugs may be thus given on 4 hourly basis. Continuous subcutaneous infusion via a syringe pump is ideal for many patients as they need not be disturbed and the injection site may only need to be changed once every 7 to 14 days. When changing from an oral to a subcutaneous route, the dose of morphine needs adjustment. Table 26.1 shows how equivalent doses can be calculated. Dosage should be titrated to the patients pain. Patients commencing opioid analgesia should be reviewed at least twice on the first day so that dosage adjustment can be undertaken without delay. In people aged over 80 years, the dose may need to be increased more slowly as there is a risk of morphine accumulation.

Table 26.1. Equivalent dosages for opioid drugs

4-hourly oral morphine (mg)	4-hourly subcutaneous diamorphine (mg)	Continuous subcutaneous infusion of diamorphine (24-hour dose)
5	2.5	15
15	5	30
20	7.5	45
30	10	60
45	15	90
60	20	120
90	30	180
120	45	270
150	60	360

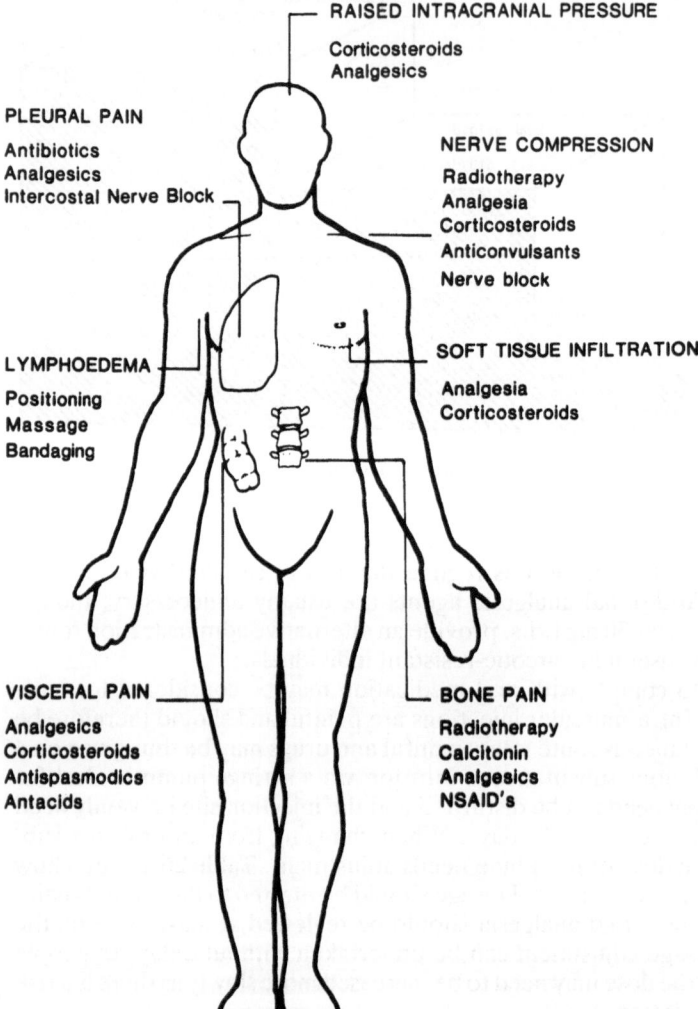

RAISED INTRACRANIAL PRESSURE

Corticosteroids
Analgesics

PLEURAL PAIN

Antibiotics
Analgesics
Intercostal Nerve Block

NERVE COMPRESSION

Radiotherapy
Analgesia
Corticosteroids
Anticonvulsants
Nerve block

LYMPHOEDEMA

Positioning
Massage
Bandaging

SOFT TISSUE INFILTRATION

Analgesia
Corticosteroids

VISCERAL PAIN

Analgesics
Corticosteroids
Antispasmodics
Antacids

BONE PAIN

Radiotherapy
Calcitonin
Analgesics
NSAID's

Fig. 26.2. Common causes of pain in patients with malignant disease and the means by which pain can be reduced.

The side effects of opioid drugs should be appreciated. Constipation is inevitable, therefore all patients receiving regular analgesia should receive regular laxatives. Many patients are nauseous with regular morphine and regular anti-emetic agents may be required for the initial 7 to 10 days. Drowsiness may be a problem for 24 hours, but should not persist if the dose is appropriate. Respiratory depression is unlikely even in patients with chronic obstructive airways disease as the dose required to relieve pain appears to be lower than that needed to affect the respiratory centre. Some patients report nocturnal perspiration while taking morphine. Hallucinations can be a problem and usually resolve with a reduction in dosage or a reduction in the frequency of administration. This is particularly the

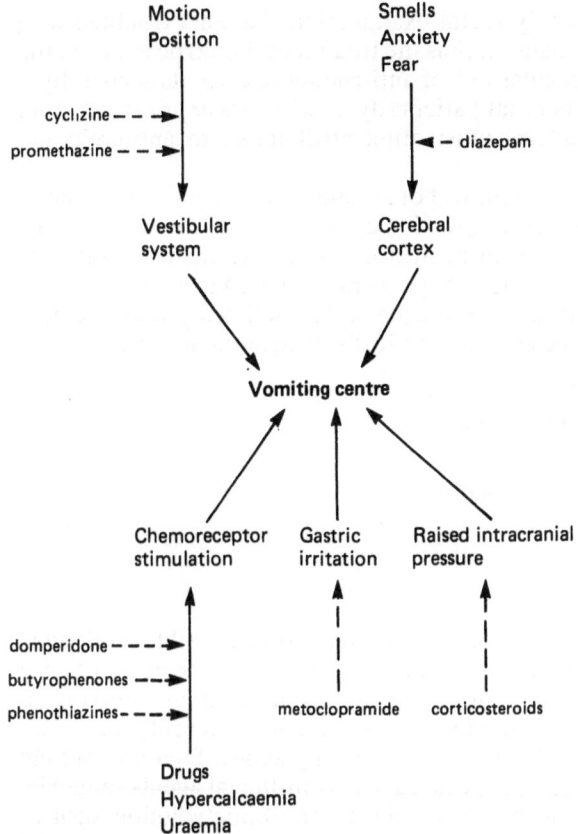

Fig. 26.3. The causes and remedies for nausea in a patient with malignancy.

case with very old people. There are certain analgesic agents which should be avoided in patients with malignant disease. Pentazocine is short-acting and is well known to cause confusion in elderly patients. Pethidine is also short-acting and has an upper limit of 300 mg after which the drug is not tolerated. Methadone is contraindicated as it accumulates in old people. Pain may be relieved by agents other than analgesics (Fig. 26.2). It is also important to realise that the emotional state of the patient will affect pain appreciation. Anxiety, fear, depression and loneliness will all reduce the pain threshold and pain control cannot be optimised without due attention to these factors.

Nausea and Vomiting

As with pain these symptoms may be due to a variety of causes and a careful history, examination and investigation is required for accurate diagnosis and optimal therapy. When the cause is multi-factorial, the effect on symptoms is often additive. Fig. 26.3 outlines some of the conditions causing nausea and vomiting and indicates the therapeutic options in dealing with them. Constipation is a cause which must always be excluded by rectal examination. Patients troubled with copious sputum can experience nausea, thus the treatment should be aimed at the reduction of the sputum with regular use of anti-cholinergic agents such as hyoscine. It is important to remember that patients dying with cancer are at risk from iatrogenic gastrointestinal problems most often attributable to antibiotic and analgesic therapy.

Management initially consists of removal of all underlying causes. When none can be identified or reversed, drug therapy will be required. It is advisable to start with one drug and if the response is unsatisfactory, to add agents from different groups in a step-wise fashion. Anti-emetic agents may be used in a syringe driver and may be used together with analgesic agents. The following drugs remain active when mixed with morphine and are physically compatible with it:

haloperidol (2.5 mg over 24 hours)
metoclopramide (30–150 mg over 24 hours)
cyclizine (50–150 mg over 24 hours)
methotrimeprazine (25–150 mg over 24 hours)

Oral Problems

Many doctors neglect to examine the oral cavity, the most accessible of all body cavities. A dry mouth is a common complaint and is usually a side effect of drug therapy. It can be helped by sucking pineapple chunks or by taking effervescent ascorbic acid or Sialivix pastilles. Monilia is common and if present, careful inspection of the oropharynx invariably reveals typical plaques. Dentures should always be removed when inspecting the oral cavity. Anti-fungal agents should be prescribed. Any dentures should be soaked in an antiseptic solution such as hypochlorite and, prior to re-use, a small quantity of the anti-fungal agent should be placed on them. Oral hygiene is important and the use of Corsodyl oral gel which contains chlorhexidine gluconate may be more acceptable than an oral rinse.

Dysphagia

Monilial infections can involve the oesophagus and present with dysphagia and the presence of oral monilia should suggest this as the cause. Anti-fungal agents will normally effect an improvement within 48 hours.

Neurological problems may give rise to disorganised, uncoordinated swallowing and can result in weight loss. This is discussed in more detail in Chapter 10. Such dysphagia can be improved by anti-cholinergic agents such as hyoscine. Dietary advice is often advantageous and the provision of liquidised meals may be required.

Squashed Stomach Syndrome

This term refers to dyspeptic symptoms associated with an inability of the stomach to distend and is normally associated with hepatomegaly and ascites. The effects are similar to those found following a gastrectomy, the patient complaining of fullness, epigastric discomfort, flatulence, nausea and post-prandial vomiting of large amounts of ingested food. The treatment consists of reassurance, antacids and the provision of small frequent meals.

Gastrointestinal Obstruction

This is almost always related to constipation, drug therapy or a bowel neoplasm. If drugs and constipation are excluded by history and examination and it appears that the cause is related to an intrinsic bowel problem, then the patient's condition should be assessed with regard to surgical intervention. If the patient's general condition is good and a reversible cause seems likely, then surgical intervention should be considered.

If previous findings preclude successful surgical intervention, then medical measures should be undertaken. This involves more than the normal "drip and suck" regime which is more appropriate as a stop-gap measure whilst considering surgery. Irreversible bowel obstruction in a patient with terminal cancer requires measures aimed at reducing the obstruction. High doses of corticosteroids should be given combined with phosphate enemas delivered high up into the colon. Stimulant laxatives should not be used, though it may be appropriate to prescribe spasmolytics and faecal softeners. Anti-emetic agents may give symptomatic relief.

Anorexia

Anorexia causes a great deal of distress to patient and relatives alike. The patient may be disheartened by his inability to eat and carers may feel that rejection of food which they prepare implies rejection of themselves. Time should be spent explaining to both the patient and his carers that food requirements are less and that a small meal on a small plate is often more appetising than a dinner plate filled to overflowing. Taste sensation is often diminished so sharp tastes may be more appreciated.

Corticosteroids may be used to improve the appetite in the initial stages. In advanced disease food and drink may not be required and the relatives may need counselling in this regard. Time taken to explain that the body may not require food and drink in the terminal stages allows the patient to die without the indignity of naso-gastric intubation and intravenous feeding.

Insomnia, Anxiety and Depression

As with any elderly patient complaining of insomnia, one should always try to identify the cause or causes. It could be secondary to other symptoms such as pain, dyspnoea or anxiety, or to physical factors such as excessive noise and light in an institutional environment. Unrelieved boredom or over-zealous sedative medication during the day are other important causes. Such underlying problems should be identified and reversed. If the patient is still experiencing sleeping difficulties then it is appropriate to prescribe hypnotics. Although counselling may be preferable to drug therapy in an otherwise well, mobile 80-year-old living at home, it is inappropriate for a severely debilitated dying patient. The geriatrician should adopt a more relaxed attitude towards the prescription of hypnotics in this particular instance. However, it is still essential to choose hypnotics such as temazepam or chlormethiazole with a short duration of action so that over-sedation is avoided.

Anxiety cannot be relieved by drug therapy alone though anxiolytic agents are a useful adjunct to treatment. The most successful form of therapy consists of psychological support and the adoption of the listening role. Allowing the patient time to express his anxieties is an important step in his treatment. If medication is requested then lorazepam is a suitable first line agent. It is addictive, but this is of minor importance in this situation. Haloperidol is a suitable alternative and can be given in small doses on a twice daily basis. Using small doses such as 1 mg b.d., it is unlikely that parkinsonian features will develop.

Many patients dying with cancer are erroneously thought to be depressed. Usually they are just manifesting their very natural sadness. Sadness will not respond to antidepressants. The diagnosis of depression in the terminally ill is exceedingly difficult as the normal symptoms cannot be used as indicators. If true depression is possible then it may be worth considering the addition of a small dose of antidepressant medication preferably taken as a single dose at bedtime. Amitriptyline has sedative properties and can be prescribed as a single daily dose. However, drowsiness and anti-cholinergic affects such as a dry mouth may be troublesome. Some old people may also be stimulated by amitriptyline and experience unpleasant dreams and restlessness and it is therefore advisable to prescribe a small initial dose. Mianserin is not as potent as amitriptyline but causes fewer side effects. It can be started at a dose of 10 mg per night, increasing by 10 mg increments to a maximum of 60 mg.

Constipation

Constipation is one of the commonest complaints experienced by elderly people and in the terminally ill it is inevitable unless laxatives are used prophylactically. Factors such as poor mobility and inadequate intake of food and fluid, which predispose to constipation in old people, are even more frequent in the terminally ill. In addition to these factors the prescribing of opiates, anti-cholinergics and aluminium antacids can worsen the condition. Constipation may give rise to other symptoms such as anorexia, nausea, pain, confusion and diarrhoea. It is perhaps appropriate to adopt the belief that every patient suffers with constipation until proven otherwise. Physical examination is essential. Faeces may be palpable as an indentable mass usually in the left iliac fossa, but occasionally involving the transverse colon. Digital examination of the rectum is mandatory, although an empty rectum does not exclude the diagnosis. A straight abdominal X-ray may be required to demonstrate impacted faeces high in the colon.

The management of constipation consists of the initial clearing of the bowel and subsequent preventative therapy (see Chap. 11). The treatment consists of both "top and tail" measures: a laxative should be prescribed on a regular basis and initially a combination of a faecal softener together with a bowel stimulant is required. A combination of danthron together with dioctyl sodium sulphosuccinate may be found useful. An alternative would be to use a titrated dose of sennoside together with dioctyl sodium sulphosuccinate. For long-term use a faecal softener or an osmotic laxative may be sufficient.

In the debilitated patient it may be adequate to clear the bowel with less aggressive measures such as a glycerine suppository. However, a high- phosphate enema may be required if more simple measures are unsuccessful. If severe faecal impaction is present then manual evacuation may be required. This is usually extremely distressing for the patient and sedative cover may be required.

Psychological factors should not be overlooked. There should be an immediate response to a patient's request to defaecate, and whenever possible the patient should be allowed to use the toilet, which should be private, clean and warm. It would benefit the debilitated patient if his feet were supported on a footstool.

In patients who have undergone colostomies for anal or rectal carcinomas a mucous discharge can be an unpleasant problem. If the skin is not broken then suppositories of Witch Hazel will provide relief. If fungating lesions are present then the use of metronidazole either topically or systemically should be considered.

Dyspnoea

Dyspnoea (see Chap. 7) may have many causes and requires careful evaluation. In the case of bronchogenic carcinoma it can be directly related to spread of disease, i.e. pleural effusion, consolidation, lymphangitis or replacement of lung tissue by tumour. It may be related to the treatment of the underlying carcinoma such as radiation fibrosis, or follow pneumonectomy. The debilitated patient is obviously at risk from pulmonary emboli and pneumonia, therefore multiple pathology has to be considered. There may be pre-existing chronic obstructive airways disease or biventricular heart failure. Reversible underlying causes such as pulmonary oedema, consolidation and pleural effusion should be treated, anaemia corrected and bronchospasm relieved. Dyspnoea related to compression of the trachea responds to high doses of corticosteroids. Should dyspnoea remain following the treatment of reversible conditions then morphine should be used for symptom control. When sputum is tenacious a nebulised solution of acetylcysteine may be useful. Hyoscine may be used to reduce the rattling noise produced by movements of secretion. Hyoscine is also a sedative and may be used in the dose of 0.3 mg subcutaneously every 4 hours.

Counselling

The ability to talk freely to a dying person is not easily acquired. Some people are more skilful than others, and an acceptance of the proximity of death can be a greater problem for the doctor than it is for the patient. It is impossible to counsel a patient unless one is aware of his mental and physical needs. These can only be elicited by proper communication and the most important step that a doctor can take towards providing good terminal care is the adoption of a listening role.

There is much debate among health workers and others regarding whether or not to inform patients of the nature and prognosis of their terminal illness. There are no rules which apply in all cases but, if given the opportunity, practically all patients will seek as much information as they want at any given time. The patient should be allowed to lead any discussion, with the doctor steering the conversation towards topics which he wishes to discuss (e.g. the diagnosis and prognosis). Asking the patient for his views on his illness may indicate that he already has a degree of insight. Phrases such as "What do you think is wrong with you?" and "What have you been told so far?" may provide a platform for further discussion. Patients appreciate the time that professionals spend with them. The fact that their problems and fears are important enough to merit discussion can restore self-esteem and be an invaluable part of symptom control. It has been shown that the pain threshold will increase if a patient is secure and confident in his carers. Ideally it should be the patient who indicates the end of a consultation, rather than the more usual scene of the doctor backing away and trying to reach the door before another question is asked. Patients often come to the realisation that they have a terminal illness gradually, so a gradual transference of awareness over a period of time is the ideal goal.

A series of interviews with the patient is usually essential; short discussions in a traditional ward round setting are inappropriate, privacy and a one-to-one relationship being essential. Counselling is not the prerogative of the doctor. All members of the multi-disciplinary team should be involved. The most appropriate person to explain the diagnosis and prognosis is the one present when the patient communicates the desire to know. Questions must be answered honestly. It is essential that every member of the team be kept informed of the patient's current state of awareness so that all replies will be appropriate. Each team member should be well versed with the stages (outlined by Kubler-Ross) which patients pass through as their awareness of their imminent death increases. Carers should anticipate emotions of denial and anger before a phase of acceptance is finally reached. Statements and behaviour will therefore not be misinterpreted and the response of the carer will be appropriate.

Support must also be given to relatives. However, it must be borne in mind that the first obligation is to the patient. The family should be guided through their desire to maintain a conspiracy of silence regarding the illness. They will need explanation and reassurance as much as the patient will. They should be aware of the phases of grieving so that they do not consider themselves abnormal. It is accepted that preparation for bereavement can reduce the incidence of pathological grief though contact with and continued support for the relatives is often necessary after the death of a loved one.

Further Reading

Kubler-Ross E (1970) On death and dying. Tavistock Publications, London
Saunders C (ed) (1984) The management of terminal malignant disease (2nd edn). Edward Arnold, London
Smith C (1982) Social work with the dying and bereaved. Macmillan, London
Stott N, Finlay I (1984) Care of the dying – a clinical handbook. Churchill Livingstone, Edinburgh

Twycross RG, Lack SA (1984) Oral morphine in advanced cancer. Beaconsfield Publishers, Beaconsfield
Twycross RG, Lack SA (1984) Therapeutics in terminal cancer. Pitman, London

Section IV
Delivery of Health Care to the Elderly

Chapter 27

Geriatric Medicine and the Law

C. Twining

The importance of the law in relation to medical practice is well recognised, particularly in respect of such matters as negligence and consent to treatment. However, there are often situations in the care of older people where special considerations may apply. In these cases confusion rather than clarity about legal matters is the norm.

This chapter will not attempt to deal with legal aspects of medicine in general. Rather it will focus on those areas which seem to give cause for special concern when trying to provide medical care for older people. One obvious example is the situation where someone, a relative, neighbour, general practitioner, social worker or even local newspaper is saying that "something must be done" about a frail elderly person, usually someone living alone. This person is in one way or another seen as being at risk. This may be because of poor physical health, some form of mental infirmity or difficult housing or other social circumstances. In other cases it may be a problem in determining the best course of action in relation to a person who might benefit from medical treatment, but where there is some disagreement, typically with the patient and/or relatives about whether such treatment is justified.

The issues involved include those of consent, vulnerability, the balance of risks and benefits, the degree to which judgement may be impaired by mental disorder and the extent to which others can be said to have the best interest of the patient at heart. That these matters do not give rise to greater public concern is due to at least two factors. First, there is the general lack of public enthusiasm for facing up to the difficulties of providing the right sort of help for older people, other matters seeming to press more urgently upon the public conscience. Second, there is the reality that the outcome for older people is less often a dramatic one than for younger people, and in most cases some other new factor intervenes which resolves the problem. In many cases this "other factor" is an acute physical illness or even death and may not be related to the original problem, though the extent of this may be underestimated.

Put crudely, if there is difficulty in providing care or treatment for a young person and he or she subsequently dies, this will be examined very carefully. In the case of an older person it will more easily be assumed that he or she died because of "old age" rather than through any fault in the system of care. Indeed that person's death may solve so many problems (e.g. for the hospital and for the family) that it is in nobody's best interests to make an issue about why things might have gone differently.

I do not suggest some form of general conspiracy against older people. Rather, there is a problem in balancing the needs of older people and those who look after them. Those who are vulnerable often have need of someone who will champion their cause. In the case of children this is most often their parents. In the case of those who suffer acute illness they themselves can seek redress once they have recovered. Neither factor acts to support the needs of frail elderly people who may themselves have unrealistic and low expectations of the service that they receive.

These are complex matters to which it is unlikely that there will in all cases be an easy solution. However, there are times when a failure to appreciate the available options, including the possible recourse to legal powers, can lead to delay or indeed complete failure to come up with any effective course of action. The outcome may not be some dramatic disaster, but will certainly result in unnecessary distress to older people and those who care for them.

Time and time again there is some conflict between the need to protect the individual and the desirability of maximising individual freedom and choice. Older people have rights to treatment as well as a right to protection from exploitation and interference. Furthermore, there may be conflict between the individual's wish to remain in his or her own home and the strain that this places on others. In the majority of cases good professional practice maintains a satisfactory balance between these opposing forces. The law should act as a back-stop, providing some formal recognition of society's ways of resolving these problems.

My intention here is to set down briefly the existing aspects of legislation which are of most relevance. I do so as a health professional, as which I am qualified, not as a lawyer, which I am not. There are therefore times when I have emphasised words or phrases which are not so emphasised in the original statute. Those who wish to study the letter of the law should look elsewhere. Those who seek to understand enough to use the law for the benefit of frail elderly people will, I hope, find this of value.

The Law in the United Kingdom

The first legal heresy which I shall commit is to talk about the law for the United Kingdom, as if this were itself unitary. In truth one must consider three parts, England and Wales, Northern Ireland and Scotland. The precise statutes and acts differ between these countries, but the principles remain broadly the same. I therefore hope that those in Scotland and Northern Ireland will forgive me if, for the sake of brevity, I use the structure of English law.

Compulsory Admission

One of the most difficult and recurrent problems in clinical practice is the case of someone who needs care or treatment, but who refuses to come into hospital or into a residential home. The system of care which has developed over the last two centuries relies on moving people to medicine rather than medicine to people. In part this is an inevitable result of developments in medical technology, although the trend towards seeing in-patient care as better than care in the home has been going on for at least 150 years. Nevertheless, it is very hard to see how we could arrange for many of the procedures commonly used in modern acute geriatric medicine to be carried out in a person's own home. Even basic care is often seen as being only available in a hospital or other institution, though this may be changing.

As with other aspects of care, there is usually an assumption of implied consent unless the person actively refuses to consider admission to a hospital or residential home. Certainly the vast majority of admissions to hospital, whether medical or psychiatric, as well as those to residential homes are voluntary. It is when someone objects to leaving their own home in the face of clear professional advice that problems can arise.

There can be several reasons why an older person may refuse to agree to admission. He may be determined to die in his own home, may be frightened of hospital or other institution because so many people do not come out alive. He may have impairment of intellect so that he cannot appreciate the risks to which his present living circumstances expose himself or others.

The first distinction to make is between the mentally alert and the mentally infirm. For those who are mentally alert there are only very few circumstances when such a person can be removed from their home against their will. Most people accept that people of sound mind must be allowed to live as they choose even if they put themselves at risk by so doing. It is a fundamental principle of our political system that our disagreeing with their decision is insufficient grounds for intervention. It is when there is some risk to others, due for example to poor hygiene or safety with gas or other appliances, that some form of compulsion is deemed appropriate.

The National Assistance Act (1948) and National Assistance (Amendment) Act 1951

Section 47 of this act allows for adults to be forcibly placed in care in order to secure necessary care and attention if:

1. he/she is suffering from grave chronic disease *or* being aged, infirm *or* physically incapacitated, is living in insanitary conditions, *and*
2. he/she is unable to devote to him/herself *and* is not receiving from other persons proper care and attention.

The community physician must certify to the local authority that a person satisfying these conditions should be put into care in his own interest or to prevent injury to health or serious nuisance to other people. The local authority (or the community physician if authorised by them) can then apply to a magistrate for an order committing that person to care.

The original Act set up this procedure with a requirement that the person being taken into care should be given 7 days' notice. Orders made under this provision are for 3 months in the first instance and can then be renewed. The individual against whom the order is made cannot apply for the order to be revoked until 6 weeks after the original application.

The 1951 amendments include provision for an immediate order, i.e. without the requirement for 7 days' notice if the community physician *and* one other doctor certify that removal without delay is necessary in the person's own interests. Such an immediate order has a maximum duration of 3 weeks.

These procedures are used about 200 times each year in Britain as a whole. There are many more cases however where the "threat" of such procedures leads to the person agreeing to go into care voluntarily and these would not appear on the formal statistics. It has been suggested that this provision, the origins of which have more to do with slum clearance than the protection of an individual's well being, should be abolished. Certainly there are considerable differences between different areas in how frequently it is used. Some local authorities, for example, have a policy of not using this legislation. In those cases where it is a matter of public hygiene which gives cause for concern, there is other legislation in the Public Health Acts which is of better use.

There can also be problems where a person is being looked after by people in the community, but these carers have reached the limit of their ability to cope. The frail elderly person may refuse other sources of help, perhaps because he or she sees it as the others' "duty" to look after them. There is no such legal obligation on families in Britain however, and the strain can be enormous.

Relatives and others may feel strongly that "something must be done", but as long as they continue to give "care and attention" there is little recourse to legal action. It requires them to shoulder an additional burden of guilt if they have to withdraw from care so that a Section 47 application can be made. All too often it is not until the situation has passed the breaking-point that anything can be done.

It has been estimated that about half of those taken into care under Section 47 are suffering from some degree of mental impairment. There may be alternatives to this under the provision of the Mental Health Act, and I shall therefore now turn to this.

The Mental Health Act (1983)

The Mental Health Act (1983) superseded the previous Act of 1959 and was yet a further attempt to balance the rights and risks of the mentally ill with regard to admission, treatment and the management of their affairs. In many respects the changes from the previous legislation affect functionally mentally ill people more than those who are afflicted by the dementias which represent the main management problems of psychiatric illness in late life. However, the Act does not draw such a distinction, although it does give separate consideration to those suffering from mental handicap and, to some extent, to those suffering from psychopathy.

The relative neglect of the specific needs of elderly people in this legislation may be seen as yet another example of the age discrimination inherent in society. Even more cynically one could also point out that as most dementias are irreversible such patients are never in a position to question what happened to them at a later date. In this respect they are among the most vulnerable people in society, having neither the capacity for self-expression afforded the intellectually normal nor the parental advocacy of those afflicted by arrested intellectual development.

It is important to note in passing that the terms "mental impairment" and "severe mental impairment" are used in the Act to refer to those suffering from mental handicap *not* those suffering from dementia, which is subsumed under the general category of "mental disorder". This can lead to some confusion for those not familiar with the terminology, especially as older people suffering from severe dementia are often referred to as the "elderly severely mentally infirm", sometimes abbreviated to ESMI.

Other terms used in the Act are also given specific definition including a definition of nearest relative. However, the term "mental disorder" is left undefined. This has advantages in terms of flexibility, but can cause some problems in the case of elderly people who may be suffering some mild degree of intellectual decline. Is someone who is aged 80 and rather forgetful showing signs of early dementia, which presumably would be considered as mental illness, or some extreme form of the slight but definite memory impairment which is associated with normal ageing? Does the advantage of legal protection outweigh the stigma of being certified mentally ill?

Even if it is clear that someone is showing some form of dementia, how far does this affect their ability to cope on a day-to-day basis? Is that person's refusal to agree to go into hospital or into a home a result of the decline in intellectual function, or merely a wish to remain independent and at home, which has nothing to do with any mental deterioration?

Each individual case must have these sorts of dilemmas resolved. This does leave scope for differences of opinion between practitioners, resolved to some extent under the legislation by requiring that more than one person be involved with acts of compulsion, whether they be for admission or treatment. Furthermore, the more serious or irreversible the action, the more opinions are required.

There are a number of categories of professionals referred to in the Act and it is as well to be clear about the differences between them. For example, there are two categories of medical staff: registered medical practitioners (who need have no special knowledge of mental disorder) and those who are in addition recognised as being specially qualified in mental illness (i.e. psychiatrists). The Act also distinguishes a particular category of social worker who has successfully completed an additional course of training and is thus recognised as being "approved" under the Act.

The 1983 Mental Health Act provides for the compulsory admission to hospital of those suffering from mental illness and/or mental impairment. As the numbers of older mentally handicapped people are small in comparison, I shall summarise briefly the sections in relation to the mentally ill. Admission to hospital may be for assessment (Section 2), for treatment (Section 3) or in the case of emergency (Section 4). The provisions may be summarised thus: compulsory admission for assessment or treatment may only take place if

1. the patient is suffering from a mental disorder warranting assessment or treatment
   and
2. would require to be detained in hospital in the interests of his/her own health or safety or that of others
   and
3. such assessment or treatment could not be undertaken outside hospital.

The application for admission is made by the nearest relative or an approved social worker and must be supported by a recommendation by two independent registered medical practitioners, one of whom must be a psychiatrist and one who knows the patient. The patient can only be detained for up to a time limit specified in the Act, unless a further application is made.

It is worth emphasising one or two points which can cause problems in relation to older people. First, the person must be suffering from a mental illness. This is no problem in the case of those who are suffering from severe dementia, depression or paraphrenia. However, there may be cases where someone is awkward, eccentric or slightly forgetful and these are not included. Secondly, the person should require admission to hospital for their own or other people's protection, not just because they can be a bit of a nuisance. Moreover, in the case of those being admitted for treatment, the treatment must be likely to benefit them and should be such as requires admission. Thus it is not simply that treatment can be more conveniently given in hospital. In the case of those suffering from dementia this raises particular issues in so far as there is no treatment which directly affects the underlying mental disorder.

It is clear therefore that these sections of the Act meet best the needs of the functionally mentally ill, especially those requiring acute treatment. For those who need care and supervision rather than treatment, the most relevant part is that relating to Guardianship (Sections 7–10).

Guardianship

The powers of guardianship under the 1983 Act are more restricted than those under the 1959 Act which it replaced. The guardian, who may be a specified individual or a local social services authority, can require the patient (again this can only be applied to those with mental disorder) to live in a specified place (which need not be a hospital), to attend for medical treatment, occupation or training and can require that the person should have access where they are living to a doctor, social worker et al.

The guardian can only require that the person attend for treatment, not that the person agree to have such treatment, so the same principles of consent to treatment apply as to other patients (see below). The guardianship order must be accepted by the local authority, so it is in effect a social services order even when the guardian appointed is a named individual. The application has to be supported by two doctors, one approved under the Act and by an approved social worker.

The application lasts for six months, may then be renewed for six months initially and annually thereafter. The patient has the right to appeal to a mental health review tribunal, and there are specified penalties for any guardian who is found guilty of neglecting or wilfully ill-treating the person for whom they act as guardian.

It was originally hoped that this form of guardianship order would be more useful than its predecessor. Indeed, it would seem to fit well the needs of some vulnerable elderly people suffering from dementia who might need care and supervision rather than hospital treatment. However, it is rarely used, about 200 times a year nationally, and this stems in part from reluctance on the part of some local authorities to take on such cases.

Consent to Treatment

The great majority of those who receive medical treatment, whether for physical or mental illness, do so with their own consent. In most cases this consent is implied, such as if the patient rolls up his or her sleeve in order to receive an injection. In some cases, notably surgical treatment, explicit consent is routinely sought and again there is usually no problem in this.

There are three factors generally deemed necessary for valid consent to treatment. First of all there should be adequate information available to the patient. There is some difference between countries in deciding how much is "adequate". In Britain, the criterion is at present similar to that in relation to negligence, namely what a reasonable practitioner would tell his or her patient. Elsewhere, there is greater emphasis on the role of the patient and the criteria depend on what a prudent patient would expect to know. Secondly, the patient should be capable of giving consent, just as in relation to testamentary capacity (see below). Thus there are special problems for the elderly patient who is confused, whether acutely or chronically. Finally, the patient should have given his or her agreement to the treatment. As we have seen, this can be implied rather than explicit.

For elderly patients problems of consent are more common for two reasons. First there is the higher incidence of both acute confusion and dementia, and secondly there are issues concerned with the acceptability of withholding treatment.

In cases of emergency treatment where the patient is unable to give consent, for example because he or she is unconscious, it is accepted that the doctor concerned may assume that the patient would consent, unless he or she has already indicated otherwise. There can be more of a problem in the situation where treatment might be beneficial, but not necessarily life-saving and the patient is partially or intermittently mentally incapable. In this sort of case the responsible medical officer will normally consult with others involved, including the next of kin.

It is, however, important to note that relative's consent has, in the case of adults, no validity in law. Clearly, it is desirable to proceed with the agreement of relatives who, in the vast majority of cases, have the patient's best interests in mind. However, this may not be the case and it is quite possible for relatives' views to be opposed. This is particularly important in respect of any decision to withhold treatment. In the care of older people with severe chronic illness, especially dementia, it is important that the responsible medical officer knows the wishes of those close to the patient. It requires a good deal of wisdom and experience to refrain from medical heroics. Thus where "on-call" junior staff are suddenly asked to attend to a severely demented elderly person who has become acutely ill they may well decide to "play safe" and treat a condition which might better be left untreated. Such dilemmas are at least as much ethical as legal. They are however much more common than the matter of euthanasia, which generally is given greater prominence.

The special provisions for the treatment of those with mental illness apply only to those treatments which are aimed at curing or alleviating the mental illness. Thus they do not apply, for example, to the patient with severe dementia who requires unrelated physical treatment. Similarly, treatments for mental illness can only be given under the Act and against the patient's consent when that person is formally detained under the Act.

The Act specifies certain different categories of treatment which require vary-ing amounts of professional involvement. For example, ECT can only be given without the patient's consent if it is supported by two independent psychiatrists. Leucotomy cannot be carried out without both the patient's consent *and* the agreement of two psychiatrists.

Management of Property and Affairs

Testamentary Capacity

As we have already seen, there are many instances where the ability of the patient to understand information and make judgements about the effects of his or her actions is central to decisions regarding care and treatment. These can be seen as particular examples of testamentary capacity; it is, however, most obviously associated with the making of a will. The situation here is fairly clear; in order to be judged capable of making a will, a person must:

1. know the nature of his actions, i.e. understand that he/she is making a will
2. be capable of understanding the nature and extent of his/her property
3. be aware of who might be the potential beneficiaries
4. be free from any delusions or obsessions which could affect his/her judgement in relation to the will
5. not be abnormally suggestible or under the influence of drugs, alcohol, etc.

Note here that there is no need for the person to be free from *all* mental illness, including dementia, provided this does not affect the items specified. Similarly, it is quite possible to leave all your money to the cats' home instead of your family provided you do so deliberately. For those concerned with the medical care of older people the possibility of the side effects of drugs is particularly pertinent.

Similar criteria would apply to entering into other legally binding agreements such as a bank loan or house sale. The extent to which a person can carry out such matters must therefore be determined according to their present function and the nature of the business to be transacted.

Where there are problems in managing affairs then there are a number of rele-vant procedures.

Agency and Appointee

There are two types of procedure which apply specifically to the collection and management of pensions or other benefits administered by the Department of Social Security (DSS). These are governed by DSS regulations and do not apply to other financial affairs.

Agency

It is quite common for an elderly person to ask someone else to collect his or her pension or other social security benefit. There are recognised procedures for this, whereby the pensioner asks someone else to act as agent. Appropriate wording appears on the pension book itself and the pensioner must sign both the pension form and the agency authorisation. The agent is only empowered to collect the money, not to spend it, unless of course the elderly person has instructed them to do so.

In cases where there is to be a long-term arrangement of this sort, a card can be supplied by the DSS which authorises the agent to collect the pension or other benefit indefinitely. The pensioner still has to sign each pension order however. Normally the agent will be the next of kin, though for a person in a residential home, it may be the local authority. It has been recommended that staff in private homes should not act as agents unless absolutely necessary.

Appointee

Where there is temporary or permanent incapacity the DSS can appoint someone to act on that person's behalf in respect of social security benefits. Thus the appointee can collect the money, spend it for the person and even appeal against benefit decisions as if he or she were the claimant. The appointee is instructed to act in the claimant's best interests.

The DSS has its own regulations for managing such applications. The officers must satisfy themselves that the claimant is incapable and that the person being appointed is suitable to act on their behalf. This will usually be a close relative, although where there is no such person able and willing to take on the task an officer of the local health or social services authority may be appointed. It is possible for a member of staff in a private home to be made the appointee, but this is usually discouraged by those responsible for registration.

As with all such procedures, the appointee system works very well most of the time. However, there is no formal mechanism for monitoring the work of the appointee and the system relies on positive reports of maladministration before action is taken.

Power of Attorney

If for reasons of physical incapacity someone is unable to perform any particular duty then he or she can appoint someone to act on his or her behalf. This is done by drawing up a legal document granting that person (the "attorney") the power to act on one's behalf. The powers specified can be as narrow or wide ranging as the person giving them sees fit and may cover one single activity or a whole range. It is necessary that the person giving the power is of sound mind and the power of attorney only remains valid as long as the person who gave it remains capable of revoking it. It is a fairly simple matter for this sort of arrangement to be drawn up and it has considerable flexibility.

What it does not cover is the eventuality that the person making the arrangement should become mentally incapable. This can however be accommodated using an alternative procedure.

Enduring Power of Attorney

This is similar to the power of attorney but specifies that the power is to continue if the person becomes mentally incapable. It has to be drawn up in a specified way and, should the worst happen and mental incapacity occur, the power must then be registered with the Court of Protection. The attorney is then accountable to the Court as is a receiver appointed by them (see below).

Once again this sort of arrangement can only be drawn up initially when the person granting the power is of sound mind. Few of us have the foresight to make plans for our mental infirmity. Once someone has become mentally disordered without making such an arrangement then there is little alternative besides the Court of Protection.

The Court of Protection

Although the present function of the Court of Protection is regulated by the provisions of the Mental Health Act (1983), there was little change in its provisions from the previous legislation. Indeed the origins of the Court of Protection lie in the Supreme court and it is an office of the Lord Chancellor's department. It is therefore a good deal older than most of the other legislation affecting mental health.

The Court is authorised to make arrangements for the management of the affairs of those who are no longer mentally capable. Application to the Court for it to take over someone's financial affairs may be made by anyone, although in practice it is usually the nearest relative acting through a solicitor. The Court requires a medical certificate that the person is no longer capable of managing his or her own affairs. This may be completed by any medical practitioner who knows the patient. It does *not* need to be completed by a psychiatrist.

The usual procedure is for the Court to give written notice to the person that an application has been made and that a date for a hearing has been set. The person has the right to appear or be represented at that hearing to contest the application. If the application is successful the Court appoints a receiver, usually the next of kin, whose job it is to manage the person's affairs in the interests of the patient and his or her family. The receiver is accountable to the Court (generally annually) which can appoint another receiver at any time. Where there is no suitable person to act as receiver this is taken on by the Management Division of the Court.

The receiver can be authorised to do anything that a person would normally do for him or herself. This includes the drawing up of a will and the filing of divorce proceedings! The receiver continues to act until the person recovers or dies. There are various fees chargeable by the Court against the patient's income, including an annual charge related to the size of that income.

There are a small number of "Visitors" employed by the Court's Management Division to make enquiries into the affairs of those under the Court's jurisdiction. The Court can also ask the Visitors of the Lord Chancellor's department to enquire concerning the well-being of those who have their own receiver. However, because of the large number of those under its care (over 22,500 people in 1985) their work is primarily confined to those who are not in a hospital or residential home. About three quarters of those under the orders of the Court are aged over 60.

There are a number of problems from the viewpoint of those trying to coordinate the care of frail elderly people. First, the procedure is somewhat cumbersome and expensive, especially for those with modest estates, and applications on behalf of those with small incomes are not encouraged. Secondly, despite recent improvements, it seems to take a very long time to complete an application and for an order to be granted; a period of several months is quite usual. Opinions differ as to the reasons for this, but in part at least it may be due to unfamiliarity with the Court on the part of both relatives and some solicitors. Thirdly, there is the assumption made that the person making the order, typically the next of kin, is the best person to act on the patient's behalf. Where this turns out not to be the case, appointing another receiver can be difficult. Finally, the Court is based only in London and there can be delays in communication which make it appear remote from the needs of those it is trying to serve.

Medical Fitness to Drive

Fitness to drive may be affected both by physical or mental disorder and by the effects of normal ageing such as increased reaction time and difficulty in dividing attention. There are, of course, many older people who continue to drive safely and each case must be assessed individually.

In Britain the great majority of licences to drive a motor vehicle are administered by the Driver and Vehicle Licensing Centre (DVLC) in Swansea on behalf of the Secretary of State for Transport. Age criteria are applied in that full licences are issued for a period of three years or until the applicant is aged 70, whichever is the longer. Applicants for a licence have to make a declaration of health and may be required to undergo a medical examination. Such an examination may also be required by an insurance company before agreeing to provide cover. Thus there are regular opportunities for older people to consider their fitness to drive. All applicants have to declare both any "relevant disability" and any "prospective disability", that is any condition which is progressive and in future might impair the ability to drive. The sorts of problems which might apply particularly to older drivers would include sensory deficits, cardiovascular disease (including stroke), joint disease and dementia. Drug side effects may also be an important factor.

For those who already hold a licence, the responsibility for informing the DVLC lies with the licence holder. He or she is bound by law to inform the authority as soon as he or she is aware of any relevant or prospective disability. This is often not appreciated by the patient who will understandably be reluctant to curtail the freedom given by driving. It is therefore appropriate to make it clear to the patient that it is up to him or her to inform the DVLC. Any advice regarding fitness to drive should be recorded in the medical notes.

There can be particular problems in the case of dementia when insight is impaired, but which of course is a "prospective disability". It is by no means uncommon to encounter cases where those who would be quite unable to find their own way around due to dementia are still driving. Often the spouse has taken on the role of navigator and sits in the passenger seat giving instructions!

Medical advice to the patient is governed by the usual rules of confidentiality. When confronted with a patient who is unfit to drive, the first step should be to explain the reason to the patient and to explain his legal obligation to stop driving. Only in exceptional circumstances and as a last resort is it appropriate to inform the DVLC without the patient's consent that he is no longer fit to drive. In most cases older people themselves decide that it is better initially to limit and then to stop driving. This is a much better option than being told by some other body that it is time to give up. Those who are very elderly are in any case likely to find it increasingly difficult to obtain even the minimum insurance cover required by law.

In cases where there is some doubt as to the right course of action by the physician, advice may be sought from a medical adviser at the Licensing Centre. A handbook on "Medical aspects of fitness to drive" is published by the Medical Commission on Accident Prevention.

The Law in Other Countries

Many of the problems and procedures which I have described in relation to the United Kingdom have their counterpart in other countries. For example, the powers conferred by the Court of Protection are enacted by a guardianship of property or a conservatorship in the United States of America.

In some cases there may be significant differences in procedure, but towards the same ends. For example, the inclusion of relative's approval on consent forms as practised in Canada.

In other cases there may be quite different approaches to a particular problem or legislation covering areas not dealt with in British Law. One example here would be the procedure for the "living will" or anticipated consent which now exists in several of the states of the USA. This provides for someone to set down the way in which they would like to be cared for should they become mentally incapable. This may include, for example, willingness to participate in research studies to develop new treatments or the desire for acute medical intervention.

The Future

Active discussion of ideas from different countries may foster further developments of the law in relation to older people. Increasing economic power among older people may also have a significant effect. Where the great majority of the very elderly have little or no capital assets, recourse to the law is likely to be minimal. However, as matters relating to inheritance and the management of property become more common the limitations of the present provision are likely to be more evident. Already there is debate as to the best way to protect the increasing numbers of vulnerable elderly people. As the range of effective interventions also grows the debate will doubtless continue to broaden.

Further Reading

Age Concern (1986) The law and vulnerable elderly people. Age Concern, Mitcham, Surrey
Bluglass RS (1984) A guide to the Mental Health Act 1983. Churchill Livingstone, Edinburgh

Gostin L (1983) The Court of Protection. MIND, London
Grimes R (1987) Law and the elderly. Croom Helm, Beckenham, Kent
Levine ML (1986) Rights for the elderly in national law around the world. International Centre for
Social Gerontology, Paris

Chapter 28

Supporting Old People in the Community

Sally Venn and G. Conlon

The twentieth century has seen a large increase in the number of people surviving to old age (see Chap. 2). As people age and become more frail they have to rely increasingly on the help of others in order to continue living in the community. In Britain, this century has also seen the birth and development of the Welfare State and the introduction of laws and policies to provide for those who have difficulty in caring for themselves. The vast majority of old people are to some extent dependent on the State. Once workers reach pensionable age, for example, the government policy of compulsory retirement from state-funded jobs leaves many people dependent on the state pension.

The importance of an elderly person retaining maximum independence and individuality by remaining in their own environment, is well recognised. The current policies of central and local government aim to ensure that old people remain safe, warm and well fed, whilst continuing to live at home. Provision is also made for those vulnerable old people who require a more supportive environment in which to live.

The sources of care available to old people can be looked at under four main headings:

Informal

Voluntary

Private Sector

Statutory

In Britain there is considerable geographical variation in the network of support available. In some places, for example, statutory services are more developed than voluntary services, while the opposite situation is found in other areas nearby. It is recognised that the various services should complement each other while avoiding duplication in some areas and inadequate provision in others. To this end some local authorities in Britain employ people to coordinate the activities of voluntary organisations and statutory bodies.

Informal Carers

Traditionally, elderly people have been supported by relatives, friends and neighbours on an informal basis. This remains the most important source of care for most disabled people and it is often delivered by dedicated carers at great personal cost. While their work is too often taken for granted, the need to provide practical and financial support for such carers is increasingly recognised. Some of the supports available are described later.

Currently about 5% of old people have no living relative and another 5% have no relatives living nearby. As potential carers become geographically more mobile this latter figure is likely to increase. Furthermore, women in Western society are moving into the work-force and away from their traditional roles, which included that of carer for dependent relatives. Thus, the availability of carers is decreasing as the number of people requiring care is increasing. For the foreseeable future, other sources of support will become more important and will require further expansion and development.

Voluntary Bodies

Voluntary organisations which aim to help old people exist in most countries, organised at a local or national level. National organisations may be active politically in publicising the problems faced by old people and proposing solutions. In Britain, such organisations include Age Concern, Help the Aged, Women's Royal Voluntary Service and the British Red Cross. A fuller list of those involved at both local and national level can be obtained from the Charities Digest which is published annually by the Family Welfare Association. At a neighbourhood level local community groups exist and will provide a variety of services which complement the statutory provision and may well include local visiting schemes ("street wardens"), carer support groups, luncheon clubs, social centres and advice centres. Funds are raised by a variety of means – private donations, legacies, donations from industry and commerce, charity shops and specific fund-raising events. Many organisations will receive additional support from central and local government sources via direct grant schemes.

The Private Sector

The private sector, encouraged by British Government policy since the late 1970s, has been involved in the development of alternatives to statutory provision. The significant growth in the number of private nursing homes, residential homes and sheltered housing schemes is evidence of this trend. Accommodation for old people is discussed later in the text.

Private domestic help has always been available to those able and willing to pay. In recent times, and particularly in urban areas, informal arrangements are giving way to agencies coordinating private home help services. For many this complements the home help services available from statutory agencies and offers additional choice to those requiring support in the home. Likewise, there has been continued growth in private nursing agencies who provide nursing care in the patient's own home.

While the 1970s have seen the development of these support services, concessions for those in receipt of a state pension have been traditionally available. Reduced fares on public transport, reduced entertainment charges and low-cost educational opportunities are some examples.

Statutory Bodies

All services provided by statutory agencies in the United Kingdom such as health, housing and social services are controlled through a framework created by Parliament. There are a number of specific Acts which empower relevant agencies to provide the various services required. These are listed and briefly described in Table 28.1.

The central government departments responsible for overseeing this framework are, in England, the Department of Health and the Department of Social Security, and elsewhere, the Welsh, Scottish and Northern Ireland Offices as appropriate. The Department of Health is particularly involved in the delivery of health and personal social services (provided by local authorities), while the Department of Social Security is principally responsible for the provision of contributory and non-contributory income support.

Health Services

Health Services are organised and funded through regional and district authorities who seek to provide adequate community and hospital services depending on the relative need in each area and on the funding available. The facilities provided vary throughout the country and it is necessary to confirm with individual health authorities which services they actually provide.

The medical care of the elderly in the community is the responsibility of the *primary health care team*, which is headed by the general practitioner. The district nurse performs nursing duties in the home setting. The importance of the health visitor in educating patients and in screening for disease is being increasingly recognised. This allows early detection of impending medical breakdown and facilitates early intervention. Geriatric liaison health visitors form an important link between hospital and community services. They identify "at risk" patients prior to discharge from hospital and ensure that they are adequately monitored once at home. A list of other health care workers, who may be available to care for old people in the community, is contained in Table 28.2.

In *hospital* elderly patients with acute medical problems are managed on acute wards in a similar way to younger patients. However, many old people are unfit

Table 28.1. Legislation governing the provision of personal services to elderly people in England and Wales

National Assistance Act (1948)
Replaces the Poor Law and enables local authorities to provide for the sick, disabled and aged, including the provision of residential accommodation for those in need of "care and attention" not otherwise available. Provides for the removal to suitable premises of those in need of care and protection and the temporary protection of property of persons admitted to hospital.

National Assistance (Amendment) Act (1951)
Amends Section 47 of the National Assistance Act (1948) to enable the removal to suitable hospital or place, persons

  a) who are suffering grave chronic disease or being aged, infirm or physically incapacitated are living in insanitary conditions
  and
  b) are unable to devote to themselves and are not receiving from other persons proper care and attention and that removal is necessary in the interests of the individual or to prevent injury or serious nuisance to other persons.

Health Services and Public Health Act (1968)
Empowers local authorities to:

  a) provide meals and recreation in the home and elsewhere
  b) inform elderly persons of the services available and to identify those in need of services
  c) facilitate transport to and from the services provided
  d) assist in finding suitable households for old people
  e) provide visiting and advisory services and social work support
  f) provide assistance (including aids and adaptations) in the home
  g) contribute to the employment of wardens for assisted housing
  h) provide warden services for occupiers of private housing.

Local Authority Social Services Act (1970)
Requires each local authority to establish a social services committee to provide specific services. A Director of Social Services to be appointed to manage the integrated department.

Chronically Sick and Disabled Person's Act (1970)
Obliges the local authority to provide services to the chronically sick and disabled, including housing and welfare services, aids and adaptations, environmental improvement (access to buildings etc.), information services and aids to mobility including the "orange badge" scheme.

National Health Services Re-organisation Act 1973
Requires the cooperation of health and local authorities and provides for the establishment of joint consultative committees.

National Health Services Act 1977
Requires health authorities and local authorities to cooperate and enables health authorities to meet expenses incurred by local authorities and voluntary bodies in the provision of services.

Health and Social Services Adjudications Act 1983
Allows health authorities to pay local authorities and other bodies for expenses incurred in the provision of housing and personal services. Provides for charging residents for the first eight weeks of stay in accommodation provided under Part III of the National Assistance Act 1948.

Residential Homes Act 1984
Lays duties on health and social services authorities for the registration and inspection of residential homes and nursing homes.

Social Security Act 1986
Provides for non-contributory financial benefits in the form of income support, social fund loans and community care grants.

for immediate discharge home after their acute medical problems have been relieved, and require a period of rehabilitation (see Chap. 25). Some patients may require long-term nursing care which cannot otherwise be provided in the com-

Table 28.2. Delivery of health services to old people

In the community

Primary health care team
    general practitioner, district nurse, health visitor, geriatric liaison health visitor
Other nursing staff
    community psychiatric nurse, stoma therapist, incontinence adviser, Macmillan nurse
Therapists
    physiotherapist, occupational therapist, speech therapist
Others
    social worker, clinical psychologist, bath attendant, chiropodist, dietician, dentist, optician

In hospital

Department of geriatric medicine
    in-patient beds (acute assessment, rehabilitation, relief admission, continuing care)
    out-patient facilities (day hospital, clinics, domiciliary assessment)
Other hospital departments
    ENT/audiology, ophthalmology, rheumatology, orthopaedics, general surgery, psychiatry, etc.

---

munity and a limited number of long-stay beds are allocated to such patients in most departments of geriatric medicine. Many disabled elderly people are cared for in the community by dedicated relatives or friends and an important function of departments of geriatric medicine is to help these carers cope with the resulting stresses. To this end, hospital beds may be made available on a short-term basis for people whose carers are going away on holiday or simply need a short break from caring. Such arrangements are known as "holiday" or "respite care" admissions. Alternatively, disabled old people may be admitted to hospital for short periods on a regular basis, for 2-week periods at 6-weekly intervals, for example; these are known as "intermittent admissions" and provide more intensive support for the carers involved. In some areas, a limited number of places may be available in the day hospital to provide relief for carers on a regular basis when the person they are looking after is not fit enough to attend a day centre.

The *day hospital* aims to provide investigation, treatment and rehabilitation for people with established rather than acute problems. It has the same facilities as a hospital ward, with input from the doctor and other members of the multi-disciplinary team (see Chap. 25). Day hospital attendance may prevent admission to or facilitate an early discharge from an in-patient bed, as patients can complete rehabilitation and treatment programmes while continuing to live at home. The frequency of attendance will depend on the underlying medical problems and can range from once to several times weekly. Meals and refreshments are provided and social interaction is as important as it is on other hospital wards. However, medical intervention rather than social stimulation is the main function of the day hospital and its role should not be confused with that of the day centre. Once the medical problems have been treated, patients should be discharged from day hospital. Should follow-up of the patient be necessary, this can be undertaken by the general practitioner, the health visitor or in the hospital out-patient clinic.

The *out-patient clinic* allows the patient to be diagnosed and treated on the hospital site where there is access to specialist facilities. Most patients should only attend for a short period as, once their problem has been dealt with, they do not require hospital facilities to monitor their progress further. It is important that those patients who can be managed by their general practitioner are promptly discharged from the clinic. This will ensure the optimal use of hospital resources and avoid overcrowding at clinics and long waiting lists for appointments. Some old people are too unwell to come to the out-patient clinic and at the request of the general practitioner they can have a *domiciliary assessment* by the geriatrician. By assessing the patient in his own home, a greater insight as to how the person copes with the demands of daily living is afforded. Appropriate treatment and further management can often be planned without needing to hospitalise the patient.

Other hospital departments, particularly those listed in Table 28.2, are widely used by old people. Psychogeriatric services are generally organised in a similar way to geriatric services with the provision of a variety of in-patient and out-patient facilities. These include acute assessment beds, long-stay hospital beds, holiday and intermittent admission beds, day hospitals, out-patient clinics and domiciliary assessments by consultants or community psychiatric nurses. Some-times, hospital beds are managed jointly by the psychogeriatrician and the geria-trician, the patient benefiting from the expertise of both.

On admission to orthopaedic units many elderly patients with limb fractures have coincidental medical problems some of which may require management by a geriatrician, and some areas now provide joint orthopaedic and geriatric rehabili-tation beds.

Social Services

Social services like education, transport and environment are funded and or-ganised by local authorities. These authorities are autonomous from district health authorities and may have slightly different geographical boundaries. Al-though the health and social services are funded and organised separately they need to function as a unit when supporting old people, health and social needs being closely interrelated.

Social services funding arrangements are complicated. However, it may suffice to say that the funds are assembled from government grants and local rates levied on householders and on businesses. This will change in the immediate future with the introduction of the Community Charge ("Poll Tax").

Social services are organised in a variety of ways. Each authority serving a par-ticular geographical area will structure its services and manpower in what is be-lieved to be the most effective way of meeting the community's needs. Local au-thorities provide services not only for the elderly, but also for children and their families, as well as for those with mental illness and physical and mental handicap. Following the Barclay report in 1982, the trend has been to locate social workers in local centres in order to improve access to services.

Along with social workers, the local authorities employ other personnel such as home helps, day centre staff, residential home staff, occupational therapists, all of whom may be involved in the provision of necessary care and support. Their varying roles are described below.

Social workers may also provide a counselling service to old people and their families to enable them to make appropriate choices about their future and to pre-pare them for any impending change in their living circumstances. The range of advice may differ from area to area, particularly in relation to options involving care in the private sector.

Depending on need, the *home help* service provides personal care in addition to domestic help in the home for a few hours each week. The degree of care given should be comparable with that which would be expected from a caring relative. This could well include help with bathing, dressing, preparation of meals, light household jobs, etc. Home helps should not do heavy work and are neither employed nor trained to undertake nursing duties. Many become close friends of their elderly clients and do far more for them than they are contracted to do. As a general rule however, this service cannot be relied upon for intense physical or social support. It is often viewed as a supervisory service geared to ensuring the safety of the frail in their own home. However, in reality, the limited hours available will of necessity mean that such supervision is limited.

Traditionally home helps provided by local authorities have not been placed in family situations where there is already somebody who could reasonably be expected to provide care. However, in recent years, the value of providing direct support to carers has been recognised and the ground rules are changing as a result.

In most local authorities, the home help service is managed by home help organisers. Some authorities are now introducing domiciliary care managers who have a wider coordinating and management role in relation to a range of community services, including home helps. Demand generally exceeds supply so that priority is given to those who in the opinion of the organiser are in greatest need. Information on local provision and priorities is generally available from the local authority.

The referral mechanism for the home help service generally involves a direct approach either from the elderly person or an agent (e.g. general practitioner, relative, neighbour). Referrals are usually received at a time of crisis such as following the death of a caring relative, acute illness or discharge from hospital. Following referral, the organiser will make an assessment visit to the home. Depending on demand this initial visit may be delayed. However there is a recognition that significant delay can have serious consequences and every effort is made to respond speedily.

Some local authorities have experimented with the provision of "super home helps", known as *home care aides*. These were intended to overcome the traditional difficulties associated with the home help service in relation to personal care. The referral mechanism is generally similar to that for home helps.

The *meals-on-wheels* service provides people at home with a hot, cooked, midday meal if they find it difficult to buy and prepare food for themselves. In some parts of the country, meals can be provided on 2 or 3 days per week only, whereas in other areas, the service is more intense though still not always available every day. The referral mechanism for this service will vary between areas, although some will have meals-on-wheels organisers who work as part of the local social services team. A charge is made which reflects the cost of the meal and may well vary between local authorities. While meals are usually cooked in central kitchens and distributed while still hot, concern about the length of time between cooking and eating has led to the development of more localised services provided from day centres and residential homes. Some local authorities have experimented with delivery of frozen meals and provide freezers and microwave ovens as a means of providing a more effective service.

Choice of menu can be limited, particularly for ethnic minority groups and those on special diets. The delivery of a meal should not lead one to assume that it is acceptable and always eaten. The delivery system varies between authorities. Some rely on voluntary organisations such as the Women's Royal Voluntary Services (WRVS) or Red Cross and others have paid drivers. The need to deliver meals quickly of necessity reduces contact-time with the recipient. Thus while the service is valuable to some people, it does not in itself guarantee that all those receiving it have an adequate diet or receive regular, effective social contact.

Luncheon clubs have in the main been established by both voluntary and statutory agencies with the help of local authorities who provide finance and advice. Church and community groups are often the focal point and the input from the WRVS is particularly noteworthy. In recent years luncheon clubs have developed in housing complexes provided for the elderly as well as in local church and community halls. Although some will prepare and cook their own midday meal, many will depend on the local authority meals-on-wheels catering service to provide and deliver meals.

The luncheon club based in a local centre offers not only food but social contact and stimulation to people with a common interest. Clubs, in addition to providing the meal will also arrange other activities which may well include entertainment, advice sessions, discussion groups and some educational activities.

People may attend several times each week, although a limiting factor may be access to appropriate transport for those with impaired mobility.

There is a significant difference between the luncheon club and the *day centre*. This difference is generally in the range of services provided and in the degree of frailty of users. However, this is not always the case. Day centres, although operated in the main by local authorities, are in some places operated by major charities (e.g. British Red Cross, Age Concern) with the financial support of the local authority.

Traditionally, local authority-run day centres have had a similar role to that of luncheon clubs in that elderly people are brought to a place where they meet friends and are provided with a hot meal. In recent years, with the increase in the numbers of the very frail elderly, this role is being questioned. A range of practical personal care services such as bathing, hairdressing and chiropody are increasingly available. Some local authorities in conjunction with health authorities are moving beyond this to develop and extend their activities into an increasingly comprehensive role incorporating aspects of remedial therapy, social interaction and respite care to relieve carers.

Day centres are generally open between 9 a.m. and 5 p.m. on five days per week, excluding bank holidays. They do not therefore address the needs of those in need of support outside of traditional "office hours". Some more enlightened authorities are now providing day services on each day of the year and increasingly for longer hours, often complementing day hospital provision. Transport to centres is provided by local authorities or voluntary agencies and its limited availability restricts the number of days on which people may attend.

Day care is increasingly available in local authority residential homes where the skills of trained staff can be utilised. This arrangement is particularly useful for those living nearby as well as for those who are awaiting permanent admission to the home. It enables the latter to become familiar with the staff and surroundings and helps to lessen the trauma of the eventual move.

Residential care and *family care* ("fostering") schemes are provided by local authorities for those elderly people who are unable to look after themselves in their own homes but are not in need of nursing care. They are discussed more fully in the section on accommodation for the elderly (see below).

The assessment of need for and provision of *aids and adaptions* in the home is generally made by an occupational therapist, employed either by the local authority or the health authority. However in some cases assessment of need is made by a specialist social worker or technician working under the supervision of an occupational therapist. Referral for these services is generally made to the local authority, although allocation of aids to patients attending hospital may also be made by occupational therapists in the hospital. The degree of difficulty in performing the activities of daily life (e.g. washing, going to the toilet, cooking, getting about the house, etc.) is evaluated and recommendations made. This may include aids which will help people to cope more easily (e.g. bath rail, raised toilet seat, mobility aids, etc.) together with minor adaptions to the house (e.g. provision of a stair rail, ramps). Incontinence aids including various types of appliances and disposable pads are provided by the health authority. Major adaptions to the home may be co-financed by district housing authorities and the local social services department.

In addition to the above, emergency alarms are provided for some disabled elderly people who generally live alone and are at high risk. Such provision is intended to facilitate a call for help in an emergency. At its simplest level this may mean the installation of a flashing exterior light to attract assistance or the provision of a telephone. However, recent advances in communication technology have resulted in the availability of more sophisticated alarm systems which link the disabled person via a personal alarm to a central computer-controlled station. These are provided either by local authorities, charities or by private enterprise.

The criteria under which various aids to daily living are provided or adaptions to housing made by the local authority are outlined in the Chronically Sick and Disabled Person's Act (see Table 28.1).

Street warden or *voluntary visiting* schemes have been promoted by local authorities as a means of providing additional support and reassurance for frailer elderly people living alone. This service is often organised by voluntary groups. There is evidence that such schemes complement statutory services in providing security and combatting isolation. The centralised alarm system mentioned above has in some areas added sophistication to this means of support. Information about the availability of these facilities can generally be obtained from the local authority. This information may also be found in advice centres, local libraries or health centres.

In some areas, a *day-sitting* or *night-sitting service* is available. This service, which is provided either by the local authority or the health authority, is aimed at providing relief for carers. This focus of activity reflects the agency providing the service – health authorities provide nursing care and supervision, whilst local authorities only undertake to provide such care as would be given by a relative. This service in the main is provided to meet short-term need and often whilst alternative longer term arrangements are being made. Increasingly however, with the concern to provide care in the community, this is being used as a longer term means of support. Day and night sitters are also available from private agencies for those willing and able to pay.

Personalised *laundry services* are available in most areas and may be provided by health authorities and/or local authorities. At its simplest level, this service is designed to help people cope with incontinence. However, the importance of clean clothes in promoting individual dignity is increasingly recognised, as is the fact that removal of the burden of laundering can help to maintain people at home and especially can relieve carers. Local authorities and health authorities are now examining opportunities for expanding this service through the use of laundry equipment in day hospitals, day centres and residential homes. A small charge is usually made by local authorities for the service whereas health authorities do not charge. Yet again, access to this service varies from area to area. However, when provided by local authorities it is generally available as an addition to home help/home care services.

Some local authorities arrange *holidays* for certain groups of people, including the old. Provision of short-stay and holiday accommodation has been offered by some local authorities as respite not only to individual elderly people living alone but also to carers.

Orange badges for disabled car users are issued free of charge by local authorities to people who are unable to walk, can only walk short distances or who are registered as blind. Such people do not have to be in receipt of mobility allowances in order to qualify. The badges are issued to disabled car owners or passengers and when displayed allow free and unlimited parking at on-street parking meters and in time-limited waiting areas. Free parking for up to 2 hours is allowed on yellow lines in England and Wales, except in the inner London area. There is no time limit on parking in Scotland. The badges also allow parking in specially designated "disabled parking" places and, in some authority areas, in pedestrianised or semi-pedestrianised streets. Holders of the badge are not allowed to park anywhere they choose and have the same obligations as other road users to ensure that they park safely and do not cause an obstruction.

Accommodation

The vast majority (97%) of old people in Britain live in the community. Their housing circumstances have been described in Chapter 2 and summarised in Figure 2.6. It is particularly relevant to focus on those dwellings in which only elderly people live. As illustrated in Figure 28.1, there is a high rate (61%) of owner occupation of "elderly-only" houses. The remaining 39% of "elderly-only" households rent from the statutory or private sector or are in sheltered housing.

While the majority of elderly people remain in their family home to the end of their days, some will choose to move to specialised accommodation more suited to an overt or anticipated increase in frailty. Such accommodation has been designed to encourage and maintain independence. The ideal living unit is accessible, on one floor, suitably small, easily maintained, warm, private, secure and geographically well located within easy reach of shops and other facilities. The accommodation may or may not be supervised.

This specific accommodation for old people takes the form of *sheltered housing* and 5% of the elderly population live in such accommodation. Living units generally consisting of a living room, bedroom, bathroom, toilet and kitchen are self-contained and grouped together in a complex supervised by a paid warden. Each living unit is connected to an alarm system which generally provides a 24-hour call service. In traditional sheltered housing the warden, who may not be trained, provides a simple "good-neighbour" service and is available to summon assistance in an emergency. Wardens do not generally provide care or domestic help and so

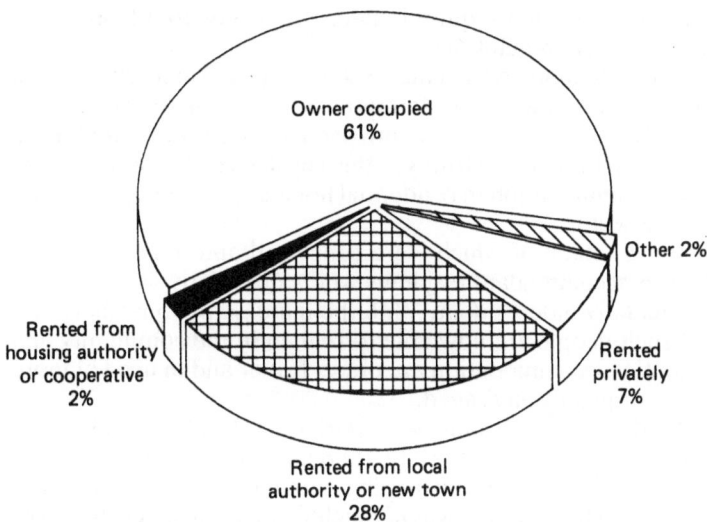

Fig. 28.1. Tenure by household type for people aged over 60 years in England and Wales.

tenants may also require the help of family or the health and social services for their personal care. Latterly however, health and social services and housing organisations have recognised the limitations of this provision and have started to develop "extra care" sheltered housing schemes. Such schemes provide more and often better trained wardens who are involved to some degree in personal care and support. The increasing development of dispersed alarm systems as already described has made many of the advantages of sheltered housing available to those in their own homes.

Along with sheltered housing, the development of "shared living schemes" has provided a form of support for some elderly people. The Abbeyfield Society in particular has been active in this area. Large houses are converted to provide several small bed-sitting units for rent where residents are supported by a house-keeper who may herself be of pensionable age. Problems can arise, however, as older residents become more frail and less mobile. The concept of shared living has been adopted by some local authorities although such schemes are often supported to a higher level by paid housekeepers and other community care workers.

Innovative *board and lodging schemes* which provide both accommodation and personal care have been developed by a number of local authorities. Family care ("fostering") schemes are modelled on fostering schemes for children and aim to provide a substitute family environment in which the elderly person is a valued member. Some local authority social service departments employ home-finding officers who manage these fostering schemes, ensuring that clients are suitably matched and supported in these surrogate families. The carers receive an allowance to cover the costs of care (currently around £70 weekly). While a number of schemes have been developed by local authorities, there is a growing number of informal private arrangements which are not controlled by legislation. As many as three elderly people may be fostered. Above this number, the residence is classified as a residential home and required under the Residential Homes Act (1984) to comply with statutory regulations.

Under Part III of the National Assistance Act 1948 (see Table 28.1), local authorities are required to "provide care and attention which is not otherwise available". In practice, this has come to mean the provision of *residential care* for old people in so-called "Part III homes". However this legislation also permits local authorities to finance accommodation in residential homes operated by voluntary agencies and the private sector.

Local authority homes, many of which were conceived and built in the late 1960s, were designed to accommodate residents who were relatively young and both physically and mentally independent. With the increase in domiciliary services the majority of such people are now able to remain in the community and those requiring residential accommodation are older, frailer and in need of more intensive care than was originally envisaged.

The homes are staffed by care-assistants who work on a shift basis and are responsible for seeing to the general welfare of the residents. Staff usually have little training in the problems of old age, have no nursing training and are not employed to carry out nursing duties. This situation was highlighted in the Wagner Report of 1988. While it is recognised that the well-being of residents requires attention to emotional and intellectual as well as physical needs, the low staff/resident ratio often found in homes imposes limitations on the quality of care given, particularly to the more dependent residents. As also stated in the Wagner Report, the physical environment of homes if often not ideal.

Some people are too frail to be cared for in local authority residential homes and yet are not in need of constant nursing care. Their need falls in between that catered for by social services and that provided by the health services. In order to fill the gap, homes jointly funded by social services and the health services are being developed in some areas. Residential homes can sometimes provide short-term accommodation for holiday relief or intermittent care. This can provide relief to carers, support to the frail living alone and maintenance for those others who may be awaiting admission to long-term care in a residential home.

In addition to local authority residential homes, many homes are operated on a commercial basis by private individuals or companies. Others are owned and run by voluntary organisations catering for specific groups (e.g. ex-service personnel, religious groups etc.). Homes operated by the private and voluntary sectors are required to register with the local authority and comply with minimum standards set by that authority. The registration and inspection of homes is the responsibility of each local authority. A scale of fees is payable by operators both for registration and the formal twice-yearly inspections. The standards set and the degree of supervision by individual authorities varies.

Elderly people requiring continuing nursing care may be cared for by the health services in a long-stay geriatric bed. Alternatively, they can move to a private *nursing home*, whose numbers are increasing to cope with demand. All homes must be registered with the Secretary of State through the local health authority under the Residential Homes Act of 1984 and it is the responsibility of the health authority to ensure that adequate standards are maintained. The fee structure for registration and inspection of these establishments is similar to that of private residential homes already described. The medical care of patients in private nursing homes is undertaken by general practitioners. Other paramedical services such as chiropody and remedial therapy are not generally provided by health authorities as it has been assumed that these services would form a normal part of nursing home activities. Such a view is increasingly questioned.

The Government funds housing for old people through grants to housing departments of district councils and metropolitan boroughs and also to housing associations via The Housing Corporation.

Housing departments within district councils function as landlords and have responsibility for allocation of tenancy, collection of rents and the maintenance of the property. They also provide an advice service through their Housing Advice Centres. The level of provision by a district council specifically for the elderly will be decided by local politicians, thus the amount of specialised housing for the elderly as a proportion of overall housing stock will vary from district to district.

The Housing Corporation, an autonomous body funded directly by central government, funds housing associations which have charitable status and are non-profit making. Housing associations provide accommodation for rent to vulnerable and disadvantaged groups (e.g. the old, physically handicapped, the mentally ill, ethnic minorities, etc.). As well as direct government funding, a number of large financial institutions, particularly building societies, have in recent years become more involved in funding housing associations.

Application for tenancy of sheltered housing either provided by the district council or housing association is made directly to that body. However, under certain circumstances district councils have nomination rights to housing association tenancies. The list of property for rent available to elderly people can be obtained from the local Housing Advice Centre. Along with provision of sheltered housing for rent, the last five years has seen the growth in purpose-built sheltered housing for sale, particularly along the south coast of England and in the major conurbations.

Information about shared living schemes is generally available through Housing Advice Centres, Citizens Advice Bureaux and from the local authority. The latter will also have information relating to local family care ("fostering") schemes.

Long-term admission to institutional care can be one of the most traumatic events in a person's life. The decision to move into a home requires very careful consideration not only of the potential advantages but more importantly the potential disadvantages. Social workers and other health professionals must provide counselling to help the person explore available options and ultimately to make the most appropriate choice. This should apply both to admission to a local authority home as well as homes in the private and voluntary sector. In general, admission to local authority residential care follows multi-disciplinary assessment involving a social worker and medical staff. Admission to private sector accommodation may not always follow such an assessment.

Specialist forms of accommodation will invariably require a specific form of application from which the individual's needs may be assessed. The application forms may vary between establishments and will be geared to matching need with provision. Applications are generally completed by the applicant with assistance from trained personnel (e.g. housing officer, voluntary visitor, social worker).

Through local councils, the government provides assistance in the form of *housing benefit* to help people on low incomes pay their rent and rates. People either in work or unemployed who pay rent to a council or to a private landlord or who even own their home may be eligible. It is not a prerequisite to be in receipt of any other social security benefit, but those with significant savings (currently in excess of £8000) are not eligible. Housing benefit can cover some or all of the rent and up to 80% of the rates payable for local services. This benefit is not available for the payment of a mortgage but home-owners may be eligible for assistance with their rates. As highlighted in Figure 28.1, 61% of "elderly-only" households are owner-occupied. Most people who get income support (see below) are entitled to housing benefit if they pay rent or rates. Application for housing benefit is made to the local council.

Income support (see below) may be payable by the Department of Social Security for elderly people accommodated in board and lodging establishments, including the family care ("fostering") schemes described above.

Accommodation and care in local authority residential homes is not free and each authority sets a charge for the service annually. The charge reflects the operational costs and will vary between authorities. Individual residents pay a weekly sum which reflects their means and will range from the minimum charge set by Central Government (currently about £33) to the full cost. In determining the charge to be levied, local authorities are required to take account of the individual's total financial circumstances, including capital, property and income. Capital below a certain level (currently £1200) is disregarded. On admission, all non-contributory benefits (e.g. income support) ceases. However the person will be left with a small personal allowance (currently about £8 weekly).

The scale of charges to be paid by individuals is determined by Central Government guidelines. The system is complicated and occasionally leads to dissatisfaction particularly when, for example, two elderly people sharing a room can be paying greatly differing amounts. Details of how charges are levied can be obtained from local authorities. This information should be available to potential residents prior to admission.

Elderly people entering private residential care negotiate a contract with the proprietor for the provision of board and lodging and personal care. As the service is a business enterprise, this charge will reflect the operational cost and allow for a profit margin. This explains the differences in both charges and in the quality of service between homes. Should a person be unable to continue to pay, application can be made for assistance to the Department of Social Security. If assets drop below a certain level (currently £6000), assistance may be given with all or part of the charge.

As with private residential homes, individuals may apply for admission to voluntary homes. However, under certain specific circumstances, in addition to the help available from the Department of Social Security, local authorities may be able to assist financially. The system of payment for private nursing home accommodation is identical to that for private residential home accommodation. Under certain circumstances, health authorities can make contractual arrangements with private nursing homes for the provision of continuing care.

People in long-stay hospital beds do not have to pay for their care, irrespective of their personal assets, but after a certain length of time their state pension is reduced to a small weekly allowance.

Financial Provision for the Elderly

A *state retirement pension* is paid to all people of retirement age (currently 65 years for men and 60 years for women) who have paid sufficient National Insurance contributions during their working life. In addition, in 1978 the State Earnings-Related Pension Scheme (SERPS) was introduced for those wishing to participate. It provides an additional pension relating to earnings and serves as an alternative to a private occupational pension scheme. This scheme is to be phased out by the end of the century, to be replaced by personal pension schemes.

The Department of Social Security sends a claim form for state pension to each citizen four months prior to reaching pensionable age. If they choose to defer retirement and continue working they may do so and their pension will be higher when they eventually do claim. Under certain circumstances, specific benefits are paid to widows where the husband although above retirement age was not drawing a state retirement pension. However, once the age of 70 (for men) or 65 (for women) is reached, citizens are automatically assumed to have retired and may draw their pension irrespective of what they earn. The state retirement pension in Britain is linked to the retail price index which has in recent years been below the average increase in earnings. The pension is normally paid weekly by an order book which is cashed at a post office by the pensioner or by an agent. The role of the agent is outlined in Chapter 27. Alternatively, the money may be paid directly into a bank or building society account, in which case it is paid monthly or quarterly in arrears.

For those who were employed in state industries or services since 1948, *occupational superannuation schemes* provide pensions on retirement. Many large employers also provide employees with similar pension opportunities. However a substantial proportion of the work-force, especially those involved in manual occupations, have rarely had such opportunity. As well as occupational pensions, *private pension schemes* available through insurance companies are available to supplement the state pension.

People who were injured while serving in the Armed Forces between 1914 and 1918 and after the 2nd September 1939 may be entitled to a *war disablement pension*. The amount of compensation depends on the disability and the rank of office. War pensioners may also be entitled to a mobility supplement or constant attendance allowance. Those widowed as a result of their husband's service in the Armed Forces may be entitled to a *war widow's pension*. The War Pensions Welfare Officer is responsible for ensuring that adequate compensation and help is given to all those bereaved or disabled as a result of military service.

People who contracted pneumoconiosis, byssinosis or certain other industrial diseases as a result of employment before 1948 may be entitled to compensation paid on a weekly basis. They must not have received any previous compensation as a lump sum payment and the amount paid depends on the severity of the disease and subsequent disability as assessed by a medical panel. Those people disabled as a result of an accident at work or industrial disease acquired after 8th July 1948 may be entitled to *industrial injuries disablement benefit*.

People who have only their state pension or have no pension at all, may have insufficient money to live on. Elderly women are particularly vulnerable as they are less likely to receive an occupational pension and may be relying on their husband's National Insurance contributions. Very elderly people are less likely to receive an occupational pension and any personal savings they may have had will diminish as they grow older. The latter group may be entitled to a weekly "over 80s pension" which does not depend on the payment of National Insurance contributions.

There are certain fixed amounts, set by Government, that the law says people in difference circumstances need to live on. Below these amounts, individuals are entitled to *income support* which in 1988 replaced supplementary benefit. Income support is intended to meet regular weekly needs. At the cessation of the supplementary benefit scheme, some 2 million elderly people were receiving benefit. It is believed that many more were eligible but did not know how to claim. Others may have been too proud to accept further state benefit for a variety of reasons, including the implied stigma of poverty and loss of independence.

An application for income support is made to the Department of Social Security. Information leaflets may be obtained from their local offices or the Citizens Advice Bureaux. House rents and rates are not considered as these are dealt with under housing benefits (see above). Eligibility for income support does not depend on National Insurance contributions. Depending on their circumstances, those receiving income support may be entitled to financial help from the Social Fund.

The *Social Fund*, introduced in 1988, is a scheme to help people with exceptional or unforeseen expenses which their regular income does not allow them to meet. Each locality has a specific budget for loans and grants administered by Social Fund Officers of the Department of Social Security. When the annual allocation to the local fund is exhausted, no further loans are made available. In practice, priorities are established at a local office level. Discretionary payments are made under three distinct headings: budgeting loans, crisis loans and community care grants. Loans are usually repaid by deduction from weekly income support payments. Where some savings (currently of over £500) are held, loans are not available. Furthermore, applicants for budgeting loans are required to have been in receipt of income support for at least 26 weeks. Crisis loans are available to help people pay for things urgently required because of an emergency or disaster. Being in receipt of income support or other social security benefit is not a requirement. Community care grants are for people in receipt of income support or who expect to receive income support when they return to the community as, for example, from hospitals or other institutions. They are also payable to enable vulnerable people to stay in the community rather than have to be placed in care or to help them cope with such problems as disability, long-term illness or family breakdown. Finally, they can be given to assist with transport costs to visit somebody who is ill or for other urgent reasons. Like budgeting and crisis loans, the possession of savings will influence eligibility. Unlike the loans, grants are not repayable. The upper limit for grants is currently in the order of £500, although this varies slightly between areas. Like the budget for loans, the budget for community care grants is limited and priority allocations are set in consultation with local authorities.

Under Social Fund arrangements, special grants formally made to old people through supplementary benefit, such as heating, laundry costs, provision of regular baths, etc., are no longer payable.

Health benefits for people who get income support take the form of free NHS prescriptions, NHS dental treatment and transport to hospital for NHS treatment. Such people also get assistance with the cost of spectacles and hearing aids.

Severe disability allowances are provided by Government for the severely disabled to help cover the extra expense involved in their being cared for at home. While some allowances are paid directly to the disabled person, others are available specifically to carers to help with increased costs (e.g. heating and laundry) and to partially compensate them for potential earnings which are lost by their remaining at home.

An *attendance allowance* is payable to anyone aged over 2 years who is so severely disabled (mentally or physically), as to require constant attention and supervision. Those eligible must have required care for 6 months before the allowance is payable, but they can apply for it after they have needed care for 3 months. It is paid directly to the disabled person after assessment by a medical officer employed by the Department of Social Security. The benefit is tax-free, is not means tested and does not depend on National Insurance contributions. The amount paid depends on whether care is needed during the day or night or throughout the 24-hour period.

A *mobility allowance* is payable to people between the ages of 5 and 75 years who are virtually immobile. An applicant must claim before his 66th birthday but have been eligible for the benefit before the age of 65 years. Once it has been granted it is payable up to the age of 75 years. There is no restriction on how the money is spent, though it is intended to encourage the recipient to be more mobile (e.g. to help pay for private or public transport). It is tax-free, is not means tested and does not depend on National Insurance contributions. It does not count as "income" when one is being assessed for supplementary or housing benefit purposes and it can be the key to other benefits (e.g. exemption from road tax and eligibility for the orange badge parking scheme).

Invalid care allowance is paid to people of working age (including married women), who are caring for a severely handicapped person at home and are therefore unable to go out to work. The applicant must be over the age of 16 and below retirement age and spend over 35 hours a week caring for someone, not necessarily a relative, who is receiving attendance allowance. They must not be in full-time education but can receive a small amount of money per week from part-time employment. The benefit is not means tested and does not depend on National Insurance contributions but is taxable and can affect entitlement to other benefits. Claimants are credited with Class I National Insurance contributions which safeguards their pension rights.

The *home responsibilities protection scheme* protects the pension rights of those who cannot work regularly as they are caring for an elderly or disabled person at home. For each tax year spent at home, the number of years of National Insurance contributions needed to qualify for a full pension is correspondingly reduced. People receiving invalid care allowance do not need home responsibilities protection because they are already accredited with Class I National Insurance contributions.

Tax allowances are granted to people who care for disabled elderly people. A *dependant relative's allowance* is available to people who support various relatives, including those aged over 64 years.

Allowances available to elderly disabled people themselves include an *age allowance*, available to all people over the age of 65 years. A *housekeeper's allowance* is available to widows or widowers who have a relative or employee living with them and acting as a housekeeper. Those over the age of 65 years who maintain a son or daughter on whom they are dependent are eligible for the *child service's allowance*.

In addition to the private pension arrangements already discussed, other sources of income for old people include those derived from private investments or savings, annuities and home income mortgage plans.

An *annuity* is a financial arrangement whereby a lump sum of money is paid to an insurance company, in return for which, the company guarantees the purchaser a monthly income for life. The income may be either fixed or rise by a certain percentage each year. Once purchased, the capital cannot be regained but the insurance company must make a minimum number of payments so that, even if the owner of the annuity dies, the capital is protected for their beneficiary. Even for those policies which give an annual increase in income, there is no guarantee that this will keep pace with inflation, so that the value of the income may fall behind the cost of living. Advice can be obtained from insurance agents and financial consultants as to which companies offer the best rates and which scheme best suits the individual client.

Home income plans may be attractive to elderly people who own their own homes. A large amount of capital is tied up in their property but they may have little money for day to day expenses. Mortgage annuity schemes enable them to mortgage part of their property and use the money to purchase a life annuity. Some of the income from the annuity pays the interest on the loan and the remainder is available as regular income. Tax relief is available on the interest and the loan is repaid when the property is sold – usually after the death of the client. Married couples should select a scheme which covers both of their lives. *Home reversion schemes* allow people to sell their own homes to a finance company but remain living in them free of charge or for a minimal rent. They still have to maintain the property and pay rates but they are able to use the capital to invest or purchase an annuity and guarantee a regular income. There is no loan on which to pay interest but the property no longer belongs to the client and cannot be bequeathed. *Interest-only loans* may be offered to retired home owners usually to help with repairs to the property. The loan is repaid when the house is later sold, before or after the owner's death.

Further Reading

Barclay PM (1982) Social workers and their tasks. Report by the National Institute of Social Work. HMSO, London

Billis D (1984) Welfare bureaucracies. Heinemann, London

Griffiths R (1988) Community care: agenda for action. Report to the Secretary of State for Social Services. HMSO, London

Kina, Lady Avebury (1986) Home life: a code of practice for residential care. Centre for Policy on Ageing, London

Levin J, Levin WC (1980) Ageism, prejudice and discrimination against the elderly. Wadsworth, California

Norman A (1980) Rights and risks. Centre for Policy on Ageing, London

Norman A (1982) Mental illness in old age. Centre for Policy on Ageing, London

Chapter 29

Care of the Elderly in Other English-Speaking Countries

G. Davison, T. E. Finucane, D. W. Molloy, K. Smith, J. B. Walsh and M. Woodward

This chapter outlines the way in which care is delivered to elderly people in other English-speaking countries. The population of the countries described together with the percentage of people aged over 65 years is summarised in Table 29.1.

Australia

M. Woodward

Geriatric services in Australia have been largely modelled on UK services, but have several important differences. Most long-term care is now provided by private nursing homes with medical care for residents being provided by their general practitioners. Pre-admission assessment of private nursing home residents by geriatricians is being increasingly developed and is encouraged by the federal government which pays most of the nursing home fee. A minority of long-term patients, usually those with high degrees of dependency, are resident in state-run geriatric hospitals.

All Australians are entitled to free public hospital care, funded through a government fee-for-service scheme called Medicare. Costs for community medical services are reimbursed by Medicare – most elderly patients are only charged the Medicare fee, resulting in little or no out of pocket expenses. Insurance for private hospital care is carried by an increasing number of citizens.

Most acutely ill elderly patients are cared for by general physicians in acute general hospitals, run either by the state, federal Department of Veterans' Affairs or by private concerns. A minority are admitted directly to geriatric units. There is much variation in the provision of acute geriatric services between different

Table 29.1. Demographic characteristics of various English-speaking countries

Country	Population (millions)	% aged over 65
Australia	15.9	10.1
Canada	25.7	10.4
Great Britain	56.1	15.1
New Zealand	3.3	10.4
Rep. of Ireland	3.5	10.9
USA	240.1	11.7

states. In some states, geriatric units are isolated from the mainstream of hospital services. These used to provide custodial long-term care only but they now provide some acute services. Other states provide all acute care in the geriatric wards of general hospitals. There is very little private geriatric care, with nearly all geriatricians receiving a state or federal salary.

The provision of rehabilitation services varies considerably between regions. Some are provided by separate geriatric hospitals, some by acute hospitals and some by separate rehabilitation hospitals.

Community services are similar to those in the UK – meals-on-wheels, day hospitals, day centres, some community rehabilitation services, community social services, lay support organisations etc. The federal Department of Community Services is encouraging more support services and support for carers as a way of reducing costly long-term care. The frail elderly unable to remain at home are frequently cared for in private "special accommodations", there being no direct equivalent to local authority residential accommodation. This leaves a considerable gap to the next level of care, the nursing home.

Psychogeriatric care is in the process of being developed, with most resources currently being expended on long-term care. The development of community assessment and support along with acute care services is also still in its infancy.

Canada

K. Smith and D. W. Molloy

The *Office for Senior Citizens Affairs* acts as a policy development agency and informs elderly citizens of the wide range of programmes and services provided by the State. Such services can be usefully classified as community, educational, financial, health and housing services, together with long-term care facilities.

Within the *community*, elderly persons' centres provide social, recreational and cultural activities. These are voluntary and non-profit making, being partially funded by provincial government. Various complementary programmes aim to coordinate the delivery of multi-disciplinary services to seniors in their own home and are designed to encourage both patient and family independence. They include the Home Care Programmes, the Homemakers and Nurses Services Programmes and Home Support Programmes. Under them, short-term rehabilitation as well as long-term care can be provided in the elderly person's own home. Input from nursing staff, remedial therapists and ancillary workers is available and where people are struggling to cope, home care staff should facilitate access to other resources not already being availed of. Homemakers may prepare meals, shop, do laundry, help with housekeeping or provide personal care. Home support programmes include the provision of meals-on-wheels, transportation, hospital equipment, day care and respite institutional care. Under New Horizons Programmes, financial aid is given to groups of 10 or more elderly people who undertake activities of benefit to themselves and their communities (e.g. through the establishment of drop-in centres, craft and hobby workshops, historical, cultural and educational groups, etc.).

Universities, colleges and other educational bodies encourage seniors to pursue *education* by providing courses free or at reduced cost. The Ministry of Education provides a free home-study programme and "open college" educational services are available through radio and television broadcasts.

The Canadian Government aids each province or territory to ensure that the *income* of those aged over 65 will not fall below a specified level. All residents aged over 65 receive an Old Age Security (OAS) pension. Those receiving the OAS may also be eligible for a guaranteed income supplement if in need of additional aid. Widowed spouse allowance and spouse allowance may be available, depending on means. In addition, the Canada Pension Plan, a compulsory contribution plan for working Canadians, is provided to those who have contributed.

All individuals aged 65 years and over and who have lived in Canada for the previous 12 months are entitled to premium-free *medical care*. Some provinces have drug benefit programmes which provide prescription drugs free of charge. Citizens requiring assistive devices, extended health care and chronic care are given financial help. Public health nursing is designed to assist seniors to maintain health and independence and may be provided at home or in institutions.

Assistance with *housing* and rent is available to those aged over 60 years. Senior citizen buildings are administered by local housing authorities with representation from federal, provincial and municipal government. Rental charges are related to income and generally approximate 25%.

In 1979, placement coordination services were established by the Ministry of Health to organise long-term institutional care. Seniors who cannot continue living at home may enter a home for the aged. These are managed by municipal government or by non-profit organisations. Accommodation is subsidised by the Ministry of Community and Social Services for those who cannot afford to pay. Nursing homes are privately run but licensed and subsidised by the Ministry of Health. They serve those individuals requiring at least 90 minutes of nursing care per day. For more independent seniors, rest or retirement homes are operated primarily by the private sector. Standards of care vary widely and at present there are no guidelines or regulations in place to govern standards.

Some 8% of people aged over 65 years in Canada are in institutional care. Comparative figures for the United States and Britain are 5% and 3% respectively. Current policies in Canada aim at maintaining people at home and at preventing inappropriate placement in institutional care.

New Zealand

G. Davison

New Zealand's population is 3.3 million of whom 10.4% are aged over 65 years (Table 29.1). Maori people make up one tenth of the population but only 4% are over 65 years. The country has National Health and Social Welfare services but private enterprise has been increasingly encouraged in recent years with an up-surge in private insurance to cover primary medical care and elective surgery. The Accident Compensation Commission is an independent body funded by levies on all employers and contributes on a "no blame" basis towards the rehabilitation and compensation of all victims of accidental injury, including fractured neck of femur in the elderly.

Services for old people are similar to those in the UK, the main differences being in the funding of general practice and in the organisation of residential homes, long-stay hospital care and domiciliary services.

Primary medical care is provided by general practitioners on a fee for service basis: the average fee is currently around NZ$28, of which 40% comes from a general medical benefit. There is no dental benefit for the elderly but they are exempt from prescription charges.

Public *hospital care* is free and provides mainly for acute illness and rehabilitation. Geriatric units are usually on general hospital sites and provide some acute medical care and most rehabilitation with variations similar to those found in Britain. Recruitment of geriatricians is rapidly improving but there are few trained psychogeriatricians and therefore a very limited psychogeriatric service. Almost all long-stay hospital care is undertaken in private or religious and welfare hospitals (nursing homes). These are funded to a ceiling of 23 beds/1000 people aged over 65 years by a Health Department income-based subsidy which is dependent on pre-admission assessment by a geriatrician.

Residential care is plentiful (e.g. 50 beds/1000 over 65 in Auckland) and is provided both by religious/welfare organisations and by the private sector. The former have purpose-built complexes including nursing homes, while the latter provide accommodation which varies from modified houses for 5–20 residents to grander homes associated with retirement villages. Subsidies are unlimited in number but are asset based (NZ$2500) and provided by the Department of Social Welfare following assessment by a geriatrician. Dependency among residents in these homes has been shown to be lower than in local authority residential homes in the UK.

Approximately 80% of non-institutionalised elderly people live in their own homes. The remainder rent privately or from local councils or the Housing Corporation. There are no housing associations for the elderly. The last five years has seen a burgeoning of large retirement villages built by finance companies. Concentration of housing facilities on the more affluent and a tendency to draw people out of the wider community is viewed with some concern.

Domiciliary services are mainly provided free by public hospitals except for a significant proportion of home help which is funded under asset test by the Department of Social Welfare. This department, in response to rapidly increasing subsidies to private residential care, has mounted a multi-million dollar project

("60 plus") to encourage voluntary organisations to initiate personal care schemes for the elderly at home.

Day care centres are organised by voluntary bodies supplemented by centres in religious and welfare homes. There is a strong network of stroke clubs (Counterstroke) and Alzheimer support groups (Alzheimer's Disease and Related Diseases Society). Age Concern NZ has a similar but lower profile than in the UK.

Universal Superannuation is 80% of the average adult weekly wage for a married couple and begins at 60 years. It is however under serious threat from taxation and asset testing.

Gerontological research of relevance to the care of the elderly includes the plight of the carers of the frail old, a study of accommodation change in old age, a population sample study and a major study of stroke incidence and prognosis.

Republic of Ireland

J. B. Walsh

As shown in Table 29.1, the population of Ireland is only 3.5 million and at 11%, the proportion who are elderly is less than in the UK and many other European countries. One third of the population lives in the Greater Dublin area.

Medical care of the elderly takes a "mid-atlantic" position in that 85% of the population benefits from a comprehensive health care structure similar to that found in the UK, while the remaining 15% have voluntary health insurance based on a tax allowable premium. Everyone is allowed free access to hospital care, but those whose income is greater than IR£15,000 are liable for consultant fees. However, it is rare for people in this income bracket to be without private health insurance. Some 85% of those aged over 65 years are entitled to free general practitioner services and to free drugs. For those without insurance, medical expenses are tax allowable.

Dublin has a well-organised geriatric medical service and is served by six full-time consultant geriatricians. All ill elderly patients are admitted to assessment wards on general hospital campuses. There is however a shortage of long-stay beds and the private nursing sector partly fills this void at present. In the cities and towns there is a very comprehensive care system similar to the NHS in Britain, with close liaison between the community and the hospital. There is a very good home-help service which is organised by voluntary bodies and funded by Central Government through the regional health boards.

In rural Ireland, institutional care facilities are well provided for with an average of 30 beds per 1000 elderly. If this figure appears large, one must consider that community support structures are more difficult to organise in sparsely populated areas than in an urban environment. In rural areas, medical care of the elderly is undertaken by general practitioners who refer patients to district general (county) hospitals where they are cared for by general physicians (internists) who have a broad general medical training.

The community nursing service is generally excellent. Public health (community) nurses receive the same training as do health visitors in the UK, but they have a nursing service commitment as well as a preventive role. Their role therefore incorporates that of the district nurse in the UK. Public health nurses serve a specific geographical area and relate to the local general practitioners.

Traditionally, *voluntary organisations* have had a major role in the provision of care in Ireland, their range of services extending to all sections of the community. They play a very important role in complementing state facilities and are usually partly funded by state grants. Examples of services run jointly by voluntary groups and health boards are the home help and meals-on-wheels services, day centres and holiday schemes. They also jointly run residential and nursing homes. In areas such as Cork city, a comprehensive sheltered housing scheme is organised by a voluntary agency and supported by the local housing authority.

Many *benefits* are available to people aged 65 years and over irrespective of means. These include free public transport on all city and rural buses and on the rail network. Other entitlements to those living alone include free electricity and free fuel vouchers during the winter, a living alone financial allowance, free television licence and telephone rental. Thus, there is a wide range of services for the well elderly person as well as a comprehensive care system for those who become ill.

Areas of development include an increase in the number of consultant physicians in geriatric medicine in rural areas. There will also be the appointment of consultant psychiatrists with a special interest in the psychiatry of old age and three such posts have recently been approved and funded for the Dublin area. It is also proposed to build a number of small "multi-purpose units", where residential accommodation will be integrated with units of extended nursing care. These are planned initially for the Dublin area where the shortage of long-term care beds is most acute.

The United States

T. E. Finucane

The United States is the wealthiest nation in the world and yet substantial numbers of its citizens are homeless, impoverished, illiterate and hungry. Analogously, while physicians compete shamelessly for "customers", tens of millions of Americans are uninsured and either cannot obtain medical care or are impoverished in so doing. An unresolved philosophical tension leads to a second central paradox in American medicine. On the one hand, the development of new technology regardless of cost is an unquestioned value. On the other, egalitarian instinct engenders reluctance to withhold treatment from patients simply because they cannot pay. Thus, the paradox: if two young women, one rich and one poor, require heart transplantation to survive, few Americans would agree to let the poor woman die, yet if asked in a different context, most would be unwilling to support a tax increase necessary to make transplantation available to the poor.

Within the context of these unresolved paradoxes, provision of health care and social services to the elderly in the USA is understandably pluralistic, replete with redundancies and large gaps. Public and private programmes support acute and chronic health care and social services for the nation's elderly. Per capita expenditures on health care are 2 to 4 times greater than those in the UK, but differences in outcome have been difficult to demonstrate.

Medicare is the centrepiece of government support for health care for the elderly. About 95% of elderly Americans, regardless of income, are insured by Medicare against acute illness and during a limited period of recovery. Many people have supplemental private insurance known as "Medi-gap" policies, to cover Medicare deductibles and co-payments. Congress has recently enacted "catastrophic illness" legislation which will require Medicare subscribers to insure further against very expensive, prolonged severe illness. In this case, the mandatory insurance is in the form of an added tax. The "catastrophic illness" law serves to underline an important dissonance in American health care. The willingness to spend, or more accurately the inability not to spend, large sums of money on critically ill elderly patients with extremely poor prognosis conflicts directly with the harsh underfunding of programmes that provide basic services and long-term care to frail, chronically ill elderly at home or in nursing homes. Only about 3% of Medicare's budget for example, is spent on long-term care. "Custodial care" for persons without prospect of recovery is excluded from Medicare reimbursement.

In contrast to Medicare, *Medicaid* spends about 50% of its budget on long-term care, mostly in nursing homes. Unfortunately, Medicaid differs from Medicare in an even more fundamental way: it is a welfare programme for poor people regardless of age. Thus, in a tragically common scenario an elderly couple must impoverish themselves in order to qualify for Medicaid benefits, most often when one of the two requires nursing home placement. The spouse remaining at home is placed in a very difficult position.

A pastiche of some 80 additional government programmes provides long-term care in some way for the elderly. Examples include the Veterans Administration, Social Security, the Administration of Ageing and the Office of Housing and Urban Development.

Private insurance programmes for long-term care are quite limited. Young people have been unwilling to pay even small premiums for insurance against possible nursing home placement decades in the future. If the risk is then divided only among older people, premiums are much higher. Potential buyers anticipate that future public programmes might obviate the need for such insurance. From the insurers point of view, uncertainties about future inflation in cost of care and about longevity of subscribers makes these policies risky. Finally, the problem of adverse selection, that is the disproportionate enrolment of people who will need prolonged care, is a serious one.

Regardless of the plethora of underfunded federal programmes or the paucity of private options, many dependent elderly Americans are cared for at home by adult daughters (29%) or wives (23%) and only about 10% of these care givers use any formal services. Several demographic trends in the USA threaten this arrangement. An ever-increasing proportion of the population is very old. Women are entering the work force. Families are having fewer children and later in life. Separation and divorce are commonplace.

In the extreme heterogeneous democracy of the United States, confronting difficult and complex policy issues has recently been difficult. The future of long-term care is such an issue, particularly since the associated costs are likely to be tremendous. The consensus that government should somehow ensure a basic minimum of services and health care for the elderly is a shaky one at best. There is no consensus about how that minimum should be defined, nor about how it should be funded. Because of the rising number of elderly Americans, the more rapidly rising costs of care and the basic inadequacies and inequities in the current system, major changes are likely.

Subject Index